Physical Therapy - Towards Evidence-Based Practice

Edited by Hideki Nakano

Published in London, United Kingdom

Physical Therapy - Towards Evidence-Based Practice
http://dx.doi.org/10.5772/intechopen.111144
Edited by Hideki Nakano

Contributors
Ibrahim Ahmad Abubakar, Sham'unu Isah Abdu, Abduljalil Hussaini Maikarfe, Hassan Bukar Gambo, Isa Muhammadu Tanko, Fatima Sada Sani, Ryosuke Yamamoto, Shun Sawai, Hideki Nakano, Marziyya Mammadova, Akira Nihonmatsu, Yoshibumi Bunno, Chieko Onigata, Toshiaki Suzuki, Shoya Fujikawa, Olubusola Johnson, Christopher Akosile, Emeka Mong, Ukamaka Mgbeojedo, Harshavardhan Sai Sadineni, Pavol Kostka, Elena Ziakova, Marek Janitor, Nina Sladekova, Martin Janitor, Daniel Vrabel, Paulina Chripkova, Monica Chiş, Ruxandra Copotoiu, Om Prakash Palanivel, Sanjay Theodore, Senthil Purushothaman, Ali Albshabshe, Nasser Mohammed Alwadai, Mohammed Abdu Rajhi, Margit Eidenberger

First published in London, United Kingdom, 2024 by IntechOpen
IntechOpen is the global imprint of INTECHOPEN LIMITED, registered in England and Wales, registration number: 11086078, 5 Princes Gate Court, London, SW7 2QJ, United Kingdom

British Library Cataloguing-in-Publication Data
A catalogue record for this book is available from the British Library

Additional hard and PDF copies can be obtained from orders@intechopen.com

Physical Therapy - Towards Evidence-Based Practice
Edited by Hideki Nakano
p. cm.
Print ISBN 978-0-85466-116-9
Online ISBN 978-0-85466-115-2
eBook (PDF) ISBN 978-0-85466-117-6

Meet the editor

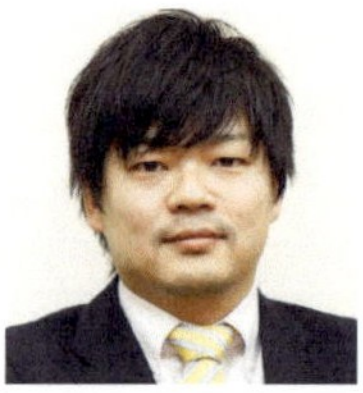

Dr. Hideki Nakano is a physical therapist and associate professor at the Neurorehabilitation Laboratory, Graduate School of Health Sciences, Kyoto Tachibana University, Japan. He received his Ph.D. in Health Science from Kio University, Japan, and has accepted research training experience as a JSPS Research Fellow at Neurorehabilitation Research Center, Kio University, Japan, and Queensland Brain Institute, University of Queensland, Australia. He specializes in neuroscience, neurophysiology, and rehabilitation science and conducts research using non-invasive brain function measurement and brain stimulation methods such as electroencephalography, transcranial magnetic stimulation, and transcranial electrical stimulation. His current main research interest is developing rehabilitation evaluation and treatment methods using visualization and manipulation methods of brain functions for healthy, elderly, and diseased patients..

Contents

Preface

The appropriateness of clinical judgment in formulating a treatment plan for physical therapy may affect the effectiveness of physical therapy treatment itself. Therefore, promoting a shift from conventional empiric-based physical therapy to evidence-based physical therapy is essential. To implement evidence-based physical therapy, it is vital to integrate not only the evidence from clinical studies but also the patient's intention and values and the physical therapist's professional knowledge and skills to make a comprehensive clinical judgment.

Toward the dissemination and practice of evidence-based physical therapy, this book consists of three sections: "Physical Therapy Theory", "Physical Therapy Assessment", and "Physical Therapy Practice".

The first section, "Physical Therapy Theory", describes the basic principles and models of physical therapy and discusses the importance of evidence in physical therapy.

The second section, "Physical Therapy Assessment", outlines how to evaluate patients in physical therapy. This section covers the basic principles of assessment and how to evaluate a patient's physical condition and function.

The third section, "Physical Therapy Practice", outlines treatment methods of physical therapy to improve a patient's physical function. This section describes the development of a physical therapy treatment plan, the actual practice of physical therapy, and the role of evidence in physical therapy.

We hope this book will be a valuable resource for physical therapists, healthcare professionals, and students.

I would like to express my great appreciation to the authors of this book and all those involved in its editing.

Hideki Nakano, Ph.D.
Associate Professor,
Neurorehabilitation Laboratory,
Graduate School of Health Sciences,
Kyoto Tachibana University,
Kyoto, Japan

Section 1

Physical Therapy Theory

Chapter 1

Stages of Evidence Based Practice in Physiotherapy

Ibrahim Ahmad Abubakar

Abstract

Each physiotherapist carries the ethical duty to practice in a holistic manner, ensuring that treatment approaches are firmly grounded in the most up-to-date evidence. Consequently, the primary objective of this chapter is to provide a comprehensive exposition of the essential stages that physiotherapists ought to adhere to when addressing patients with deformities. Additionally, it seeks to empower physiotherapists by offering practical insights into formulating precise and pertinent queries during patient interactions. This includes effective strategies for sourcing and evaluating evidence, which can then be judiciously applied to inform optimal decisions regarding patient care and treatment strategies. Throughout the course of this chapter, I will illustrate these concepts through the lens of a stroke patient scenario, facilitating a more accessible grasp of the material. However, it is crucial to note that the insights and instances presented within this chapter possess applicability that extends to various other neurological conditions within the domain of physiotherapy.

Keywords: evidence based practice, neurological conditions, physiotherapist, patients, stroke, treatment

1. Introduction

1.1 Meaning of evidence based practice

Evidence-based practice (EBP) holds a crucial role in the fields of rehabilitation and physiotherapy, progressively gaining significance. EBP is defined as the dedicated use of the most reliable evidence available to guide decisions regarding individual management, involving a fusion of clinical expertise, professional judgment, and systematic research [1]. Sackett et al. [2] further refined the concept, describing it as the fusion of top-tier research evidence, clinical proficiency, and patient preferences. The National Institute of Public Health (NIPH) in 1996 characterized evidence-based as the latest credible facts derived from pertinent, valid research. These encompass the effects of healthcare approaches, potential treatment risks, diagnostic precision, and prognostic foresight [3].

In essence, evidence-based practice in physiotherapy encompasses a methodical process of locating, evaluating, and applying current preeminent evidence to guide clinical actions. Practicing evidence-based physiotherapy involves integrating contemporary research findings with clinical skill and patient values, resulting in the most pertinent and effective care [4]. Despite its evident benefits in physiotherapy and broader healthcare, the adoption of EBP remains inconsistent in terms of quality [5]. Researchers and clinicians have voiced concerns about the compatibility of EBP elements and the scarcity of relevant, substantiated research [6, 7]. Bridging the gap between research and clinical insights can heighten the competence of physiotherapists' practice [8], guarding against inappropriate healthcare utilization [9].

Given the rising accountability of healthcare professionals, including physiotherapists, this framework gains significance as a guiding principle. Some argue that a moral obligation exists for practitioners to base decisions on research findings [7]. Physiotherapists can enhance patient management outcomes by integrating three distinct forms of evidence into their decision-making process.

1.1.1 Scientific research

Scientific research stems from rigorous hypothesis testing and observation, providing valuable experiential insights. When communicating research evidence to patients, it's essential to use clear and straightforward language and encourage open-ended questions to ensure patient comprehension. Physiotherapists are responsible for identifying, evaluating, and summarizing research evidence pertinent to patient care.

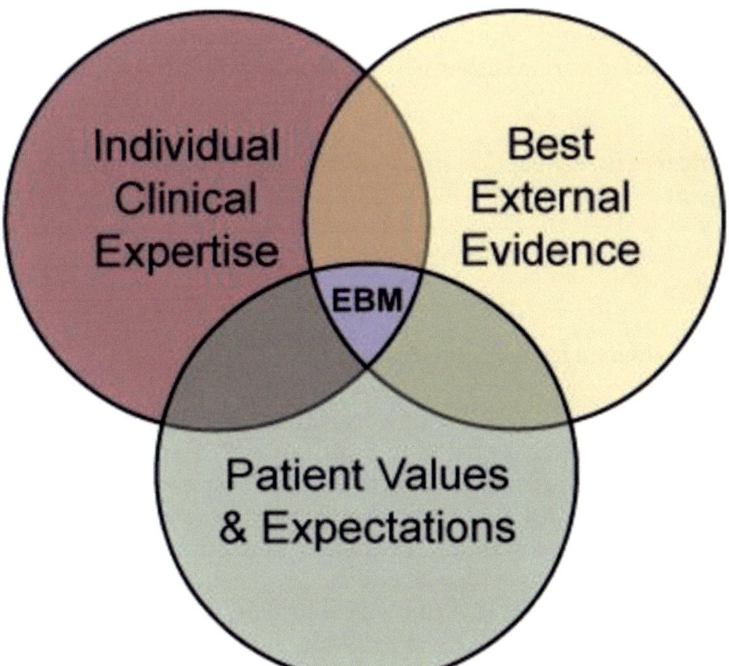

Figure 1.
Evidence based medicine (EBM).

1.1.2 Clinical expertise

Clinical expertise encompasses both implicit and explicit knowledge gained from experience in diagnosing, intervening, preventing, and predicting outcomes for patients with physical conditions. This knowledge is accumulated over time and contributes to refining patient care.

1.1.3 Patient values

The foundation of decision-making and management lies within the caregivers, patient relatives, and the patients themselves. Patient values can be categorized as values and circumstances. Values include the patient's beliefs, preferences, expectations, and cultural identity, which significantly influence their life choices and decisions [10].

In the original framework (depicted in **Figure 1** above), to summarize, the most reliable evidence often emerges from clinically significant research carried out with robust methodological procedures. Clinical expertise encompasses the amassed knowledge, experience, and clinical skills of the Physiotherapist. Patient values encompass the distinct preferences, concerns, and expectations that each patient brings when engaging in a clinical interaction. The integration of these three elements constitutes the foundation of making evidence-based clinical decisions [11].

2. Aim of evidence based practice

The primary goal is to empower healthcare professionals, including Physiotherapists, to make well-considered choices regarding clinical practice by employing the 'thoughtful, clear, and prudent utilization of the most current and reliable evidence within the healthcare system' [11].

3. The stages of evidence-based practice (EBP)

In their work [12], a set of six stages outlining evidence-based practice was delineated. Physiotherapists are advised to adhere to these stages in order to provide optimal care for their patients (**Figure 2**).

3.1 How to formulate a clear and answerable clinical question

The time allocated for assessment and diagnosis in a clinic is often limited for a Physiotherapist. As a result, efficiently searching for the most suitable available evidence requires mastering the skill of formulating well-structured questions within a short timeframe. Questions posed by a Physiotherapist to their patients can be categorized into these groups [11]:

1. **Etiology**: How can I identify potential causes of a problem? For instance, what leads to limited shoulder range of motion among stroke survivors?

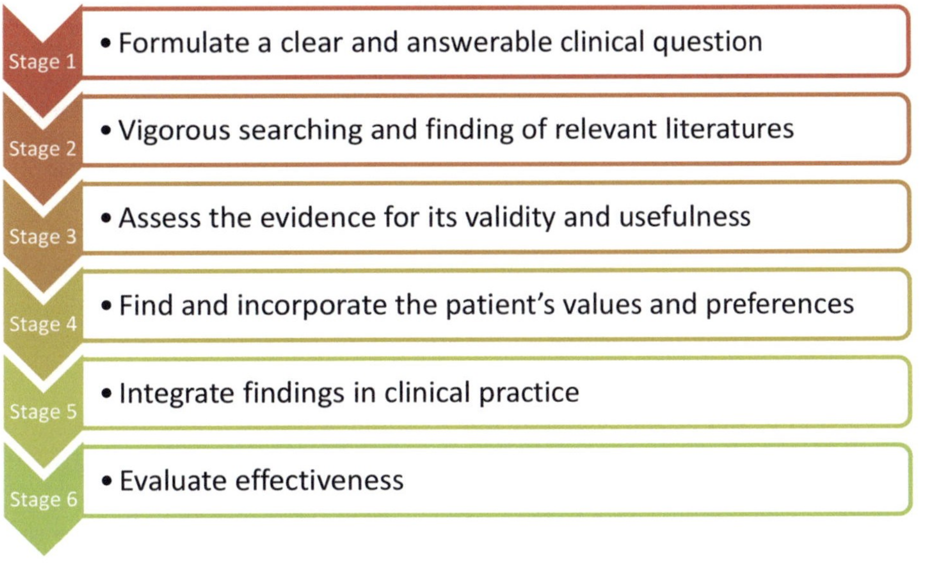

Figure 2.
Stages of EBP.

2. **Assessment/Diagnosis:** What crucial information should I collect? How can I obtain that information and correctly interpret the results? For example, what's the optimal method for evaluating balance in stroke patients?

3. **Treatment:** Which intervention or procedure will be most beneficial for my patient? For instance, what are the outcomes of applying the Proprioception Neuromuscular Facilitation concept in post-stroke patients compared to other physiotherapy approaches?

4. **Prognosis:** What's the recovery pattern over time and what potential complications might arise? As an illustration, if my patient had a stroke two months ago, when can they expect to regain independent walking ability?

5. **Prevention:** How can I avert emerging problems and enhance my patient's well-being? As an example, what's the most effective approach to prevent shoulder pain in post-stroke patients?

6. **Differential diagnosis:** When symptoms point to various potential diagnoses, how do I determine the most probable one? For example, in a young man with knee swelling, stiffness, pain, crepitus, quadriceps atrophy on examination, pain on palpation, and resistance during extension, what's the likely underlying cause?

3.1.1 PICO framework

The PICO framework holds great importance in shaping a precise question. This framework identifies and outlines the crucial components of a well-organized question. It's important to remember that a focused question should address a single issue at a time (**Figure 3** and **Table 1**).

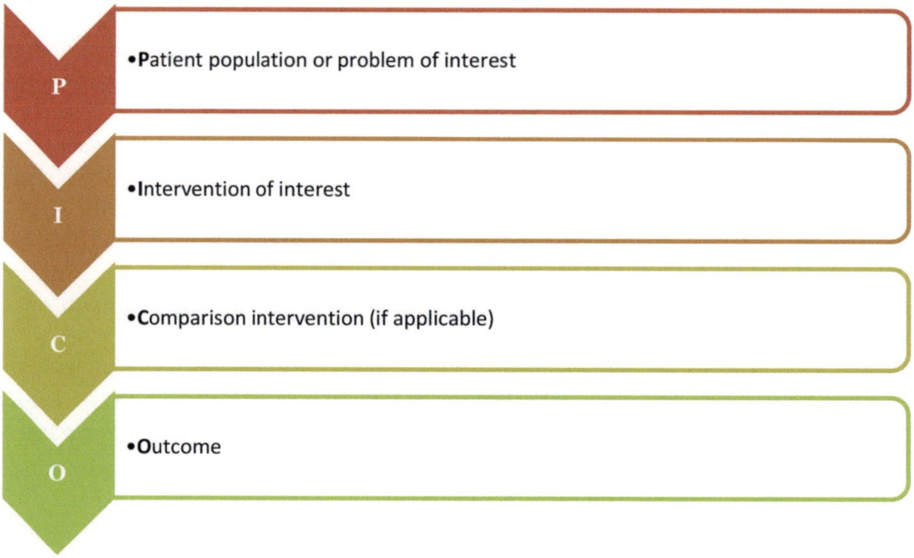

Figure 3.
PICO framework.

		Example
Patient population or relevant issue	What is the specific disease or condition under consideration?	A 60-year-old woman dealing with shoulder pain post-stroke
Intervention	What particular treatment, modality, or procedure is being focused on?	Transcutaneous Electrical Nerve Stimulation (TENS)
Comparison	What is the alternative to the current treatment being administered? For instance, placebo or medication.	Non-steroidal anti-inflammatory drugs
Outcome	What are the goals in terms of measurement, enhancement, or impact?	Reduction in the level of experienced pain

Table 1.
Using the PICO framework to develop a clear question.

An example of clinical question from the above table could be 'Is TENS better than non-steroidal anti-inflammatory drugs at reducing the intensity of post stroke shoulder pain?'

3.2 Searching and finding the best evidence

Once you have carefully formulated a precise clinical question addressing the disease or condition presented by your patient, your next step involves sourcing the most reliable evidence to address this query. A range of resources exists to aid your quest for answers. These encompass personal experience, logical reasoning, and intuition, inquiring with a fellow practitioner, referring to textbooks, accessing pertinent scientific papers from your personal collection, utilizing bibliographic databases such as Medline or Embase, and consulting literature that's clinically assessed or grounded in evidence, along with established healthcare guidelines.

However, a caveat exists when relying on personal experience and subjective opinions. Such an approach might not yield the most efficient, effective, and economically viable treatment pathways. Conversely, seeking advice from a seasoned colleague can be an expedient approach, especially when grappling with unique or infrequent scenarios. It's worth noting that textbooks, while informative, often become outdated even before their publication, necessitating a cautious approach when consulting them.

The specific type of evidence you seek hinges on your question's scope. Navigating the different types of research available will direct you toward attaining the utmost level of evidence relevant to your specific clinical inquiry. By discerning the nature of your question, you can methodically select the research avenue that aligns with your inquiry, leading you to the most robust evidence available to inform your clinical decisions effectively and accurately.

3.2.1 Levels of evidence

'Levels of evidence' refer to frameworks for categorizing research designs. These systems rank research designs based on intervention assessment, evaluating their reliability, validity (protection against bias and error), and truthfulness. Systematic reviews, meta-analyses of randomized controlled trials, and evidence-based clinical practice guidelines hold the highest status on the evidence hierarchy (illustrated

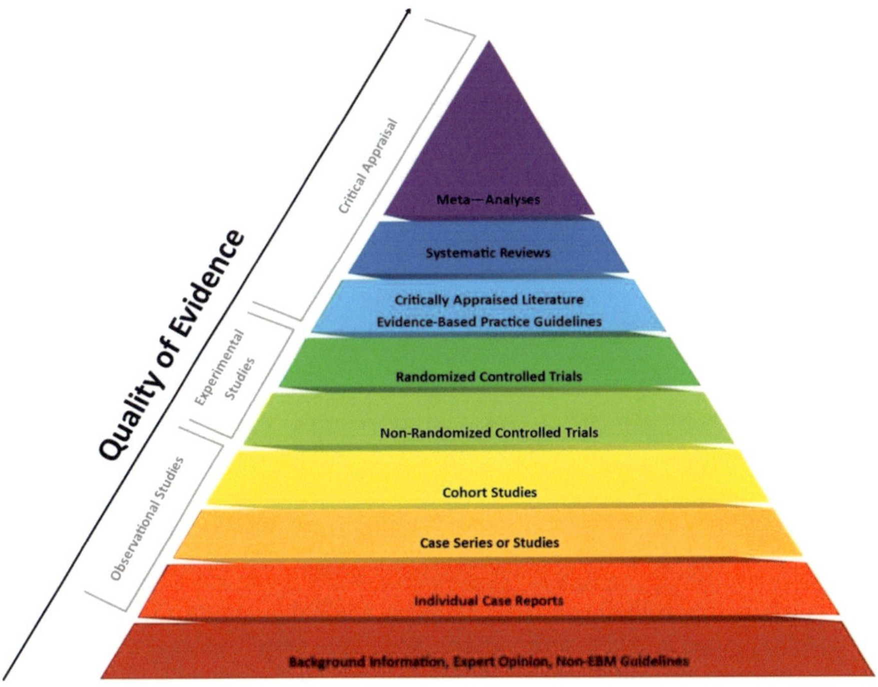

Figure 4.
Level of evidence pyramid.

as a pyramid in **Figure 4**), forming a robust foundation for treatment decisions. Conversely, expert opinion is widely considered the least robust evidence category in this hierarchy.

3.2.2 Observational studies: Understanding research design

Research design encompasses two main approaches: qualitative and quantitative. Both methods, if properly executed, are rigorous and valuable for addressing significant clinical inquiries [13, 14]. Employing both designs within a single study is especially advantageous for extensive trials assessing clinical practices. This comprehensive approach is particularly beneficial for large-scale trials aimed at evaluating clinical practice.

3.2.3 Quantitative design

The quantitative design focuses on robustly examining hypotheses related to predefined variables. Examples of such designs encompass clinical trials, comparative studies, and epidemiological investigations. These studies primarily address queries like "whether" (evaluating whether Physiotherapy treatment yields more benefits than harm) and "how much" (measuring the strength of the correlation between a specific risk factor, like hypertension, and the occurrence of a particular disease or condition, such as stroke) [15].

3.2.4 Qualitative design

Qualitative studies delve into inquiries involving "how," "what," and "why" [15]. These studies often employ detailed interviews and focus group interactions to investigate and gain insight into "social, emotional, and experiential phenomena" within healthcare contexts. Examples encompass exploring the significance of the stroke experience for survivors and their families, offering a deeper understanding of these individuals' perspectives.

4. Critical appraisal

Critical appraisal constitutes a crucial aspect of evidence-based practice (EBP), involving the meticulous and systematic evaluation of research evidence to gauge its credibility, significance, and relevance to clinical application [16]. It's pivotal to recognize that diverse research designs entail distinct methodological procedures and levels of validity. This distinction underscores the significance of comprehending how findings can be translated into practical use within specific clinical contexts.

5. Implementing evidence-based into clinical practice

Incorporating optimal evidence-based practices into your daily routine as a Physiotherapist is challenging. However, identifying barriers specific to your setting can aid in devising a more efficient strategy, enhancing the likelihood of successful patient management [17].

Barriers	Example
Structural	Policies and Financial disincentives
Organizational	Lack of staff skills, poor working environment or lack of equipment/diagnostic tools
Peer group	Local standard of care not standard
Individual	inadequate knowledge, quackery, attitudes or skills
Professional-patient interaction	Problems with information processing, lack of communication skills
Consumers	Wrong information and illiteracy

Table 2.
Barriers to implementing evidence-based practice [21].

6. Barriers to evidenced based physiotherapy

Barriers to evidence-based Physiotherapy can impede optimal patient care. The challenges of a busy clinical setting may make accessing current, relevant evidence difficult [18]. Reluctance to alter established practices in light of new evidence can impede progress. Limited familiarity with research resources and a lack of confidence in interpreting findings are common obstacles [19]. Moreover, the absence of conclusive evidence might discourage practitioners, though it should not deter them from engaging in evidence-based processes [20]. Overcoming these barriers through education, enhanced resource accessibility, and fostering adaptability is vital for advancing evidence-based Physiotherapy and ensuring informed, effective patient management (**Table 2**).

7. Conclusion

Embracing evidence-based practice within Physiotherapy necessitates a resolute commitment to furnishing optimal care for patients. Amid the bustling hospital milieu, the initial stride toward effective evidence-based practice in Physiotherapy lies in discerning where to access the most current, fitting, and superior evidence, ideally in a readily accessible format. Equally vital is the determination and self-assuredness to recalibrate practices in light of evidence.

Occasionally, the sought-after answers to inform clinical practice may remain elusive. It's essential to internalize that the absence of evidence does not imply an absence of impact. The absence of conclusive evidence should not hinder Physiotherapists from participating in the evidence-based process; instead, it should fuel the impetus to galvanize fresh research endeavors in pursuit of the requisite evidence within the domain of Physiotherapy. This resilience underscores the dynamic nature of evidence-based practice as a driver for continuous improvement and growth in the field.

Author details

Ibrahim Ahmad Abubakar
Federal Medical Centre, Nguru, Yobe State, Nigeria

*Address all correspondence to: ibrahimcsskd@gmail.com

References

[1] World Confederation for Physical Therapy—European Region. Evidence Based Physiotherapy. Brussels: The Confederation; 2015. Available from: http://www.erwcpt.eu/education/evidence_based_physiotherapy_evidence_and_research

[2] Sackett DL, Strauss SE, Richardson WS. Evidence-Based Medicine: How to Practice and Teach EBM. London: Churchill-Livingstone; 2000

[3] National Institute of Public Health (NIPH). First Annual Nordic Workshop on How to Critically Appraise and Use Evidence in Decisions about Healthcare. Oslo, Norway: NIPH; 1996

[4] Haynes RB, Devereaux PT, Guyatt GH. Clinical expertise in the era of evidence based medicine and patient choice. Evidence-Based Medicine. 2002;**7**:36-38

[5] Caldwell K, Coleman K, Copp G, Bell L, Ghazi F. Preparing for professional practice: How well does professional training equip health and social care practitioners to engage in evidence-based practice. Nurse Education Today. 2007;**27**:518-528

[6] Chan S, Clough A. A critical evaluation of evidence-based practices of physiotherapy in musculoskeletal medicine. IMM. 2010;**32**:163-166

[7] Dannapfel P, Peolsson A, Nilsen P. What Supports Physiotherapists' Use of Research in Clinical Practice? A Qualitative Study in Sweden Implementation Science. 2013. p. 8. Available at: http://www.implementationscience.com/content/8/1/31/prepub [Accessed: January 31, 2012]

[8] Bello A. Utilizing research findings in physiotherapy: A call for gap bridging. Nigerian Postgraduate Medicine. 2011;**18**(19):54-58

[9] Kumar S, Grimmer-Somers K, Hughes B. The ethics of evidence implementation in health care. Physiotherapy Research International. 2010;**15**:96-102

[10] Linda F, Julie T. Evidence Based Physical Therapy. FA Davis; 2008

[11] Sackett DL, Rosenberg WMC, Gray JAM, Haynes RB, Richardson WS. Evidence based medicine: What it is and what it isn't. BMJ. 1996;**312**:71-72

[12] Greenhalgh T, Toon P, Russell J, et al. Transferability of principles of evidence based medicine to improve educational quality: Systematic review and case study of an online course in primary health care. BMJ. 2003;**326**:142-145

[13] Marshall DC, Rossman DB. Designing Qualitative Research. Thousand Oaks CA: Sage Publications; 2006

[14] Portney LG, Watkins MP. Foundations of Clinical Research: Applications to Practice. 2nd ed. London: Prentice-Hall Health; 2000

[15] Giacomini M, Cook DJ. Users' guides to the medical literature: XXIII. Qualitative research in health care. Are the results of the study valid? JAMA. 2000;**284**:357-362

[16] Greenhalgh T. How to read a paper: Papers that summarise other papers (systematic reviews and meta-analyses). BMJ. 1997;**315**:672-675

[17] Grimshaw JM, Shirran L, Thomas R, et al. Changing provider behaviour:

An overview of systematic reviews of interventions. Medical Care. 2001;**39**(8):II-2-II-45

[18] Smith A, Johnson B, Williams C. Challenges in evidence-based practice for physiotherapists. Physical Therapy Reviews. 2019;**24**(4):203-208

[19] Jones R, Davies D, Green J. Barriers and facilitators to evidence-based practice in physiotherapy. Physiotherapy. 2020;**106**:e134-e135

[20] Brown L, Green J. Challenges and barriers to implementing evidence-based practice in physiotherapy. International Journal of Physiotherapy and Research. 2018;**6**(1):2677-2680

[21] Grimshaw JM. Changing Professional Behaviour: Empirical, Theoretical and Pragmantic Perspectives. Sydney, Australia: Australasian Cochrane Collaboration Course; 2003

Section 2

Physical Therapy Assessment

Chapter 2

Clinical Measurement as a Resource for Evidence-Based Practice in Physiotherapy

Sham'unu Isah Abdu, Abduljalil Hussaini Maikarfe, Hassan Bukar Gambo, Isa Muhammadu Tanko and Fatima Sada Sani

Abstract

Evidence-based practice (EBP) is the cornerstone of the twenty-first century. It is an approach to healthcare that emphasizes making decisions based on the best available evidence, combined with clinical expertise and patient values. The main goal of every healthcare professional is to have credible and reliable justification for the treatment of an individual patient. Scientific evidence should be used to influence practice in physiotherapy. The need to measure outcomes in physiotherapy practice is undisputed with the growing pressure on physiotherapy to embrace evidence-based practice. An outcome measure gives baseline data before giving any intervention, and initial outcomes may assist in establishing the path of therapy intervention. To evaluate and enhance patient care, uphold professional standards, and "do the right thing," clinical audit is crucial.

Keywords: evidence-based practice, clinical measurement, clinical assessment tools, outcome measures, clinical audit

1. Introduction

Evidence-based practice (EBP) is the cornerstone of twenty-first century. It is an approach to healthcare that emphasizes making decisions based on the best available evidence, combined with clinical expertise and patient values [1]. The goal of every healthcare professional is to have a credible and reliable rationale for treating an individual patient. Physical therapists participate in an assessment process that includes taking a medical history, conducting a systems review, and performing clinical tests and measurements to identify potential and existing problems, as well as to establish diagnosis and prognosis. In more recent times, there has been pressure on physiotherapist from the government and other health insurers to become more accountable for their practices and justify what they do. The need to measure outcomes in physiotherapy is undisputed with the growing pressure on physiotherapy to embrace EBP [2].

Herbert and colleagues provided further guidance for using the principles of EBP in physiotherapy, which is informed by relevant, high-quality clinical research (evidence), coupled with physiotherapist practice-generated knowledge and patient preference and perspectives. Integrating research results with the patient's values, circumstances and preferences, the physical therapist's practical expertise, and the clinical setting constitutes evidence-based physical therapy practice [3]. Despite the obvious advantages of EBP, its implementation in physical therapy (and other medical disciplines) has been poor and variable in terms of quality [4]. Concerns about the compatibility of aspects of EBP and the lack of clinically relevant research were of concern [2]. Clinical measurement plays a vital role in generating such evidence in order to promote the best possible clinical outcomes and offer patients/colleagues with reliable information (**Figure 1**).

1.1 High quality clinical research

The term clinical research is usually used to mean a comprehensive research of the safety and effectiveness of the most promising advances in patient care that generate knowledge with either experiment or observation conducted in a clinical environment [5].

1.2 Patient values and preference

Values and preferences relate to the belief that patients place on health outcomes. Traditionally, healthcare professionals make decisions about treatment for their patients. Recently, there has been a shift toward patient involvement in making decisions. These concepts see patient values as a central part of quality healthcare practices and highlight the importance of considering aspects that people value in healthcare practices be taken seriously [6–9].

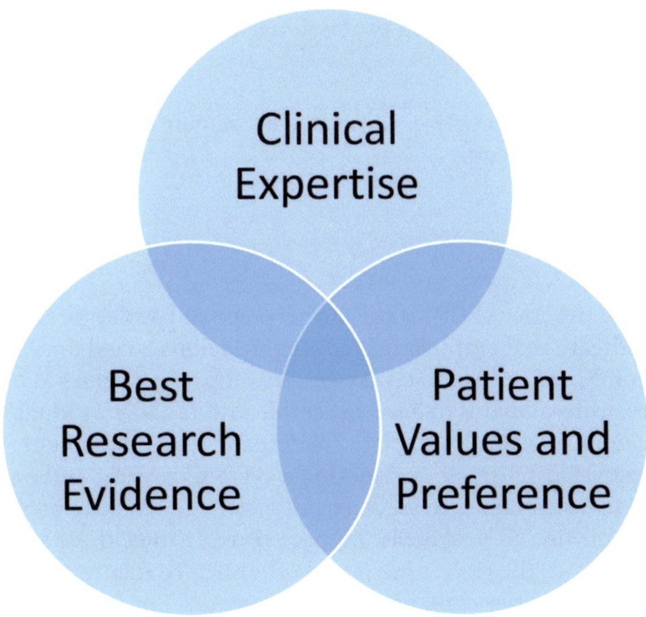

Figure 1.
Core concept of evidence based practice.

1.3 Clinical expertise/clinical knowledge

Any knowledge that comes from professional practice and experience, which includes the general basic skills of clinical practice as well as the experience of the individual practitioner [10]. Practice knowledge should always be incorporated into the decision-making process and thus contribute to professional judgments that must be made together with patients. To achieve positive and gratifying outcome, clinical expertise must take into account and harmonize the patient clinical condition and context, pertinent research findings, as well as the patient's preferences and actions.

1.3.1 Process of clinical decision-making

Clinical decision-making is a continuous and evolving process in which data is collected, interpreted, and evaluated to make an evidence-based action decision [11]. Clinical decision-making brings together information from high-quality clinical research, patient preferences, and information from therapists in a specific context. Practice knowledge alone is not evidence. It only contributes to judgment that has to be made in day-to-day practice. Decision has to interact with research evidence, patient values, and practice knowledge.

Five steps for evidence-based Physiotherapy [12].

1. Ask question Converting the need for information into answerable question (questions related to diagnosis, prognosis or therapy etc.).

2. Find information/evidence to answer question Track down the best evidence with which to answer that question.

3. Critically appraise the information/evidence Critically appraising that evidence for its validity and applicability.

4. Integrate appraised evidence with own clinical expertise and patient's preferences Integrating the critical appraisal with our clinical expertise and with our patient's unique biology, values, and circumstances.

5. Evaluation Evaluating our effectiveness and efficiency in executing Steps 1–4 and seeking ways to improve them both for next time.

1.3.2 Advantages of evidence-based practice

Engaging with both research and clinical findings can enhance the proficiency of physiotherapists' clinical practice [1] and help prevent the misuse, overuse, and underuse of healthcare services [13]. In an era of growing accountability of healthcare practitioners, this may provide a useful framework within which to work. Indeed, this has led some to argue that there is a moral obligation to base decision-making on research findings [2]. Overall, Evidence-Based Practice provides a systematic and structured approach to decision-making that benefits both practitioners and the individuals they serve. It combines the best available evidence with clinical expertise and patient preferences, leading to improved outcomes and higher quality care. EBP improves patient/client outcomes, provides higher quality of care, ensures cost effectiveness, encourages professional development and transparency and accountability, reduces variation in practice, integrates research and practice, enhances communication among interdisciplinary teams, and emphasizes the importance of considering patient preferences, values, and needs when making treatment decisions. This helps ensure that interventions align with patients' goals and promote shared decision-making.

2. Clinical measurement

Measurement is a key element of evidence-based practice that gives clinicians the data they need to make decisions regarding patient care [14]. Questioning one's own practice is the beginning and end of the evidence-based physiotherapy process. It is vital to constantly consider if the evidence-based procedure being used is yielding the optimum results for the patient. The main goal of every healthcare professional is to have credible and reliable justification for treatment on an individual patient. In recent years, due to the escalating expenses of health care, providers have been under more and more pressure to account for how their services are used. Concurrently, increased competition in the market has made it necessary for practitioners to offer evidence of treatment success to clients, insurance companies, and other funding sources. Given these elements, there is a critical need to precisely identify cost-effective treatments from the standpoint of the patient, their family, the healthcare provider, and society at large [15]. Scientific evidence should be used to influence practice in physiotherapy, and appropriately assessing health outcomes is a key tactic for accomplishing this.

An outcome can be considered as the consequences of care, a substantial change in the health condition of a patient [16], while outcome measures are tools used for measuring changes in patients' functioning, performance, or participation over time following an intervention [17–19]. Using outcome measure to monitor patient health status is seen as a crucial component of excellent clinical practice in physiotherapy [20]. There are many practical concerns that must be taken into account when implementing the day-to-day use of OMs, including the use and interpretation of OMs in the clinical setting and the psychometric properties.

2.1 Selecting an outcome measure

Choosing the right outcome measure is one of the most crucial steps in its use in clinical practice. When selecting an outcome measurement tool, the clinician must consider the purpose for which the outcomes will be used and the key health areas to be measured in the context of age, stage and patient status, and the clinical environment [21]. The need to decide which are the most relevant should be based upon sound psychometric properties, which should be quick and easy to complete and score and most importantly be intuitive to interpret (**Table 1**).

2.2 Types of outcome measures used in clinical practice

Generic: These are questionnaires designed to evaluate perceived change in the wide domain of general health and well-being across various medical conditions, populations, or interventions, for example, SF-12 and Sickness impact profile (SIP) [26].

Psychometric	Concern
Validity	Validity is often defined as the extent to which an instrument measures what it purports to measure [22].
	Content validity: is the degree to which the content of the tool adequately reflects the construct of interest [23].
	Construct validity: is the degree to which the scores of a tool are consistent with hypotheses based on the abstract concept [23].
	Criterion Validity: when the measurement of one tool can be used as a substitute measurement, for an established reference standard (gold standard) [23].
	Concurrent validity: establishes the validity of two measurements taken at the same time (perhaps one tool is considered more efficient than the Gold Standard) [23].
Reliability	is the reliability of an outcome measure is the extent to which the outcome measure scores remain consistent over repeated tests of the same patient under identical conditions. (intra class correlation coefficient (ICC)) [24].
	Test-retest reliability: indicates consistency of measures over time, (i.e., with more than one application).
	Intra-rater reliability: indicates agreement of repeated measures obtained by the same person.
	Interrater reliability: indicate agreement between two or more examiners.
Responsiveness	is the ability instruments have to measure small changes that are clinically important, where participants or patients respond to effective therapeutic interventions [25].

Table 1.
Psychometric properties of outcome measures.

Dimension-Specific: focuses on how the patient perceives aspects like pain, locus of control, anxiety, or coping pain rating scale and the Borg scale of perceived exertion (limited to a single dimension of health) [27].

Condition-specific outcome measurement tools are questionnaires that have been devised for specific diseases. Eg Arthritis impact mea-surement scale (AIMS), and Western Ontario Rotator Cuff Index (WORC) [28].

Region-Specific: These are questionnaires that have been devised for specific regions of the body, for instance, lower limb task questionnaire, Neck disability index (NDI), and Disabilities of the arm shoulder and hand (DASH) [28, 29].

Patient-Specific: rely on the experiences of each patient rather than on predetermined queries.

These center on the functional limitations status of the specific determined at the time of questioning. Questions and answers are specific to individual patients, for example, Patient specific functional scale (PSFS) [30].

3. Barriers toward evidence-based practice among physiotherapist

Evidence-based practice barriers can be thought of as modifiable elements that prevent the implementation of EBP, and understanding them could help to improve the environmental and organizational context as well as education [31]. In a recent systematic review by Matteo Paci and colleagues that investigated the barriers to evidence-based physiotherapy. The review included 29 studies reporting the opinions of nearly 10,000 physiotherapists. Lack of time was the most frequently encountered barrier and was reported by 53% of physiotherapists. This was followed by language (36%), lack of access (34%), and lack of statistical skills (31%). Herbert et al. [32] report that even in most evidence-based practice settings, implementing an evidence-based approach to clinical decision-making and practice faces significant practical challenges. Many studies have identified several barriers to evidence-based practice in physiotherapy and other health professionals. In a cross-sectional survey conducted in Columbia, 56% of the respondents indicated that the most common barrier was lack of research skills as being the most important barrier to using EBP. The next two highest rated barriers that were rated as significant barriers were lack of understanding of statistical analysis and inability to apply findings to individual patients having unique characteristics [33]. Hannah C, [34], conducted a survey among the members of the Malaysian Physiotherapy Association and other practicing therapists in Malaysia to identify the knowledge, attitude, and barriers toward the implementation of EBP among physiotherapists. Time constraints, limited access to databases, and lack of generalizability of studies result are the three major barriers to implementing EBP [34]. Another survey carried out in Pakistan identified lack of availability of resources to access information as the biggest barrier followed by lack of time and lack of support among physiotherapists [35]. In a well-conducted study carried out in New South Wale, United Kingdom, 60% of survey participants reported that perceived impacts on the therapeutic alliance is a barrier to applying evidence, followed by skills and environmental context and resources [36]. These reported barriers are similar to

Domain	Barrier	Facilitator
Competence/skills	Lack of knowledge, education, routine, and experience Diagnosis focused on International classification of function domain: body functions	Sufficient knowledge and education Measurement instruments are already used in daily routine
Attitude	Resistance to change No conviction of additional value on the plan of care Being overloaded with information	Readiness to change Positive attitude toward the use of measurement instruments Conviction of contribution to quality of physical therapy care
Practice	Takes too much time Absence of practice policy	Patient computer system Presence of practice policy
Colleagues	Lack of discussions, meetings, and feedback from colleagues No adherence to the agreements made	Regular meetings and feedback from colleagues Innovative teamwork and cooperative colleagues
Patient	Different expectations and preferences: needs no measurement instruments, wants only therapy, and puts pressure on therapist	Patient wants objectives to evaluate outcome of therapy
Measurement instrument	Poor availability Difficult choice Feasibility: extensive, difficult interpretation, and unclear instructions	Good availability

Table 2.
Stevens, J. G. A., identifies some physical therapist barriers to and facilitators of the use of measurement instruments.

those reported from other similar studies conducted by other healthcare disciplines such as nursing [37–41], internal medicine [42], emergency medicine [43], and dentistry (**Table 2**) [44].

4. Audit of clinical practice in physiotherapy

Audit of treatment is an accepted technique for assessing the effectiveness and efficiency of a practice as well as the accuracy of record keeping that should be based upon high-quality clinical research. A clinical audit is an approach of quality improvement that strives to enhance patient care and outcomes by a systematic evaluation of treatment based on specific criteria. Changes will be undertaken as appropriate, and additional monitoring will be employed to validate healthcare improvements [45].

4.1 Why audit the clinical practice?

Clinical auditing is a valuable tool for assessing and enhancing patient care, maintaining professional standards, and promoting ethical practices. Healthcare professionals can use this approach to identify and track areas of risk in their services. Additionally, auditing fosters a culture of quality improvement within the healthcare industry, increases job satisfaction, and improves healthcare quality and efficiency. Completion of the audit cycle establishes the effectiveness of the audit in improving the care of patients [46]. The practice audit can be carried out by the individual clinician; however, it is better to have someone else collect the data methodically and without bias. The patient's physiotherapy record is the primary source of data that the auditor examines to check if the practice recorded tallies with set evidence-based criteria. If there was a discrepancy between the practice and the criteria, an action plan should be implemented against the established discrepancies. Repeating the audit cycle is mandatory to ensure adherence is greater.

The cyclical process of clinical audit can be outlined in five stages.

- Planning for audit
- Setting standards/criteria
- Measuring performance
- Making improvement
- Sustaining Improvement

Stage 1. Planning for audit: The success of an audit project's outcome depends on proper planning and preparation. In this stage stakeholder engagement, choosing the audit topic and planning the delivery of audit fieldwork are crucial for the success of the audit [45].

Stage 2. Selection of standards and criteria: Following the selection of the audit topic, the next critical step is to analyze the available evidence to define the standards and audit criteria against which the audit will be conducted. Evidence-based standards are preferred [47].

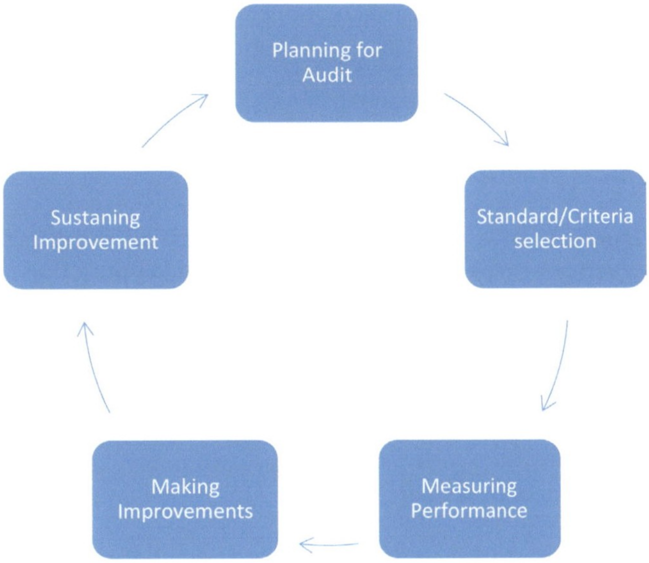

Figure 2.
Cycle of clinical audit.

Stage 3. Measuring performance: This stage involves collection of data, analysis of data, drawing conclusions, and presenting results. It is essential that the data collected during a clinical audit is accurate and relevant to the audit being conducted. The audit team should specify and approve the data source. Deciding which source to use depends on various factors, including accessibility, accuracy, and completeness [48].

Stage 4. Making improvement: Changes should be put into effect in this stage, and to ensure that necessary changes are made, all effective audit programs must include a program of change activities and post-identification of the audit results to ensure that the required changes take place [49].

Stage 5. Sustaining improvements is also crucial: This stage involves monitoring the quality improvement plan, performance indicators, dissemination and celebrating success, and reauditing. The audit cycle is a continuous process that involves two data collections and a comparison of that data after the change has been implemented after the first data collection to determine whether the desired improvements have been achieved (**Figure 2**) [50].

5. Conclusion

Measurement is a fundamental component of evidence-based physical therapy that provides most of the essential information clinicians need to make decisions in patient management. Effort to enhance the utilization of outcome measure in physiotherapy practice through the use of best available research evidence have resulted in the wide spread use of the term "evidence-based practice." Physiotherapists should be better equipped to integrate data from high-quality research with patient preferences and professional expertise.

Author details

Sham'unu Isah Abdu[1]*, Abduljalil Hussaini Maikarfe[2], Hassan Bukar Gambo[3], Isa Muhammadu Tanko[3] and Fatima Sada Sani[4]

1 Department of Physiotherapy, General Hospital Kazaure, Jigawa State, Nigeria

2 Department of Physiotherapy, General Hospital Birnin Kudu, Jigawa State, Nigeria

3 Department of Physiotherapy, University of Maiduguri Teaching Hospital, Borno State, Nigeria

4 Department of Physiotherapy, BarauDikko Teaching Hospital, Kaduna State, Nigeria

*Address all correspondence to: ask4saf@gmail.com

References

[1] Bello AI. Utilizing research findings in physiotherapy: A call for gap bridging. Journal of the Nigeria Society of Physiotherapy. 2011;**18**:54

[2] Dannapfel P, Peolsson A, Nilsen P. What supports physiotherapists' use of research in clinical practice? A qualitative study in Sweden. Implementation Science. 2013;**8**:31. DOI: 10.1186/1748-5908-8-31

[3] Herbert R, Jamtvedt G, Hagen KB, Mead J. Practical Evidence-Based Physiotherapy. 2nd ed. London: Elsevier; 2011

[4] Caldwell K, Coleman K, Copp G, Bell L, Ghazi F. Preparing for professional practice: How well does professional training equip health and social care practitioners to engage in evidence-based practice? Nurse Education Today. 2007;**27**(6):518-528. DOI: 10.1016/j.nedt.2006.08.014

[5] Antman EM, Lau J, Kupelnick B, Mosteller F, Chalmers TC. A comparison of results of meta-analyses of randomized control trials and recommendations of clinical experts. Treatments for myocardial infarction. JAMA. 1992;**268**(2):240-248

[6] Bernhardsson S, Larsson MEH, Johansson K, Öberg B. "In the physio we trust": A qualitative study on patients' preferences for physiotherapy. Physiotherapy Theory and Practice. 2017;**33**(7):535-549. DOI: 10.1080/09593985.2017.1328720

[7] Entwistle V, Firnigl D, Ryan M, Francis J, Kinghorn P. Which experiences of health care delivery matter to service users and why? A critical interpretive synthesis and conceptual map. Journal of Health Services Research & Policy. 2012;**17**(2):70-78. DOI: 10.1258/jhsrp.2011.011029

[8] Schoot T, Proot I, Meulen RT, Witte L. Recognition of client values as a basis for tailored care: The view of Dutch expert patients and family caregivers. Scandinavian Journal of Caring Sciences. 2005;**19**(2):169-176

[9] Skea Z, MacLennan S, Entwistle V, N'dow J. Communicating good care: A qualitative study of what people with urological cancer value in interactions with health care providers. European Journal of Oncology Nursing. 2014;**18**(1):35-40

[10] Higgs J, Titchen A. Practice Knowledge and Expertise in the Health Professions. Oxford: Butterworth-Heinemann; 2001

[11] Tiffen J, Corbridge SJ, Slimmer L. Enhancing clinical decision making: Development of a contiguous definition and conceptual framework. Journal of Professional Nursing. 2014;**30**(5):399-405. DOI: 10.1016/j.profnurs.2014.01.006

[12] Kumar S, Grimmer-Somers K, Hughes B. The ethics of evidence implementation in health care. Physiotherapy Research International. 2010;**15**:96-102

[13] Sackett DL, Straus SE, Richardson WS, et al. Evidence Based Medicine: How to Practice and Teach EBM. Edinburg: Churchill Livingstone; 2000

[14] Antunes B, Harding R, Higginson IJ. Implementing patient-reported outcome measures in palliative care clinical practice: A systematic review of

facilitators and barriers. Palliative Medicine. 2014;**28**(2):158-175. DOI: 10.1177/0269216313491619

[15] Beattie P. Measurement of health outcomes in the clinical setting: Applications to physiotherapy. Physiotherapy Theory and Practice. 2001;**17**(3):173-185. DOI: 10.1080/095939801317077632

[16] Duffy JR, Hoskins LM. The quality-care model blending dual paradigms. Advances in Nursing Science. 2003;**26**:77-88

[17] Copeland JM, Taylor WJ, Dean SG. Factors influencing the use of outcome measures for patients with low back pain: A survey of New Zealand physical therapists. Physical Therapy. 2008;**88**:1492-1505. DOI: 10.2522/ptj.20080083

[18] Duncan EAS, Murray J. The barriers and facilitators to routine outcome measurement by allied health professionals in practice: A systematic review. BMC Health Services Research. 2012;**12**:96. DOI: 10.1186/1472-6963-12-96

[19] MacDermid JC, Walton DM, Côté P, Santaguida PL, Gross A, Carlesso L, et al. Use of outcome measures in managing neck pain: An international multidisciplinary survey. The Open Orthopaedics Journal. 2013;**7**(Suppl. 4: M10):506-520

[20] Stevens JGA, Beurskens AJMH. Implementation of measurement instruments in physical therapist practice: Development of a tailored strategy. Physical Therapy. 2010;**90**(6):953-961. DOI: 10.2522/ptj.20090105

[21] Hefford C, Abbott JH, Baxter GD, Arnold R. Outcome measurement in clinical practice: Practical and theoretical issues for health related quality of life(HRQoL) questionaires. Physical Therapy Review. 2011;**16**(3):155-167. DOI: 10.1179/1743288X11Y.0000000004

[22] Mokkink L, Terwee C, Patrick D, Alonso J, Stratford P, Knol D, et al. The COSMIN study reached international consensus on taxonomy, terminology, and definitions of measurement properties for health-related patient-reported outcomes. Journal of Clinical Epidemiology. 2010;**63**(7):737-745

[23] Portney L, Watkins M. Chapter 4: Principles of Measurement, within Foundations of Clinical Research: Applications to Practice. 3rd ed. Pennsylvania, United States: F.A. Davis Company; 2015. ISBN10 0803646577

[24] Deyo RA, Diehr P, Patrick DL. Reproducibility and responsiveness of health status measures. Statistics and strategies for evaluation. Controlled Clinical Trials. 1991;**12**(Suppl. 4):142S-158S

[25] Lohr KN. Assessing health status and quality-of-life instruments: Attributes and review criteria. Quality of Life Research. 2002;**11**(3):193-205

[26] Ware J, Sherbourne C. The MOS 36-item short-form health survey (SF-36). I. Conceptual framework and item selection. Medical Care. 1992;**30**:473-483

[27] Brockow T, Cieza A, Kuhlow H, Sigl T, Franke T, Harder M, et al. Identifying the concepts contained in outcome measures of clinical trials on musculoskeletal disorders and chronic widespread pain using the international classification of functioning, disability and health as a reference. Journal of Rehabilitation Medicine. 2004;(Suppl. 44):30-36. DOI: 10.1080/16501960410015371. PMID: 15370745

[28] McNair PJ, Prapavessis H, Collier J, Bassett S, Bryant A, Larmer P. The lower-limb tasks questionnaire: An assessment of validity, reliability, responsiveness, and minimal important differences. Archives of Physical Medicine and Rehabilitation. 2007;**88**:993-1001

[29] Beaton DE, Wright JG, Katz JN, Upper Extremity Collaborative Group. Development of the QuickDASH: Comparison of three item-reduction approaches. The Journal of Bone and Joint Surgery–American Volume. 2005;**87**:1038-1046

[30] Stratford P, Gill C, Westaway M, Binkley J. Assessing disability and change on individual patients: A report of a patient specific measure. Physiotherapy Canada. 1995;**47**:258-263

[31] Paci M, Faedda G, Ugolini A, Pellicciari L. Barrier to evidence based practice implementation in physiotherapy: A systematic review and meta-analysis. International Journal for Quality in Health Care. 2021;**33**(2):mzab093. DOI: 10.1093/intqhc/mzab093. PMID: 34110410

[32] Herbert RD, Sherrington C, Maher C, Moseley AM. Evidence-based practice -- imperfect but necessary. Physiotherapy Theory and Practice. 2001;**17**(3):201-211. DOI: 10.1080/095939801317077650

[33] Ramírez-Vélez R, Bagur-Calafat MC, Correa-Bautista JE, et al. Barriers against incorporating evidence-based practice in physical therapy in Colombia: Current state and factors associated. BMC Medical Education. 2015;**15**:220. DOI: 10.1186/s12909-015-0502-3

[34] Yahui HC, Swaminathan N. Knowledge, attitude, and barriers towards evidence-based practice among physiotherapists in Malaysia. Hong Kong Physiotherapy Journal. 28 Feb 2017;**37**:10-18. DOI: 10.1016/j.hkpj.2016.12.002. PMID: 30931041; PMCID: PMC6385151

[35] Jesrani P, Sarfraz M, Kumar K, Imtiaz F, Kanwal R, Hasnain F, et al. Barriers to implementation of evidence-based practice in physiotherapy. International Journal of Endorsing Health Science Research (IJEHSR). 2019;**7**(1):22-32. DOI: 10.29052/IJEHSR.v7.i1.2019.22-32

[36] Gleadhill C, Bolsewicz K, Davidson SRE, et al. Physiotherapists' opinions, barriers, and enablers to providing evidence-based care: A mixed-methods study. BMC Health Services Research. 2022;**22**:1382. DOI: 10.1186/s12913-022-08741-5

[37] Adamsen L, Larsen K, Bjerregaard L, Madsen JK. Danish research-active clinical nurses overcome barriers in research utilization. Scandinavian Journal of Caring Sciences. 2003;**17**:57-65

[38] McKenna HP, Ashton S, Keeney S. Issues and innovations in nursing practice: Barriers to evidence-based practice in primary care. Journal of Advanced Nursing. 2004;**45**(2):178-189

[39] Melnyk BM. Strategies for overcoming barriers in implementing evidence-based practice. Pediatric Nursing. 2002;**28**(2):159-161

[40] Young JM, Ward JE. Evidence-based medicine in general practice. Beliefs and barriers among Australian GPs. Journal of Evaluation in Clinical Practice. 2001;7(2):201-210

[41] Kader P. Barriers to, and facilitators of, research utilization among nurses in northern Ireland. Journal of Advanced Nursing. 2000;**31**(1):89-98

[42] Straus SE, McAlister FA. Evidence-based medicine: A commentary on common criticisms. Canadian

Medical Association Journal. 2000;**163**(7):7837-7842

[43] Horsley C, Kelly A, Epstein J. Evidence-based practice and emergency medicine. A mismatch? Emergency Medicine. 1999;**11**(3):188-193

[44] McGlone P, Watt R, Sheiham A. Evidence-based dentistry: An overview of the challenges in changing professional practice. British Dental Journal. 2001;**190**(12):636-639

[45] NICE. Principles for Best Practice in Clinical Audit. Oxford: Radcliffe Medical Press; 2002

[46] Mungford M, Banfield P, O'Hanlon M. Effects of feedback of information on clinical practice: A review. BMJ. 1991;**303**:398-402

[47] Potter J, Fuller C, Ferris M. Local clinical audit: Handbook for physicians. In: Healthcare Quality Improvement Partnership. 2010. Available from: http://www.hqip.org.uk/assets/Guidance/Local-clinical-audit-handbook-forphysicians-August-2010-FINAL.pdf

[48] Quality & Patient Safety Directorate. A Practical Guide to Clinical Audit. HSE Quality and Patient Safety Division Report for 2013. 2013. Available from: http://hdl.handle.net/10147/628437

[49] Ashmore S, Ruthven T, Hazel-wood L. Stage 3: Implementing change. In: Burgess R, editor. NEW Principles of Best Practice in Clinical Audit. Healthcare Quality Improvement Partnership (HQIP). Abingdon, Radcliffe Medical Press. 2011c. pp. 81-92

[50] Ashmore S, Ruthven T, Hazelwood L. Stage 4: Sustaining improvement. In: Burgess R, editor. New Principles of Best Practice in Clinical Audit. Healthcare Quality Improvement Partnership (HQIP). Abingdon: Radcliffe Medical Press; 2011d. pp. 93-106

Chapter 3

Assessment Indicators for Determining Walking Independence

Ryosuke Yamamoto, Shoya Fujikawa, Shun Sawai and Hideki Nakano

Abstract

Walking disorders not only significantly reduce activities of daily living and lower the quality of life, but also increase the burden on caregivers and the use of social resources. Therefore, an appropriate assessment of walking independence is very important in physiotherapy practice. Several indices have been reported to assess walking independence in stroke patients. Most of them are evaluated with a focus on physical function and balance ability, and the cut-off values for each indicator have been reported. This chapter describes the validity, relevance, and cut-off values of the balance and walking indices used to assess walking independence in stroke patients, and outlines their clinical applications.

Keywords: physiotherapy, evaluation, level of walking ability, balance, stroke

1. Introduction

Aging is often associated with a decline in physical function, which ultimately leads to a loss of independence while performing activities of daily living (ADL). Walking is a general ADL and is important as a major determinant of the quality of life (QOL) in older people. Walking velocity has been called the 'sixth vital sign' because it is a central indicator of health and function in older people [1]. There is also a significant difference in the walking velocity and ADL dependence between those with sarcopenia and healthy older people [2]. Furthermore, walking velocity indicates neuromuscular quality and is an important determinant of aging [2]. Algorithms involving walking velocity measurement that have been developed to determine sarcopenia in older adults are simple and reliable [3]. They have also been used to diagnose functional impairments and dependency disorders in older adults [3–5]. Similarly, a decrease in walking velocity because of reduced muscle mass is associated with aging [1]. These factors raise the concern that the likelihood of developing a walking disorder increases with age, even in the absence of specific diseases. Walking disorders are accompanied by limitations in mobility and activity and they restrict ADL and lower the QOL. Therefore, maintaining and improving the walking ability during rehabilitation is an important goal for physiotherapists. In this chapter, the

 IntechOpen

evaluation indices that are generally used to determine walking independence and those used to determine walking independence in stroke patients are described in sections.

2. The various assessment indicators in the determination of walking independence

Most measures of walking independence are based on walking ability, physical function [disease and motor function in the region of the impairment], and balance ability. This section describes various assessment indices used to determine walking independence.

2.1 General assessment indicators for determining walking independence

There are a wide range of diseases that require physiotherapy. Therefore, physiotherapists need to consider the characteristics of individual diseases and the stage of the disease to appropriately assess the degree of walking independence. The most commonly used evaluation indices for walking independence are those that assess balance and walking indicators. The Functional Reach Test (FRT), Berg Balance Scale (BBS), and Mini-Balance Evaluation Systems Test [Mini-BESTest] are commonly used as evaluation indices for balance ability, and their reliability and validity have already been reported [6, 7]. The 10-meter walking test [10MWT] [8] and the Timed Up and Go (TUG) test are generally used as walking indicators. This section summarizes the assessment indicators commonly used in walking independence assessment and their details (**Table 1**).

TUG is reportedly a reliable assessment, strongly correlating with balance, postural control, walking ability, and fall risk [8, 13]. TUG ≥13.5 s and BBS < 46 points are the cut-off values for a balance disorder [9]. In frail older adults, the cut-off value of the FRT to determine the risk of falling is ≥18.5 cm [6]. Furthermore, the cut-off value of the Mini-BESTest to determine walking independence in patients admitted

	Evaluation indicator	Detail
Balance ability	Functional Reach Test (FRT) [6]	The cut-off value for discriminating the risk of falls in frail elderly people is ≥18.5 cm.
	Berg Balance Scale (BBS) [9]	Balance impaired the cut-off value of 46 points.
	Mini-Balance Evaluation Systems Test (Mini-BESTest) [10]	In patients admitted to recovery units, the Mini-BESTest cut-off value for determining walking independence is 18 points.
Walking ability	10-meter Walking Test (10MWT) [11, 12]	In patients admitted to recovery wards, the cut-off value for walking independence is 0.8 m/s. In community-dwelling elderly, indoor walking independence is 0.5 m/s; outdoor walking independence is 1 m/s.
	Timed up and Go Test (TUG) [9]	The cut-off value for determining a balance disorder is ≥13.5 s.

Table 1.
Generally used assessment indicators for determining walking independence.

to rehabilitation wards is 18 points [10]. The BBS score of hip fracture patients admitted to rehabilitation wards helps to predict walking independence at discharge and determine treatment according to the predicted level of independence [14]. The reported cut-off value for the 10MWT, a walking indicator, for walking independence in patients in recovery wards is 0.8 m/s, indoor walking independence in older adults living in the community is 0.5 m/s, and outdoor walking independence is 1 m/s [11, 12]. As described above, several previous studies have reported on the use of general balance and walking indicators to identify cut-off values for determining walking independence and fall risk.

2.2 Indicators for assessing walking independence based on walking ability in stroke patients

Walking disorders are one of the most serious consequences associated with stroke, and approximately 30% of stroke patients have difficulty walking independently even in the chronic phase [15]. In addition, 38% of stroke patients are unable to walk at 6 months after stroke onset [16]. Stroke is a neurological disease and its sequelae are associated with physical disability. Walking disorders are observed in more than 50% of stroke patients. Walking disorders may be due to motor or sensory disorders, spasticity, or balance disorders [17]. It is necessary to assess the factors involved in walking disorders to improve walking independence. Walking ability includes walking independence, velocity, and endurance. The Functional Ambulation Categories (FAC) are used to assess walking independence, the 10MWT to assess walking velocity, and the 6-minute walk test (6MWT) to assess endurance. Stroke patients suffer problems such as motor paralysis and sensory impairment [17, 18]. Moreover, impaired balance is due to reduced motor control of the limbs, pelvis, and trunk, sensory impairment, and impaired spatial perception of the body [19]. Furthermore, impaired balance has been reported to lead to reduced mobility [20]. Therefore, it is essential to assess gait ability from multiple perspectives using the above assessment indices to appropriately assess stroke patients' gait ability (**Figure 1**).

The FAC is a walking indicator that classifies walking ability on a 6-point scale from 0 to 5 based on the amount of care required while walking and has been reported to have excellent reliability in patients with post-stroke hemiplegia [21]. The FAC at 4 weeks after stroke onset has been reported to have predictive validity for walking ability at the regional level 6 months after stroke onset [21]. In addition, walking velocity is one of the most sensitive measures to assess walking independence, using an assessment index related to walking indicators, walking velocity being one of the walking ability indicators [22]. It has also been reported that the comfortable walking velocity for the 10MWT is a valid walking indicator for assessing walking ability in stroke patients [23]. Another study reported that the trunk control test (TCT) and FAC can predict walking independence 45 days after stroke onset [24]. Previous studies have compared the BBS, Mini-BESTest, and Functional Gait Assessment (FGA) in terms of reactivity, floor effect, and ceiling effect at different levels of walking: The BBS showed the highest relative effect in the FAC2-3 group and the Mini-BESTest showed the highest relative effect in the other two groups (FAC 4-5 and 6) [25]. In patients with FAC 2-3, the floor effect occurred with the FGA, and in patients with FAC 6, the floor effect occurred with the BBS [22]. The BBS is suitable for stroke patients with FAC 2 to 5, while the MBT and FGA are suitable for stroke patients with FAC 4 to 6 [25]. The cut-off values for the 10MWT in stroke patients are

<0.4 m/s for those with walking independence at home, 0.4–0.8 m/s for those with walking independence in a limited area, and > 0.8 m/s for those with walking independence in the community [26]. Furthermore, walking endurance and velocity are good predictors of whether subacute stroke patients will reach community walking levels at 6-month post-discharge. The cut-off values are 195 m and 0.56 m/s, respectively [27]. The 10MWT and 6MWT have different cut-off values depending on which level of walking independence is targeted, so the meaning of the measured times and distances should be interpreted according to the needs of the individual patient.

2.3 Indicators for determining walking independence based on physical function in stroke patients

Patients present with a wide range of clinical symptoms following stroke. Post-stroke motor function impairment appears as muscle weakness, abnormal muscle tone, and impaired motor coordination, and mobility is also impaired with these symptoms. Voluntary neurological recovery of post-stroke motor function progressively improves over the first 3–6 months after stroke onset, before reaching the ceiling [28]. In physiotherapy, it is necessary to quantitatively assess physical function and plan intervention methods tailored to the patient, with the aim of improving the patient's physical function.

Various assessment indices, such as the Fugl-Meyer Assessment (FMA), Brunnstrom recovery stage, Motor Assessment Scale (MAS), and Stroke Impairment Assessment Set, have been developed to evaluate motor function in stroke patients.

The reliability and validity of these assessment measures have been reported [29–31]. Stroke also reduces the ability of the trunk coordination immediately after stroke onset. In particular, reduced trunk muscle activity reduces pelvic movement, affecting trunk asymmetry and causing reduced balance ability [32]. The TCT and Trunk Impairment Scale (TIS) are reliable and valid as assessment indices of trunk function in stroke patients [33–35]. It has also been reported that in stroke patients, the TIS score on admission is strongly correlated with the National Institutes of Health Stroke Scale, upper limb FMA, and lower limb FMA scores [29]. Furthermore, trunk function has been shown to influence stroke severity and upper and lower limb motor function. The cut-off values for determining walking independence in stroke patients using each index to assess motor function are described below. Patients with a lower limb MAS score of ≥5 within 4 weeks after stroke onset can walk independently [36]. In addition, patients with a TCT score of ≤50 at 14 days after stroke onset have a FAC < 4 [34]. Thus, previous studies have shown that the motor function of the paralyzed lower limb and trunk function affect the physical functional factors involved in the degree of walking independence in stroke patients.

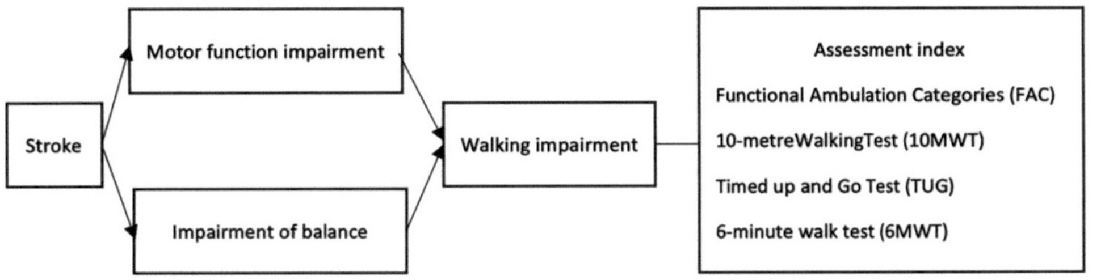

Figure 1.
Assessment index for gait ability in stroke patients.

2.4 Indicators for the assessment of walking independence based on balance ability in stroke patients

Stroke causes a variety of complications, including muscle weakness, sensory impairment, and cognitive decline [35]. Sensory impairment, in particular, affects balance and postural control in stroke patients and is important for keeping the body upright and stable under different conditions [37]. Reduced balance ability after stroke is associated with reduced ADL [38] and limited social participation [39]. Decreased balance ability is caused by reduced motor control of the limbs, pelvis, and trunk, sensory impairment, and reduced spatial cognition of the body [19]. It has also been reported that reduced balance ability increases the risk and fear of falling [20] and leads to reduced ADL and a lower QOL [40]. After stroke, patients present with a wide variety of clinical symptoms. It is, therefore, essential to assess motor function as described in the previous section and balance function in detail (**Figure 2**).

The commonly used balance assessment indices in stroke patients include the BBS, FRT, TUG, and one-leg standing (OLS). Their role in determining treatment strategy is limited, but their effectiveness in stroke patients has been reported [41]. The cut-off value of the FRT to determine the presence of falls in stroke patients is 15.0 cm [42]. The BBS, one of the typical assessment indices, has also been found to be a very valid and reliable means of assessment of balance ability in stroke patients [43]. This section provides a table summarizing the assessment measures used in gait independence assessment in stroke patients and their details (**Table 2**).

The BBS has been reported to have a cut-off value of 31 points as a discriminatory criterion between the falls and non-fall groups in hospitalized stroke patients [44]. In addition, stroke patients with a BBS score of ≥29 points on admission recover to community ambulation or walking ability without walking aids after 4 weeks. It has been reported that if the BBS score on admission is ≥12 points, non-ambulatory patients can reach walking independence [45]. Furthermore, the cut-off value for the BBS score in chronic stroke patients based on walking at the community level (>0.8 m/s) has been reported to be 47.5 points [46]. However, because the BBS, OLS, and FRT

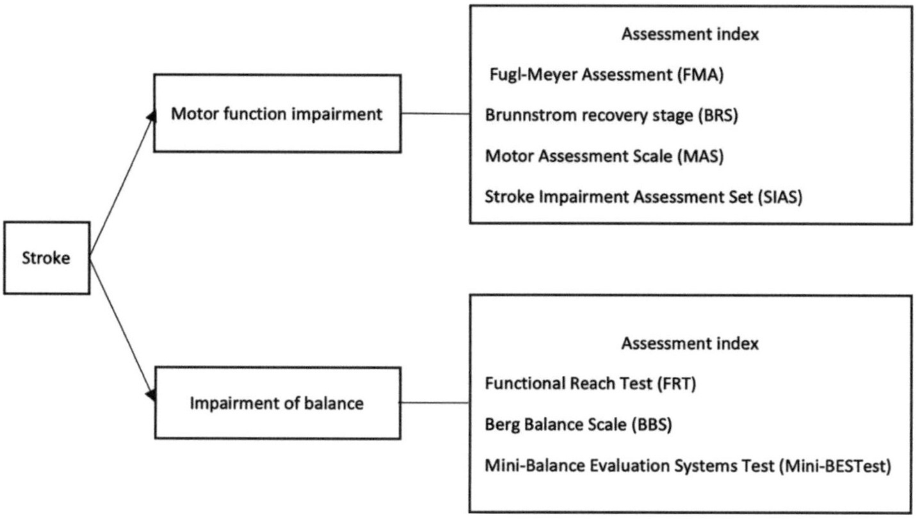

Figure 2.
Assessment indices for physical function and balance in stroke patients.

	Evaluation indicators	Detail
Balance ability	Berg Balance Scale (BBS) [22, 44–46]	Suitable assessment measure for stroke patients with FAC 2 to 5. Stroke patients with a score of 29 or more on admission will recover to community ambulation or no walking aids after 4 weeks. A score of 12 or more on admission leads to ambulatory independence for non-ambulatory patients. The cut-off value for predicting falls and the non-fall group for stroke patients on admission is 31 points. The cut-off value for community walking (>0.8 m/s) is 47.5 points.
	Mini-Balance Evaluation Systems Test (Mini-BESTest) [46–48]	Reliable assessment indicator at any stage of the disease. The assessment indicator is suitable for stroke patients with FAC 4–6. Cut-off values for the walking independence assessment are not known. The cut-off value for community walking (>0.8 m/s) is 18.5 points.
Walking ability	10-meter Walking Test (10MWT) [26]	In patients admitted to recovery wards, the cut-off value for walking independence is 0.8 m/s. In community-dwelling elderly, indoor walking independence is 0.5 m/s; outdoor walking independence is 1 m/s.
	Ambulation Categories (FAC) [26]	The assessment of FAC at 4 weeks after stroke onset is reported to provide predictive validity for the ability to walk at the community level 6 months after stroke onset.
	6-minute walk test (6MWT) [27]	In subacute stroke patients, the cut-off value for predicting whether the community walking level will be reached at 6 months after discharge from the hospital is 195 m.

Table 2.
Indicators for the assessment of walking independence in stroke patients.

have floor and ceiling effects [49–51], the Mini-BESTest was newly developed as a balance assessment indicator for patients with neurological disorders. The Mini-BESTest is an evaluation index that calculates scores for six factors related to balance function (biomechanical constraints, stability limits, postural change—predictive postural control, reactive postural control, sensory function, and walking stability). It is also a useful indicator for clarifying therapeutic intervention strategies for patients with balance disorders by identifying problems in individual balance functions by the element [47, 48]. The Mini-BESTest has also been tested for reliability and validity at all stages of stroke patients. Furthermore, the cut-off value of the Mini-BESTest in stroke patients based on walking at the community level (>0.8 m/s) has been reported to be 18.5 points [46]. In summary, walking independence and fall risk can be better determined by assessing the balance ability using the BBS, Mini-BESTest, and FRT (**Table 2**).

3. Determining walking independence based on brain imaging in stroke patients

Pathophysiological changes in motor recovery after stroke mainly occur within the first 15 weeks after stroke, regardless of the severity of the initial motor impairment [52]. Motor impairments stabilize after 6 months, which is considered as the chronic phase [53]. However, it has been reported that motor function continues to improve during the chronic phase through various mutually complementary brain plasticities [52]. Brain imaging showing the structure and function of the motor cortex has also been reported to help predict both motor recovery and motor outcome after stroke [54]. Specifically, it has been suggested that the measurement of the corticospinal tract (CST) in the acute phase may predict motor function. Early measurement of the number of fibers in the CST predicts motor outcome (FMA score) at 12 months, especially in patients with first stroke [55]. The number of fibers in the ipsilateral and contralateral CST (FA value) in the acute phase suggests a good recovery of motor function after stroke [56]. Moreover, neuroimaging and neurophysiology CST biomarkers can predict the prognosis of motor function and response to treatment after stroke and are recommended for use in clinical trials, including patient stratification [57]. The CST can be elucidated using magnetic resonance imaging, and the FA values of diffusion tensor imaging in particular have been identified as a reliable tool to identify the structural integrity of CST after stroke [58, 59]. In summary, brain imaging is a clinically important indicator when planning individualized rehabilitation of patients. Recently, several studies have reported the use of brain imaging to predict recovery of motor paralysis in stroke patients. It has been suggested that the FA value of the ipsilateral CST on day 14 after stroke onset is significantly correlated with improvement in motor paralysis [60–63]. However, the association with an index to assess walking independence is not clear and is a subject for subsequent studies.

4. Conclusion

In this chapter, each section describes an index to determine the degree of walking independence in stroke patients. It is clear that not only the reliability and validity of individual assessment indices but also the degree of brain damage, motor paralysis, trunk function, balance, and walking ability correlate with each other. Therefore, physiotherapists must assess the disability caused by stroke from multiple perspectives. In addition, it is important to match the cut-off values for balance and walking ability to determine the degree of walking independence. In the future, it will be important to clarify the relationship between the results of brain imaging analysis and indices of physical function, balance, and walking ability to improve the accuracy of prognostic prediction and establish evidence for walking independence in stroke patients.

Acknowledgements

This work was supported by JSPS KAKENHI Grant Number JP23K10417. We would like to thank Editage (www.editage.com) for English language editing.

Conflict of interest

The authors declare no conflict of interest.

Author details

Ryosuke Yamamoto[1,2], Shoya Fujikawa[1,2], Shun Sawai[1,2] and Hideki Nakano[1*]

1 Neurorehabilitation Laboratory, Graduate School of Health Sciences, Kyoto Tachibana University, Kyoto, Japan

2 Department of Rehabilitation, Tesseikai Neurosurgical Hospital, Osaka, Japan

*Address all correspondence to: nakano-h@tachibana-u.ac.jp

References

[1] Bortone I, Sardone R, Lampignano L, Castellana F, Zupo R, Lozupone M, et al. How gait influences frailty models and health-related outcomes in clinical-based and population-based studies: A systematic review. Journal of Cachexia, Sarcopenia and Muscle. 2021;**12**(2):274-297. DOI: 10.1002/jcsm.12667. Epub 2021 Feb 16

[2] Perez-Sousa MA, Venegas-Sanabria LC, Chavarro-Carvajal DA, Cano-Gutierrez CA, Izquierdo M, Correa-Bautista JE, et al. Gait speed as a mediator of the effect of sarcopenia on dependency in activities of daily living. Journal of Cachexia, Sarcopenia and Muscle. 2019;**10**(5):1009-1015. DOI: 10.1002/jcsm.12444. Epub 2019 May 8

[3] Cruz-Jentoft AJ, Baeyens JP, Bauer JM, Boirie Y, Cederholm T, Landi F, et al. Sarcopenia: European consensus on definition and diagnosis: Report of the European working group on sarcopenia in older people. Age and Ageing. 2010;**39**(4):412-423. DOI: 10.1093/ageing/afq034. Epub 2010 Apr 13

[4] López-Teros T, Gutiérrez-Robledo LM, Pérez-Zepeda MU. Gait speed and handgrip strength as predictors of incident disability in Mexican older adults. The Journal of Frailty & Aging. 2014;**3**(2):109-112. DOI: 10.14283/jfa.2014.10

[5] Graham JE, Fisher SR, Bergés IM, Kuo YF, Ostir GV. Walking speed threshold for classifying walking independence in hospitalized older adults. Physical Therapy. 2010;**90**(11):1591-1597. DOI: 10.2522/ptj.20100018. Epub 2010 Aug 12

[6] Thomas JI, Lane JV. A pilot study to explore the predictive validity of 4 measures of falls risk in frail elderly patients. Archives of Physical Medicine and Rehabilitation. 2005;**86**(8):1636-1640. DOI: 10.1016/j.apmr.2005.03.004

[7] Tsang CS, Liao LR, Chung RC, Pang MY. Psychometric properties of the mini-balance evaluation systems test (mini-BESTest) in community-dwelling individuals with chronic stroke. Physical Therapy. 2013;**93**(8):1102-1115. DOI: 10.2522/ptj.20120454. Epub 2013 Apr 4

[8] Hiengkaew V, Jitaree K, Chaiyawat P. Minimal detectable changes of the Berg balance scale, Fugl-Meyer assessment scale, timed "up & go" test, gait speeds, and 2-minute walk test in individuals with chronic stroke with different degrees of ankle plantarflexor tone. Archives of Physical Medicine and Rehabilitation. 2012;**93**(7):1201-1208. DOI: 10.1016/j.apmr.2012.01.014. Epub 2012 Apr 12

[9] Liwsrisakun C, Pothirat C, Chaiwong W, Bumroongkit C, Deesomchok A, Theerakittikul T, et al. Exercise performance as a predictor for balance impairment in COPD patients. Medicina (Kaunas, Lithuania). 2019;**55**(5):171. DOI: 10.3390/medicina55050171

[10] Hasegawa S, Kouchi H, Usuda S. Accuracies of the balance evaluation systems test (BESTest), mini-BESTest, and brief-BESTest in discriminating the ambulatory Independence of patients in a convalescence rehabilitation Ward. Rigakuryoho Kagaku. 2017;**32**(4):477-481. Submitted Jan. 23, 2017. Accepted Mar. 11, 2017

[11] Iida S, Aoki C. Reliability of the 10-meter walking test [part 1]: Influence

of different measurement orders on the fastest walking and Normal walking. Rigakuryoho Kagaku. 2017;**32**(1):81-84. Submitted Aug. 17, 2016. Accepted Sep. 14, 2016

[12] Sugihara T. Intra-assessor reliability of the 10 m walk time measurement. Specialised Rehabilitation. 2004;**3**:13-15

[13] Podsiadlo D, Richardson S. The timed "up & go": A test of basic functional mobility for frail elderly persons. Journal of the American Geriatrics Society. 1991;**39**(2):142-148. DOI: 10.1111/j.1532-5415.1991.tb01616.x

[14] Tamura S, Miyata K, Kobayashi S, Takeda R, Iwamoto H. Development of cut-off values on the Berg balance scale for predicting walking Independence in older adults with hip fracture. Progress in Rehabilitation Medicine. 2022;**7**:20220043. DOI: 10.2490/prm.20220043

[15] Park HJ, Oh DW, Kim SY, Choi JD. Effectiveness of community-based ambulation training for walking function of post-stroke hemiparesis: A randomized controlled pilot trial. Clinical Rehabilitation. 2011;**25**(5):451-459. DOI: 10.1177/0269215510389200. Epub 2011 Jan 18

[16] Kollen B, Kwakkel G, Lindeman E. Longitudinal robustness of variables predicting independent gait following severe middle cerebral artery stroke: A prospective cohort study. Clinical Rehabilitation. 2006;**20**(3):262-268. DOI: 10.1191/0269215506cr910oa

[17] Belda-Lois JM, Mena-del Horno S, Bermejo-Bosch I, Moreno JC, Pons JL, Farina D, et al. Rehabilitation of gait after stroke: A review towards a top-down approach. Journal of Neuroengineering and Rehabilitation. 2011;**8**:66. DOI: 10.1186/1743-0003-8-66

[18] Benjamin EJ, Blaha MJ, Chiuve SE, Cushman M, Das SR, Deo R, et al. Heart disease and stroke Statistics-2017 update: A report from the American Heart Association. Circulation. 2017;**135**(10):e146-e603. DOI: 10.1161/CIR.0000000000000485. Epub 2017 Jan 25. [Erratum in: Circulation. 2017 Mar 7;135(10):e646. Erratum in: Circulation. 2017 Sep 5;136(10):e196]

[19] Oliveira CB, Medeiros ÍR, Greters MG, Frota NA, Lucato LT, Scaff M, et al. Abnormal sensory integration affects balance control in hemiparetic patients within the first year after stroke. Clinics (São Paulo, Brazil). 2011;**66**(12):2043-2048. DOI: 10.1590/s1807-59322011001200008. Erratum in: Clinics (Sao Paulo). 2012;67(2):203

[20] Schmid AA, Rittman M. Consequences of poststroke falls: Activity limitation, increased dependence, and the development of fear of falling. The American Journal of Occupational Therapy. 2009;**63**(3):310-316. DOI: 10.5014/ajot.63.3.310

[21] Yoo YJ, Lim SH. Assessment of lower limb motor function, ambulation, and balance after stroke. Brain Neurorehabil. 2022;**15**(2):e17. DOI: 10.12786/bn.2022.15.e17

[22] Lee KB, Lim SH, Kim YD, Yang BI, Kim KH, Lee KS, et al. The contributions of balance to gait capacity and motor function in chronic stroke. Journal of Physical Therapy Science. 2016;**28**(6):1686-1690. DOI: 10.1589/jpts.28.1686. Epub 2016 Jun 28

[23] Kollen B, Kwakkel G, Lindeman E. Time dependency of walking classification in stroke. Physical Therapy. 2006;**86**(5):618-625

[24] Duarte E, Marco E, Muniesa JM, Belmonte R, Aguilar JJ, Escalada F. Early

detection of non-ambulatory survivors six months after stroke. NeuroRehabilitation. 2010;**26**(4):317-323. DOI: 10.3233/NRE-2010-0568

[25] Rudolf M, Vidmar G, Goljar N. A comparison of three balance-assessment scales for patients after stroke with various levels of balance disorder. International Journal of Rehabilitation Research. 2020;**43**(4):337-341. DOI: 10.1097/MRR.0000000000000431

[26] Bowden MG, Balasubramanian CK, Behrman AL, Kautz SA. Validation of a speed-based classification system using quantitative measures of walking performance poststroke. Neurorehabilitation and Neural Repair. 2008;**22**(6):672-675. DOI: 10.1177/1545968308318837

[27] Igarashi T, Takeda R, Tani Y, Takahashi N, Ono T, Ishii Y, et al. Predictive discriminative accuracy of walking abilities at discharge for community ambulation levels at 6 months post-discharge among inpatients with subacute stroke. Journal of Physical Therapy Science. 2023;**35**(3):257-264. DOI: 10.1589/jpts.35.257. Epub

[28] Jørgensen HS, Nakayama H, Raaschou HO, Vive-Larsen J, Støier M, Olsen TS. Outcome and time course of recovery in stroke. Part I: Outcome. The Copenhagen stroke study. Archives of Physical Medicine and Rehabilitation. 1995;**76**(5):399-405. DOI: 10.1016/s0003-9993(95)80567-2

[29] Hsueh IP, Hsu MJ, Sheu CF, Lee S, Hsieh CL, Lin JH. Psychometric comparisons of 2 versions of the Fugl-Meyer Motor scale and 2 versions of the stroke rehabilitation assessment of movement. Neurorehabilitation and Neural Repair. 2008;**22**(6):737-744. DOI: 10.1177/1545968308315999. Epub 2008 Jul 21

[30] Brunnstrom S. Motor testing procedures in hemiplegia: Based on sequential recovery stages. Physical Therapy. 1966;**46**(4):357-375. DOI: 10.1093/ptj/46.4.357

[31] Sato A, Okuda Y, Fujita T, Kimura N, Hoshina N, Kato S, et al. Cognitive and physical functions related to the level of supervision and dependence in the toileting of stroke patients. Physical Therapy Research. 2016;**19**(1):32-38. DOI: 10.1298/ptr.e9904

[32] Karatas M, Cetin N, Bayramoglu M, Dilek A. Trunk muscle strength in relation to balance and functional disability in unihemispheric stroke patients. American Journal of Physical Medicine & Rehabilitation. 2004;**83**(2):81-87. DOI: 10.1097/01.PHM.0000107486.99756.C7

[33] Verheyden G, Nieuwboer A, Mertin J, Preger R, Kiekens C, De Weerdt W. The trunk impairment scale: A new tool to measure motor impairment of the trunk after stroke. Clinical Rehabilitation. 2004;**18**(3):326-334. DOI: 10.1191/0269215504cr733oa

[34] Kong KH, Ratha KR. Truncal impairment after stroke: Clinical correlates, outcome and impact on ambulatory and functional outcomes after rehabilitation. Singapore Medical Journal. 2021;**62**(2):87-91. DOI: 10.11622/smedj.2019153. Epub 2019 Dec 2

[35] Liao LY, He XH, Li XZ, Ge YL, Gao Q. Effects of kinesiology taping on trunk function, balance, and mobility in stroke patients: A pilot feasibility study. Journal of Physical Therapy Science. 2020;**32**(6):359-364. DOI: 10.1589/jpts.32.359. Epub 2020 Jun 2

[36] Kwah LK, Harvey LA, Diong J, Herbert RD. Models containing age and NIHSS predict recovery of ambulation

and upper limb function six months after stroke: An observational study. Journal of Physiotherapy. 2013;**59**(3):189-197. DOI: 10.1016/S1836-9553(13)70183-8. Erratum in: J Physiother. 2013;59(4):218

[37] Balaban B, Tok F. Gait disturbances in patients with stroke. PMR. 2014;**6**(7):635-642. DOI: 10.1016/j.pmrj.2013.12.017. Epub 2014 Jan 19

[38] Yu HX, Wang ZX, Liu CB, Dai P, Lan Y, Xu GQ. Effect of cognitive function on balance and posture control after stroke. Neural Plasticity. 2021;**2021**:6636999. DOI: 10.1155/2021/6636999

[39] Desrosiers J, Noreau L, Rochette A, Bravo G, Boutin C. Predictors of handicap situations following post-stroke rehabilitation. Disability and Rehabilitation. 2002;**24**(15):774-785. DOI: 10.1080/09638280210125814

[40] Galeoto G, Iori F, De Santis R, Santilli V, Mollica R, Marquez MA, et al. The outcome measures for loss of functionality in the activities of daily living of adults after stroke: A systematic review. Topics in Stroke Rehabilitation. 2019;**26**(3):236-245. DOI: 10.1080/10749357.2019.1574060. Epub 2019 Feb 18

[41] Pollock C, Eng J, Garland S. Clinical measurement of walking balance in people post stroke: A systematic review. Clinical Rehabilitation. 2011;**25**(8):693-708. DOI: 10.1177/0269215510397394. Epub 2011 May 25

[42] Acar M, Karatas GK. The effect of arm sling on balance in patients with hemiplegia. Gait & Posture. 2010;**32**(4):641-644. DOI: 10.1016/j.gaitpost.2010.09.008

[43] Berg K, Wood-Dauphinee S, Williams JI. The balance scale: Reliability assessment with elderly residents and patients with an acute stroke. Scandinavian Journal of Rehabilitation Medicine. 1995;**27**(1):27-36

[44] Maeda N, Urabe Y, Murakami M, Itotani K, Kato J. Discriminant analysis for predictor of falls in stroke patients by using the Berg balance scale. Singapore Medical Journal. 2015;**56**(5):280-283. DOI: 10.11622/smedj.2015033

[45] Louie DR, Eng JJ. Berg balance scale score at admission can predict walking suitable for community ambulation at discharge from inpatient stroke rehabilitation. Journal of Rehabilitation Medicine. 2018;**50**(1):37-44. DOI: 10.2340/16501977-2280

[46] Madhavan S, Bishnoi A. Comparison of the mini-balance evaluations systems test with the Berg balance scale in relationship to walking speed and motor recovery post stroke. Topics in Stroke Rehabilitation. 2017;**24**(8):579-584. DOI: 10.1080/10749357.2017.1366097. Epub 2017 Aug 21

[47] Otaka E, Otaka Y, Morita M, Yokoyama A, Kondo T, LIU M. Validation of the Japanese version of the mini-balance evaluation systems test(mini-BESTest). The Japanese Journal of Rehabilitation Medicine. 2014;**51**:673-681

[48] Miyata K, Hasegawa S, Iwamoto H, Otani T, Kaizu Y, Shinohara T, et al. Comparing the measurement properties and relationship to gait speed recovery of the mini-balance evaluation systems test and the Berg balance scale in ambulatory individuals with subacute stroke. Physical Therapy Research. 2020;**23**(1):72-78. DOI: 10.1298/ptr.E10004

[49] Mao HF, Hsueh IP, Tang PF, Sheu CF, Hsieh CL. Analysis and comparison of the psychometric properties of

three balance measures for stroke patients. Stroke. 2002;**33**(4):1022-1027. DOI: 10.1161/01.str.0000012516.63191.c5

[50] Tyson SF, DeSouza LH. Development of the Brunel balance assessment: A new measure of balance disability post stroke. Clinical Rehabilitation. 2004;**18**(7):801-810. DOI: 10.1191/0269215504cr744oa

[51] Blum L, Korner-Bitensky N. Usefulness of the Berg balance scale in stroke rehabilitation: A systematic review. Physical Therapy. 2008;**88**(5):559-566. DOI: 10.2522/ptj.20070205. Epub 2008 Feb 21

[52] Stinear CM. Prediction of motor recovery after stroke: Advances in biomarkers. Lancet Neurology. 2017;**16**(10):826-836. DOI: 10.1016/S1474-4422(17)30283-1. Epub 2017 Sep 12

[53] Langhorne P, Bernhardt J, Kwakkel G. Stroke rehabilitation. Lancet. 2011;**377**(9778):1693-1702. DOI: 10.1016/S0140-6736(11)60325-5

[54] Symms M, Jäger HR, Schmierer K, Yousry TA. A review of structural magnetic resonance neuroimaging. Journal of Neurology, Neurosurgery, and Psychiatry. 2004;**75**(9):1235-1244. DOI: 10.1136/jnnp.2003.032714

[55] Bigourdan A, Munsch F, Coupé P, Guttmann CR, Sagnier S, Renou P, et al. Early fiber number ratio is a surrogate of corticospinal tract integrity and predicts motor recovery after stroke. Stroke. 2016;**47**(4):1053-1059. DOI: 10.1161/STROKEAHA.115.011576. Epub 2016 Mar 15

[56] Riley JD, Le V, Der-Yeghiaian L, See J, Newton JM, Ward NS, et al. Anatomy of stroke injury predicts gains from therapy. Stroke. 2011;**42**(2):421-426. DOI: 10.1161/STROKEAHA.110.599340. Epub 2010 Dec 16

[57] Burke Quinlan E, Dodakian L, See J, McKenzie A, Le V, Wojnowicz M, et al. Neural function, injury, and stroke subtype predict treatment gains after stroke. Annals of Neurology. 2015;**77**(1):132-145. DOI: 10.1002/ana.24309. Epub 2014 Dec 4

[58] Auriat AM, Borich MR, Snow NJ, Wadden KP, Boyd LA. Comparing a diffusion tensor and non-tensor approach to white matter fiber tractography in chronic stroke. NeuroImage. Clinical. 2015;7:771-781. DOI: 10.1016/j.nicl.2015.03.007

[59] Nakashima A, Moriuchi T, Mitsunaga W, Yonezawa T, Kataoka H, Nakashima R, et al. Prediction of prognosis of upper-extremity function following stroke-related paralysis using brain imaging. Journal of Physical Therapy Science. 2017;**29**(8):1438-1443. DOI: 10.1589/jpts.29.1438. Epub 2017 Aug 10

[60] Marumoto K, Koyama T, Hosomi M, Takebayashi T, Hanada K, Ikeda S, et al. Diffusion tensor imaging predicts the outcome of constraint-induced movement therapy in chronic infarction patients with hemiplegia: A pilot study. Restorative Neurology and Neuroscience. 2013;**31**(4):387-396. DOI: 10.3233/RNN-120285

[61] Koyama T, Tsuji M, Nishimura H, Miyake H, Ohmura T, Domen K. Diffusion tensor imaging for intracerebral hemorrhage outcome prediction: Comparison using data from the corona radiata/internal capsule and the cerebral peduncle. Journal of Stroke and Cerebrovascular Diseases. 2013;**22**(1):72-79. DOI: 10.1016/j.jstrokecerebrovasdis.2011.06.014. Epub 2011 Jul 26

[62] Koyama T, Marumoto K, Miyake H, Domen K. Relationship between diffusion tensor fractional anisotropy and motor outcome in patients with hemiparesis after corona radiata infarct. Journal of Stroke and Cerebrovascular Diseases. 2013;**22**(8):1355-1360. DOI: 10.1016/j.jstrokecerebrovasdis.2013.02.017. Epub 2013 Mar 17

[63] Puig J, Blasco G, Daunis-I-Estadella J, Thomalla G, Castellanos M, Figueras J, et al. Decreased corticospinal tract fractional anisotropy predicts long-term motor outcome after stroke. Stroke. 2013;**44**(7):2016-2018. DOI: 10.1161/STROKEAHA.111.000382. Epub 2013 May 7

Chapter 4

Assessment of Brain Inhibitory Function in Physical Therapy

Shoya Fujikawa, Shun Sawai, Ryosuke Yamamoto and Hideki Nakano

Abstract

Interhemispheric inhibition is an inhibitory function of the brain that enables complex human locomotion and plays an important role in motor control. Traditionally, interhemispheric inhibition has been assessed using transcranial magnetic stimulation, functional magnetic resonance imaging, and electroencephalography. However, motor overflow and bimanual coordinated movements have recently attracted attention as behavioral indices involving interhemispheric inhibition. Motor overflow is defined as the presence of involuntary movements or weak muscle activity that appears with voluntary movements and has been found to occur mainly in the elderly, children, and those with central nervous system diseases. In addition, interhemispheric inhibition is involved in bimanual coordinated movements associated with interhemispheric motor control and information processing. This chapter outlines motor overflow and bimanual coordinated movements as new behavioral indices of interhemispheric inhibition and proposes assessment methods that can be performed in physiotherapy clinics.

Keywords: brain inhibitory function, interhemispheric inhibition, motor overflow, bimanual coordinated movement, elderly

1. Introduction

Interhemispheric inhibition is the mechanism by which the left and right cerebral hemispheres inhibit the activity of the other hemisphere and is believed to occur during voluntary one-handed movements [1]. Interhemispheric inhibition has also been shown to be associated with motor control in humans [2]. In 1956, Creutzfeldt et al. first reported the presence of inhibition in the cerebral cortex of cats [3]. Subsequently, in 1993, experimental evidence of inhibitory effects on the cerebral cortex in humans was demonstrated using transcranial magnetic stimulation (TMS), which non-invasively modulates brain activity [4]. Since the 1980s, several studies have provided supportive evidence for the existence of interhemispheric inhibition [5–7]. However, using two TMS devices, Ferbert et al. reported particularly reliable evidence for the presence of interhemispheric inhibition in healthy adults [8]; in this study, the effects of conditioning magnetic stimulation applied to the hand area of one primary motor cortex and test magnetic stimulation applied to the hand area of the contralateral primary motor cortex on electromyographic (EMG) responses evoked in the first dorsal interosseous muscle were examined. The results showed that the test response elicited in the contralateral hemisphere was suppressed when the interval between the application of conditioning stimuli to one hemisphere, and the next test stimulus was more than 5–6 ms. The researchers termed this suppression "interhemispheric inhibition" and hypothesized that it was induced via the corpus callosum.

The measurement of interhemispheric inhibition has also been used to elucidate the pathophysiology of movement disorders from a central nervous system perspective [5]. However, recent studies have demonstrated a link between age-related alterations and interhemispheric inhibition [9]. Therefore, in the context of an increasingly elderly population worldwide, interhemispheric inhibition may serve as a predictive indicator of motor and cognitive decline in the elderly [9–11]. In this chapter, we review the latest assessment indices for interhemispheric inhibition and assessment methods for potential application in the clinical physiotherapy setting.

2. Interhemispheric suppression and conventional measurement methods

The presence of interhemispheric inhibition has been known since the 1990s, and many studies have elucidated its mechanism as a cortical inhibitory function necessary for motor control. Notably, studies on interhemispheric inhibition in humans have employed functional magnetic resonance imaging (fMRI) and electroencephalography (brain) when evaluating unilateral upper limb movements. In addition, some studies have used noninvasive modulation of the brain activity using TMS to evaluate interhemispheric inhibition instead of unilateral upper limb motor tasks. This section reviews the traditional methods used to evaluate interhemispheric inhibition, differences between the measurement methods, and the results of the associated studies.

2.1 Interhemispheric suppression and TMS

TMS is a noninvasive tool that modulates the excitability of the motor cortex by generating a magnetic field that passes through the scalp using a wire coil [12]. It has been used as a rehabilitation treatment for stroke, spinal cord injury, traumatic brain injury, and multiple sclerosis, as well as for neurophysiological diagnoses [13]. TMS interventions for assessing interhemispheric inhibition have been reported since the 1990s. In 1998, Mayer et al. investigated the mechanisms underlying the development of interhemispheric inhibition and tested whether a TMS-based approach could be used to diagnose interhemispheric inhibition [14]. Fourteen patients with lesions in the corpus callosum were included in this study. Of all the participants, four had lesions in the cerebral corpus callosum, two in the anterior trunk, six in the middle trunk, and two in the vastus callosum. TMS was applied to the hand regions of the primary motor cortex at an intensity of 80% of the maximum voluntary contraction (MVC) force. Surface electrodes were placed on the bilateral first dorsal interosseous muscles, and EMG activity was measured. The results showed that interhemispheric inhibition did not occur in one participant with a lesion in the corpus callosum nor in six participants with a lesion in the corpus callosum trunk. The other participants showed interhemispheric inhibition, leading to the conclusion that the majority of fibers mediating interhemispheric inhibition passed through the corpus callosum. Other studies have provided evidence corroborating the notion that interhemispheric inhibition occurs *via* the corpus callosum [15, 16]. Therefore, TMS can modulate brain activity to induce interhemispheric inhibition. The corpus callosum has also been suggested as a useful neurophysiological target for assessing interhemispheric inhibition.

2.2 Interhemispheric inhibition and fMRI

fMRI, based on MRI, is used to evaluate dynamic changes in the brain tissue resulting from variations in neurometabolism [17]. In 2000, Allison et al. used fMRI to examine interhemispheric interactions during a unilateral motor task compared to during a resting state [18]; in this study, 13 healthy participants with a mean age of 36 years performed one-handed tapping exercises of the thumb and fingers from the index to the little finger, in turn, for four sets of 30 s each. The tapping speed advised to participants was to tap each of the four fingers and thumb, approximately every 2 s. During the tapping task, brain activity was captured every 3 s using MRI, and 128 sets of brain images were acquired in total. Data on regional changes in blood oxygenation were extracted from the acquired brain images. The results revealed activation of the sensorimotor cortex and subcortical regions contralateral to the hand movements, as well as the ipsilateral cerebellum. In contrast, finger movements were shown to cause significant inactivation (reduced blood oxygenation) in the ipsilateral sensorimotor cortex, subcortical areas, and contralateral cerebellum. Thus, this study suggests that the ipsilateral cerebral hemisphere and contralateral cerebellar hemisphere are inactivated due to interhemispheric inhibition mediated *via* the corpus callosum.

Interhemispheric inhibition has also been shown to be related to aging. Gröschel et al. examined age-related differences in the interhemispheric inhibition process, with negative changes in the blood oxygenation level-dependent (BOLD) signal [19]. In this study, 14 individuals from the younger group (mean age 23.3 years) and 13 from the older group (mean age 73.2 years) were included. Peripheral electrical stimulation was applied to the right median nerve in all participants, and the BOLD signal of the somatosensory system was measured during stimulation. Peripheral electrical stimulation was delivered at 40 Hz, a level that produces effective fMRI responses, and two sets of stimulation for 30 seconds each were applied. The results showed negative changes in BOLD signals across all participants in the right primary somatosensory cortex, primary motor cortex, thalamus, and basal ganglia. When comparing the two age groups, a significant difference in the inactivation of the right primary somatosensory cortex was identified in the one set, indicating that the elderly group had significantly less cortical inactivation during endogenous electrical stimulation. Thus, this suggests that the inhibitory function in the brains of elderly individuals is reduced compared to that in the young. In addition, a previous study reporting age-related changes in brain structure using fMRI reported that the corpus callosum degenerates and interhemispheric inhibition is reduced in the elderly [20]. This indicates that the measurement of interhemispheric inhibition using fMRI mainly assesses regional changes in cerebral blood oxygenation and morphological changes in the corpus callosum in response to hand motor tasks and TMS. It has also been suggested that interhemispheric inhibition is reduced in the elderly owing to age-related degeneration of the corpus callosum.

2.3 Interhemispheric inhibition and electroencephalogram (EEG)

EEG is a reliable, inexpensive, and useful tool for investigating electrophysiological brain activity [21]. EEG measurements of motor tasks typically involve temporally aligning repetitive motor events and averaging motor/event-related potentials that indicate cortical activity. Studies on interhemispheric inhibition have shown that cortical activity is often narrowed to the beta frequency band (14–30 Hz) [22], which is involved in the execution of movement, and to the alpha frequency band (8–13 Hz) [23], which is involved in inhibitory processes within the brain [24]. The association between the alpha frequency band and age-related decline in motor performance control was examined in a previous study by Bönstrup et al. using EEG signal measurement during hand motor tasks [25]. The participants included 15 young individuals with an average age of 25.0 years and 15 elderly individuals with an average age of 70.0 years. The specific fingermovement task consisted of ten consecutive tapping movements with four fingers of the right hand. Tapping movements were performed at 1 Hz intervals in a randomized, complex sequence. Based on the fact that inhibitory control over motor performance depends on motor memory formation, EEG was measured 1 h and 24 h after the task. The results, shown in **Figure 1**, revealed that 1 h after the task, there was an increase in the alpha frequency band in the younger group; however, this was not statistically significant. A significant decrease was observed in the alpha frequency band in the older group. However, 24 h after the task, there was a significant increase in the alpha frequency band in the younger group but not in the older group. This study suggests that the age-related impairment of inhibitory neurotransmission may explain the reduced alpha frequency band activity observed in the elderly group. It has also been suggested that corticocortical interactions in the motor control networks may be reduced in the aging brain.

In a combined EEG and TMS study, Ishibashi et al. [26] assessed interhemispheric coupling during a motor task in 11 healthy male individuals (mean age, 24.9 years) using interhemispheric signal propagation (ISP), recognized as a reliable method for assessing interhemispheric coupling. The participants performed an experimental task consisting of visual stimulation and TMS with simultaneous measurement of motor-evoked potentials (MEPs) and EEG. In the experimental task, 100 trials were performed for each of the four conditions in a randomized sequence: (1) TMS was administered in the left primary motor cortex at rest, (2) TMS was administered in

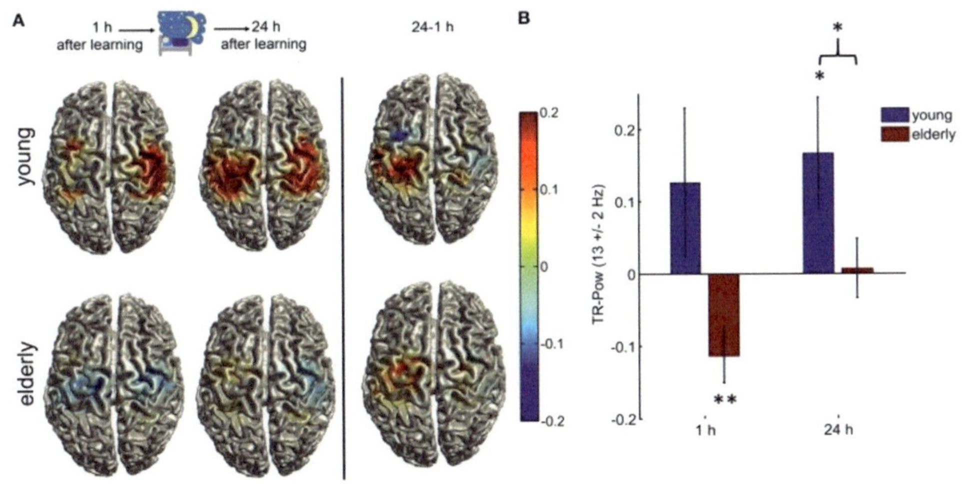

Figure 1.
(A) task-related spectral power (TR-Pow) topography diagram of the alpha frequency band of the sensorimotor cortex in the young and elderly groups at 1 and 24 h post-task [25]. Only the TR-Pow located on the central coordinates of the bilateral sensorimotor cortex is shown. In the right-hand diagram, the difference between the two measurements (24 h and 1 h later) is plotted, and (B) bar chart showing the relative change in TR-Pow for the alpha frequency band of both the groups. Error bars = 1 SEM ($^{*}p < 0.05$; and $^{**}p < 0.01$).

the left primary motor cortex at rest during a rapid abduction movement of the right index finger, (3) TMS was administered in the right primary motor cortex at rest, and (4) TMS was administered in the right primary motor cortex at rest during a rapid abduction movement of the left index finger. The occurrence of EMG activity was defined as the point at which the rectified EMG response in the first dorsal interosseous muscle exceeded 100 μV. A 19-channel recording electrode was used for EEG measurements, and a reference electrode was placed at the earlobe. The sampling frequency was recorded at 5 kHz. The results showed that the ISP from the left to the right hemisphere during right-handed fast movements was higher than that from the right to the left hemisphere. The results of this study suggest that the left primary motor cortex strongly inhibits the right primary motor cortex. Thus, EEG-based methods assess the functional connectivity between hemispheres, suggesting that interhemispheric inhibition is involved in motor control.

3. Motor overflow

Recently, motor overflow has attracted attention as a new index for evaluating interhemispheric inhibition. Motor overflow is said to be the spread of motor system output, causing muscular activity in muscles that are supposed to be at rest, as well as in target muscles [27] and an umbrella term used to describe the involuntary movements that sometimes accompany the generation of voluntary movements [28]. This refers to the involuntary movements or weak muscle activities that appear in conjunction with voluntary movements. When motor overflow occurs on the contralateral side in target muscles of the same group, it is referred to as a mirror movement [28, 29]. Regarding the relationship between interhemispheric interactions and mirror movements, it has been reported that the connectivity of the corpus callosum fibers connecting the bilateral primary motor cortices is directly involved in the mirror movement that occurs during dominant hand movements [30].

In humans, motor overflow is caused by abnormal corticospinal tracts [31]. Both transcallosal and ipsilateral corticospinal tract hypotheses have been proposed to explain the abnormal induction of corticospinal tracts. The ipsilateral corticospinal tract hypothesis states that motor overflow is caused by the functional activation of ipsilateral corticospinal projections due to the appearance of independent corticospinal neurons and the abnormal branching of crossing corticospinal fibers [32]. Hence, motor overflow is believed to occur in the ipsilateral hemisphere. In contrast, the transcallosal hypothesis states that inhibition *via* the corpus callosum is reduced and motor overflow is facilitated in the contralateral hemisphere [33]. Thus, motor overflow is believed to occur in the contralateral hemisphere. Previous studies have not yet determined which hypothesis is applicable, and both theories have been treated independently [32]. Further investigations are required to elucidate the mechanisms underlying motor overflow. Motor overflow occurs mainly in the elderly, children, and in central nervous system diseases. This section reviews the relationship between motor overflow and diseases of the elderly, children, and the central nervous system, as well as the evaluation methods and clinical significance of motor overflow.

3.1 Motor overflow in the elderly

Motor overflow in elderly individuals is primarily treated as an index reflecting motor characteristics associated with age-related alterations in interhemispheric inhibition. In 2003, Bodwell et al. evaluated the magnitude and incidence of motor overflow in the contralateral finger using a finger movement task in elderly individuals [27]. The participants of this study were 20 healthy adults aged 18–25 years and 20 healthy older adults aged 65–85 years. The finger movement task was a finger-tapping task performed in response to auditory stimuli, and measurement parameters comprised the EMG of the first dorsal interosseous muscle and the extensor and flexor muscles of the wrist during the finger movement task. The results revealed that elderly participants with greater manual dexterity exhibited greater motor overflow in the right hand. These results suggest that motor overflow is not a sign of a decline in the systems that control movement but instead reflects events that compensate for compensatory brain activity. Similarly, motor overflow observed during finger movement tasks has been reported to be caused by the increased activation of bilateral cerebral hemispheres with advancing age [34, 35]. Recently, Morisita et al. reported a relationship between interhemispheric inhibition and motor overflow using TMS [11]. In this study, 22 individuals were included in a group of young individuals with a mean age of 26.1 years and a group of elderly individuals with a mean age of 65.0 years. TMS was applied to induce isometric abduction of the right index finger at 15% MVC. The magnitude of the interhemispheric inhibition was assessed based on the MEPs produced in the primary motor cortex contralateral to the primary motor cortex to which TMS was applied, based on the dual-site paired-pulse TMS paradigm. In addition, the participants performed an anti-phase tapping task in which they alternated between synchronized tapping of the left index finger and right middle finger and synchronized tapping of the left middle finger and right index finger. The magnitude of motor overflow was assessed using the EMG waveform of the left first dorsal interosseous muscle. The results showed that older adults performed better in antiphase tapping as interhemispheric inhibition decreased due to higher motor overflow. Additionally, the lower the interhemispheric inhibition, the higher the incidence of motor overflow. Thus, it has been suggested that older adults may mobilize extensive bilateral regions of the brain to improve or maintain performance. Therefore, the prevalent theory is that motor overflow in older adults appears as a result of decreased interhemispheric inhibition to compensate for the loss of motor capacity associated with age-related changes.

3.2 Motor overflow in children

Children experience motor overflow in the same manner as older adults. However, the factors contributing to motor overflow in children have been shown to be different from those in older adults, who have reduced interhemispheric inhibition to compensate for their reduced motor skills. Specifically, Adamo P K et al. examined this factor by comparing children and adults [36]. The study included 17 children aged 8–11 years and 17 adults aged 18–35 years. The participants performed flexion exercises of the index finger at 33 and 66% MVC. The results showed that children had significantly greater motor overflow than adults, especially in the dominant hand, when exercising with the nondominant hand. These results suggest that motor overflow in children may serve as a stabilization strategy for movement, especially when exercising with the nondominant hand. A follow-on study comparing three generations, comprising 17 children aged 8–11 years, 17 adults aged 18–35 years, and 16 elderly individuals aged 60–80 years was performed [37]. The participants performed the same flexion exercises as the prior study [36]. The results revealed that motor overflow occurs to a greater extent in children and the elderly than in adults and that the neurological processes generated are age-dependent. These results suggest that children have immature motor systems and therefore, mobilize a wider network of regions when exerting maximum force. Simon-Martinez et al. reported a relationship between interhemispheric inhibition and motor overflow in children with unilateral cerebral palsy (uCP) [38]. Children are known to be able to reorganize the corticospinal tracts projecting to the paralyzed side from the contralateral, ipsilateral, or bilateral cerebral cortices. The reorganization of these three pathways varies between individuals; in this study, of the 49 individuals included 17 individuals were recruited with the contralateral pattern, 16 with the ipsilateral pattern, and 16 with the bilateral pattern. Of all the participants, 30 uCP children had periventricular leukomalacia, and nine had cortical-subcortical lesions. The participants performed 10 grip exercises on the non-paralyzed side of the cylindrical transducer. Motor overflow was measured in the paralyzed hand opposite to the moving side. Hand movements were performed bilaterally. The results indicated that motor overflow appeared more frequently on the paralyzed side of children with uCP and an ipsilateral pattern than in those with a contralateral pattern. These results suggest that the primary motor cortex contralateral to the working hand activates the ipsilateral corticospinal tracts innervating the nonworking hand, indicating that unilateral finger movements in children are executed or maintained through bilateral cerebral cortex mobilization. Therefore, it is highly likely that motor overflow appears due to bilateral cerebral hemispheric mobilization in children because their motor systems remain underdeveloped. It suggests that interhemispheric inhibition emerges with the development of the motor system.

3.3 Central nervous disorders and motor overflow

In central nervous system diseases, motor overflow is believed to be an indicator of the recovery process in patients following stroke [39]. In 1998, Nelles et al. examined the association between motor disability severity and motor overflow after stroke in 23 stroke patients and nine healthy elderly individuals [39]. The participants performed a series of exercises in which they held a grip-type dynamometer strongly and rapidly for 10 s. All participants performed this exercise on both the left and right sides, and motor overflow was measured on the nonmoving side. The results showed that motor overflow on the non-paralyzed side of the left hemiplegic patients was significantly greater than that on the paralyzed side in the healthy elderly group. Therefore, this study suggests that motor overflow, which occurs in healthy elderly individuals, may be enhanced after stroke. In addition, it has been suggested that motor overflow may be a clinical indicator of the recovery process of motor function after stroke. In addition, a correlation between motor overflow occurring on the non-operating side and muscle activity on the operating side has been reported for unilateral upper limb movements after stroke [40]; in this study, EMG was used to assess motor overflow in 60 patients with stroke. The participants performed unilateral elbow flexion exercises for 5 seconds on both sides. EMG was performed on the biceps brachii bilaterally, and a reference electrode was placed on the left humeral lateral epicondyle. In addition, the participants underwent Fugl-Meyer assessment (FMA) for the assessment of proximal and distal upper and lower limb motor function. The results showed that motor overflow occurred significantly on the non-paralyzed side when the motor task was performed on the paralyzed side, as shown in **Figure 2**. The FMA results also showed that motor overflow in the biceps brachii not only negatively correlated with motor function in the proximal upper limb but also with motor

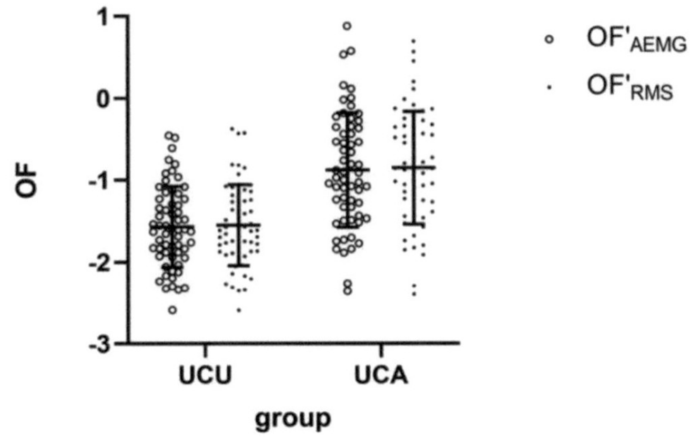

Figure 2.
Comparison between OF'AEMG and OF'RMS of bilateral biceps brachii during a unilateral contraction task [40]. AEMG represents the mean amplitude of the electromyography waveform. OF'AEMG indicates the overflow rate calculated by dividing the AEMG value of the nonoperating side by the AEMG value of the operating side. RMS is the root mean square. OF'RMS indicates the overflow rate calculated by dividing the RMS value of the nonoperating side by the RMS value of the operating side. On the vertical axis, OF indicates the overflow rate. On the horizontal axis, UCU represents the group performing the behavioral task on the non-paralyzed side, and UCA is the group performing the behavioral task on the paralyzed side. When the motor task was performed on the paralyzed side (UCA), motor overflow significantly increased on the non-paralyzed side.

function in the distal upper limb or lower limb. Thus, the results of this study suggest that the proximal muscles of the upper limbs can be used to measure motor overflow and largely reflect interhemispheric interactions.

The developmental mechanisms by which motor overflow occurs after stroke and whether cortical or subcortical triggers are responsible were examined in a study of 53 patients with stroke and 14 healthy elderly individuals [41]. In this study, participants performed 40 exercise trials in which each of the 10 fingers was flexed with four patterns of force: 20, 40, 60, and 80% MVC. Measurements were performed at 2, 4, 12, 24, and 52 weeks after stroke onset. In this study, motor overflow was defined as the difference between the force generated by the nonmoving and resting finger forces. Brain activity during motor tasks was measured using fMRI. The results showed that the pattern of motor overflow in stroke survivors was similar to that in healthy elderly individuals and was enhanced. Therefore, this study indicated that motor overflow may occur because of increased activity in the ciliary spinal system after stroke. This suggests that motor overflow is induced subcortically after stroke. In conclusion, motor overflow after stroke is often observed on the non-paralyzed side when the paralyzed upper limb is moved, suggesting that motor overflow occurring in the elderly may be amplified. Recent studies have also highlighted that poststroke manifestations are of subcortical origin, which could help elucidate the recovery mechanisms of motor function after stroke.

4. Bimanual coordinated movement

Fingers are a body part responsible for essential movements in daily life that require highly coordinated movements. It has been shown that motor control by interhemispheric inhibition is involved in the execution of hand movements [4]. Furthermore, it has been reported that, during the preparatory phase, hand

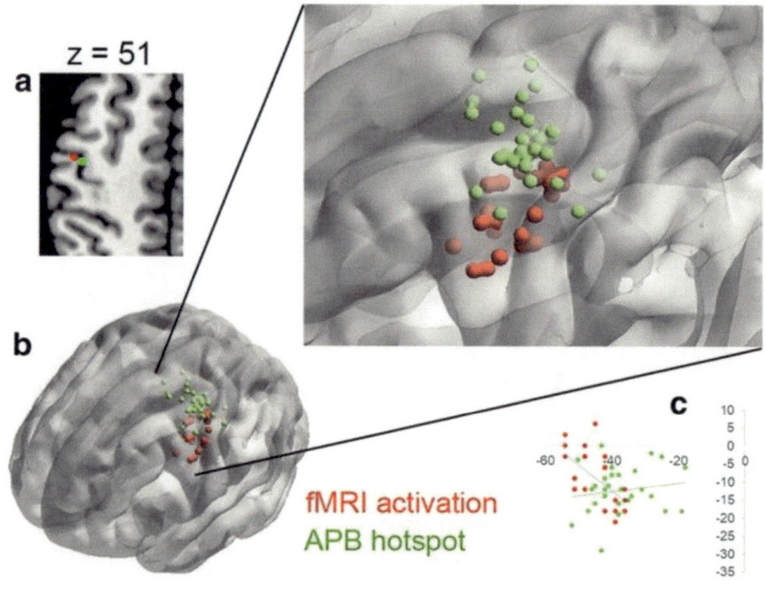

Figure 3.
Functional magnetic resonance imaging (fMRI) activation of premotor cortex and localization by transcranial magnetic stimulation (TMS) hotspots [44]. (a) red ellipses represent mean Montreal neurological institute (MNI) coordinates (± standard deviation [SD]) of the fMRI activation peak voxels. Green ellipses represent mean MNI coordinates (± SD) of the TMS hotspots. All coordinates are located in the left hemisphere, (b) individual locations are projected onto the three-dimensional brain template, and (c) scatterplot showing individual locations. It can be seen that the TMS hotspot differs from the fMRI activation area in the premotor cortex.

movements in the elderly are more dependent on the premotor cortex than those in the adults [42]. In addition, a study examining interhemispheric inhibition in the elderly showed that the quality of finger movement performance was lower than that in adults with bilateral primary motor areas activated, while premotor areas tended to be inactive [43]. As discussed in Section 2, modulating brain activity by applying TMS to the hand regions of the primary motor cortex is commonly used to assess interhemispheric inhibition. However, it has recently been reported that the hotspot of TMS in the hand region of the primary motor cortex is different from the fMRI activation area generated during finger-tapping movements [44]. **Figure 3** shows that the TMS hotspot assigned to the hand region differed from the activation area corresponding to the premotor cortex measured using fMRI during hand-tapping exercises. Hence, finger movements may be the best way to induce interhemispheric inhibition. In other words, hand-tapping exercise may be optimal for inducing and evaluating interhemispheric inhibition. Thus, the optimal evaluation method for interhemispheric inhibition is still in the process of establishment, and future research is expected. This section reviews the current methods used for assessing hand-tapping movements that reflect interhemispheric inhibition.

4.1 Measurement of bimanual coordinated movements

Recently, magnetic sensor finger-tapping devices have gained attention as a new method for measuring bimanual coordinated movements (**Figure 4**) [45]. These devices consist of a magnetic induction coil, sensing coil, and circuit unit [46]. To obtain measurements, a coil voltage is induced between the two coils based on the

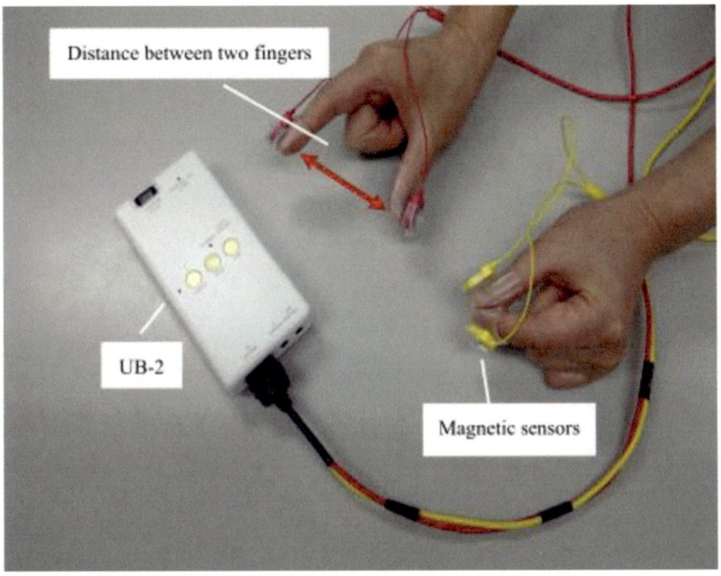

Figure 4.
Magnetic sensor finger-tapping device (UB-2, Maxell Ltd. Tokyo, Japan) [45]. A yellow cable is attached to the left thumb and index finger and a red cable to the right thumb and index finger. Magnetic sensors are attached to each fingertip, and the waveform of finger tapping can be determined using a personal computer.

law of electromagnetic induction. The induced voltage has a nonlinear modeling relationship with the distance between the coils; therefore, the distance between the fingertip and attached coil can be estimated based on the voltage [47]. The finger movement tasks using the magnetic sensor finger-tapping device include a unilateral finger-tapping task (left and right), an in-phase task in which both fingers are tapped simultaneously, and an antiphase task in which both fingers are tapped alternately (**Figure 5**) [45]. From the above four types of finger-tapping tasks, 44 measurement parameters can be extracted using a measuring instrument [48]. The 44 measurement parameters can be classified into five categories (**Table 1**):

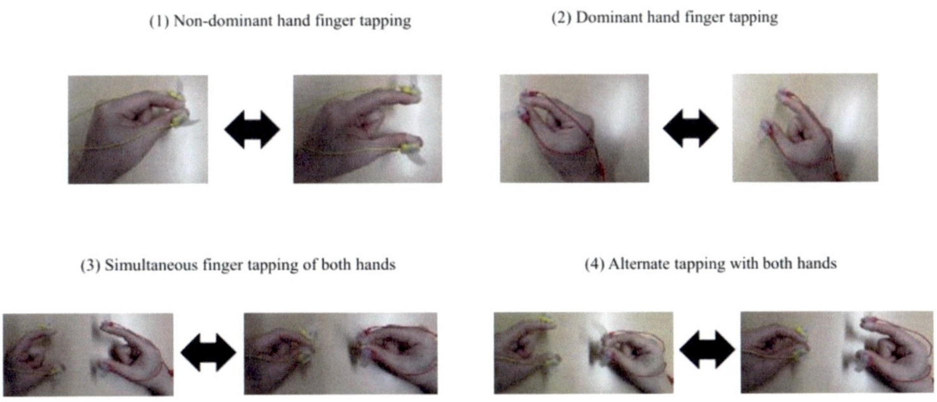

Figure 5.
Movement tasks using a magnetic sensor finger-tapping device [45]. (1) unilateral finger-tapping task performed with the nondominant hand, (2) unilateral finger-tapping task performed with the dominant hand, (3) In-phase task with simultaneous bilateral finger tapping, and (4) antiphase task with alternating bilateral finger tapping.

Distance	No. 1	Max of distance amplitude
	No. 2	Total traveling distance
	No. 3	Avg. of local max. distance
	No. 4	SD of local max. distance
	No. 5	Slope of approximate line of local max. points
	No. 6	CV of local max. distance
	No. 7	SD of local max. distance in three adjacent taps
Velocity	No. 8	Max. of velocity amplitude
	No. 9	Avg. of local max. velocity
	No. 10	Avg. of local min. velocity
	No. 11	SD of local max. velocity
	No. 12	SD of local min. velocity
	No. 13	Energy balance
	No. 14	Total energy
	No. 15	CV of local max. velocity
	No. 16	CV of local min. velocity
	No. 17	Number of freezing calculated from velocity
	No. 18	Avg. of distance rate of velocity peak in extending movement
	No. 19	Avg. of distance rate of velocity peak in flexing movement
	No. 20	Ratio of distance rates of velocity peak in extending and flexing movements
	No. 21	SD of distance rate of velocity peak in extending movement
	No. 22	SD of distance rate of velocity peak in flexing movement
Acceleration	No. 23	Max of acceleration amplitude
	No. 24	Avg. of local max. acceleration in extending movement
	No. 25	Avg. of local min. acceleration in extending movement
	No. 26	Avg. of local max. acceleration in flexing movement
	No. 27	Avg. of local min. acceleration in flexing movement
	No. 28	Avg. of contact duration
	No. 29	SD of contact duration
	No. 30	CV of contact duration
	No. 31	Number of zero crossover points of acceleration
	No. 32	Number of freezing calculated from acceleration
Taping interval	No. 33	Number of taps
	No. 34	Avg. of intervals
	No. 35	Frequency of taps
	No. 36	SD of inter-tapping interval
	No. 37	CV of inter-tapping interval
	No. 38	Inter-tapping interval variability
	No. 39	Skewness of inter-tapping interval distribution
	No. 40	SD of inter-tapping interval in three adjacent taps

Phase difference between the left hand and right hand tapping	No. 41	Avg. of phase difference between the left hand and right hand tapping
	No. 42	Standard deviation of phase difference between the left hand and right hand tapping
	No. 43	Similarity of hands
	No. 44	Time lag of similarity of hands

Abbreviations: Max: maximum; Min: minimum; Ave: average; SD: standard deviation; and CV: coefficient of variation.

Table 1.
Forty-four measurement parameters were obtained from four different finger-tapping tasks [48].

(1) distance, to evaluate the distance and magnitude of hand movements (n = 7), (2) velocity, to evaluate the velocity of hand movements and the speed of hand flexion/extension movements (n = 15), (3) acceleration, to evaluate the momentum of hand movements and the differences between hand flexion and extension movements (n = 10), (4) tap interval, to evaluate the average speed of hand movements and variations in tapping (n = 8), and (5) phase difference, to evaluate the difference in timing of tapping between the two hands (n = 4). Many recent studies using magnetic sensor finger-tapping devices have been performed on elderly people and children. However, of the 44 parameters measured, those that differed significantly in interhemispheric inhibition varied widely from study to study. **Table 2** presents the conditions of the hand-tapping task, measured parameters, individuals compared with the measured parameters, method of comparison, and parameters for which significant differences were found and reported in the studies from the PubMed database [45, 49–54], in which elderly individuals and children were the participants and a magnetic sensor-type finger-tapping device was used. Future studies identifying at least one promising measurement parameter from the aforementioned 44 parameters for evaluating interhemispheric inhibition using the magnetic sensor finger-tapping device are warranted.

4.2 Bimanual coordinated movements and aging

Bimanual coordinated movements are controlled by interhemispheric inhibition, and many studies have reported the effects of age-related changes on these movements. In particular, improved finger movement ability leads to improved activities of daily living in older adults with dementia [55], and studies investigating the relationship between bimanual coordination movements and cognitive function have gained attention in recent years. Several studies have compared individuals with Alzheimer's disease (AD) or mild cognitive impairment (MCI) with healthy elderly individuals [49, 50, 54]. In one such study, Suzumura et al. compared and verified the motion characteristics of bimanual coordinated movement in 173 MCI patients and 173 healthy elderly subjects using a magnetic sensor finger-tapping device [54]. In this study, four tasks comprise the motor tasks: unilateral finger tapping, in-phase, and antiphase (**Figure 5**). In the flow of the study, each task was practiced for 5 seconds as a pre-practice. The subject performed only one pre-practice and was instructed to "go as fast as possible." After that, only one 15-second measurement was performed. The outcome was 44 measurement parameters (**Table 1**) that indicate the kinematic characteristics of bimanual coordinated movement. The results showed that MCI patients had a significantly higher number of hand freezes calculated from acceleration than

DOI: http://dx.doi.org/10.5772/intechopen.1003275

		Task condition							
	Patient: n number (mean age)	**Tapping task**	**Tapping velocity**	**Hand distance (mm)**	**Tapping time (s)**	**Measurement parameters**	**Comparator**	**Comparison method**	**Parameter with significant differences.**
Suzumura S, et al. 2016 [48]	AD/MCI group: 14 (Ave 72.5 ± 6.1) Healthy elderly group: 13 (Ave 71.7 ± 7.9)	Dominant hand task Non-dominant hand tasks In-phase tasks Anti-phase tasks	fastest	30–40	15	44 parameters measurable from the task.	1. between-group comparison 2. MMSE	1. t-test without correspondence 2. Spearman's correlation coefficient	1. Anti-phase task (left): Total traveling distance, SD of inter-tapping interval In-phase task (left), Anti-phase task (left): SD of contact duration 2. Anti-phase task (left): Total traveling distance, SD of contact duration, SD of inter-tapping interval, Energy balance Anti-phase task (left and right): Standard deviation of phase difference between the left hand and right hand tapping
Sugioka J, et al. 2020 [49]	AD:44 (Ave74 ± 7.0) MCI:20 (Ave74 ± 7.0) Normal elderly: 57 (Ave74 ± 7.0)	Dominant hand task Non-dominant hand tasks In-phase tasks Anti-phase tasks	fastest		15	Total traveling distance Energy balance SD of inter-tapping interval SD of phase difference between the left hand and right hand tapping	Between-group comparison	Multiple comparisons Tukey-Kramer test	AD x healthy elderly Dominant hand task, non-dominant hand task, in-phase task (left/right): Total traveling distance, SD of inter-tapping interval In-phase task (left/right): SD of inter-tapping interval In-phase task: Standard deviation of phase difference between the left hand and right hand tapping MCI x healthy elderly Dominant hand task, In-phase task (left): Avg. of contact duration

		Task condition							
	Patient: n number (mean age)	**Tapping task**	**Tapping velocity**	**Hand distance (mm)**	**Tapping time (s)**	**Measurement parameters**	**Comparator**	**Comparison method**	**Parameter with significant differences.**
Tomita Y, et al. 2020 [50]	Low cognitive function group: 60 (Ave78.3 ± 6.3} Healthy Age Group: 42 (Ave74.4 ± 4.1)	In-phase tasks Anti-phase tasks	fastest	50	15	Total traveling distance Number of taps CV of inter-tapping interval	Between-group comparison	Univariate analysis	In-phase task (left/right), Anti-phase task (left/right): Number of taps
Suzumura S, et al. 2020 [45]	Cognitive impairment (AD/MCI): 69 [Internal translation] 44 patients with AD (Ave73.8 ± 7.0) 20 patients with MCI {Ave76.7±4.2)	Dominant hand task Non-dominant hand tasks In-phase tasks Anti-phase tasks	fastest		15	Parameters with similar meaning 36 parameters eliminated	Independent variable: measurement parameters Dependent variable: MMSE score	Multiple regression analysis	Dominant hand task, non-dominant hand task, in-phase task (right): Avg. of local max. acceleration in flexing movement Non-dominant hand task, in-phase (left): SD of inter-tapping interval In-phase task (left): Slope of approximate line of local max. points
Enokizo T, et al. 2020 [51]	Typically developing children: 100 (Ave 10 years ± 1 year and 7 months)	In-phase tasks Anti-phase tasks	fastest	Maximum distance	10	23 parameters measurable from the task.	Independent variables: age, gender Dependent variable: measurement parameters	Two-way ANOVA	Independent variables: age Total traveling distance, SD of local max. distance, Avg. of local max. velocity, Total energy, Max of acceleration amplitude, Avg. of local max. acceleration in extending movement, Avg. of local min. acceleration in extending movement, Avg. of local min. acceleration in flexing movement. Number of taps, Avg. of intervals, Frequency of taps, Avg. of phase difference between the left hand and right hand tapping Independent variable: gender Slope of approximate line of local max. points, Max. of velocity amplitude, SD of local min. velocity, Max of acceleration amplitude, Avg. of local max. acceleration in flexing movement, Avg. of local min. acceleration in flexing movement

		Task condition							
	Patient: n number (mean age)	**Tapping task**	**Tapping velocity**	**Hand distance (mm)**	**Tapping time (s)**	**Measurement parameters**	**Comparator**	**Comparison method**	**Parameter with significant differences.**
Enokizo T, et al. 2022 [52]	ADHD children: 14 (Ave 9 years 8 months ± 1 year 4 months)	In-phase tasks Anti-phase tasks	fastest		10	21 parameters measurable from the task.	children with stereotyped developmental characteristics	two-way ANOVA	In-fase task (dominant hand). Anti-phase task (left / right): Max of distance amplitude, Avg. of local max. distance, Number of taps, Avg. of intervals, Frequency of taps In-fase task (dominant hand): Avg. of local min. velocity, Avg. of local max. acceleration in flexing movement In-fase (dominant hand), Anti-phase (non-dominant hand): Energy balance
Sugioka J, et al. 2022 [53]	AD patients: 62 (Ave 76.7 ± 7.7)	Dominant hand task Non-dominant hand tasks In-phase tasks Anti-phase tasks	fastest	30–40	15	44 parameters measurable from the task.	Severity of medial temporal lobe atrophy assessed by VSRAS.	Pearson's product-moment correlation coefficient	Non-dominant hand task, in-phase task (left): SD of distance rate of velocity peak in extending movement
Suzumura S, et al. 2022 [54]	MCI group: 173 (Ave 77.2 ± 6.8) Healthy elderly Group: 173 (Ave 77.1 ± 6.8)	Dominant hand task Non-dominant hand tasks In-phase tasks Anti-phase tasks	fastest		15	44 parameters measurable from the task.	between-group comparison	unpaired t-test	Anti-phase task (left): Number of taps, Avg. of intervals, SD of inter-tapping interval Number of freezing calculated from acceleration

Abbreviations: AD: Alzheimer's disease; MCI: Mild cognitive impairment; ADHD: attention deficit hyperactivity disorder; MMSE: mini-mental state examination; SD: standard deviation; Avg: average; CV: coefficient of variation; Max: maximum; Min: minimum; ANOVA: analysis of variance; and VSRAS: voxel-based regional analysis system for Alzheimer's disease.

Table 2.
Comparison of studies in which magnetic sensor finger-tapping devices were used.

healthy elderly subjects. This study excluded subjects with tremors or Parkinsonian symptoms. Thus, since atrophy of the corpus callosum seems to be an early change in dementia, it is suggested that MCI patients show decreased in movements requiring bimanual coordination and rhythm-related parameters. Whereas, Sugioka et al. reported a relationship between atrophy of the medial temporal region of the brain and finger-tapping movements [53]; medial temporal atrophy was assessed using a voxel-based specific region analysis system, which is a well-known early diagnostic tool for AD. The results showed a significant correlation between the standard deviation of the distance rate of the velocity peak in extending movements in the left hand during a nondominant hand task, as well as the in-phase task and the degree of medial temporal atrophy. Therefore, the standard deviation of the distance rate of the velocity peak in extending movements from finger-tapping movements may be a useful parameter for the early detection of AD and for grading its severity.

In addition, bimanual coordinated finger movements in the elderly have been evaluated not only as a measure of interhemispheric inhibition but also as an initial treatment for MCI and for training to improve hand dexterity [56, 57]. Naito et al. performed a study on 48 right-handed elderly individuals (65–78 years) with bimanual finger training or right-hand training for 2 months [57]. In this study, interhemispheric inhibition was assessed through fMRI acquired pre-and post-training. The results revealed that individuals who underwent bimanual finger movement training exhibited improved hand dexterity, which correlated with reduced ipsilateral motor cortical activity. Therefore, bimanually coordinated hand movements appear to activate interhemispheric inhibition and could be used in training paradigms to improve hand dexterity in the elderly.

5. Conclusion

This chapter reviews conventional assessment methods and recently developed assessment indices for interhemispheric inhibition with respect to motor control. Interhemispheric inhibition is one of the most important assessment indices in physical therapy as it reflects the decline in motor ability associated with age-related alterations and is involved in the mechanisms of motor function recovery in central nervous system disorders. Conventional methods for assessing interhemispheric inhibition have used fMRI and EEG to visualize brain activity during finger movement tasks or during brain activity modulation using TMS. Motor overflow and bimanual coordinated movements have recently gained attention as new indices for evaluating interhemispheric inhibition. In particular, a magnetic sensor tapping device can measure bimanual coordinated movements and evaluate interhemispheric inhibition in a wide range of age groups from children to the elderly. However, there is a need to establish further evidence to support the widespread use of bimanual coordinated movements to assess interhemispheric inhibition in clinical practice. The use of bimanual coordinated movements to assess interhemispheric inhibition in individuals could facilitate our understanding of the pathophysiology of motor control.

Acknowledgements

This work was supported by JSPS KAKENHI Grant Number JP23K10417. We would like to thank Editage (www.editage.com) for English language editing.

Conflict of interest

The authors declare no conflict of interest.

Appendices and nomenclature

TMS	transcranial magnetic stimulation
EMG	electromyographic
fMRI	functional magnetic resonance imaging
MVC	maximum voluntary contraction
BOLD	blood oxygenation level-dependent
EEG	electroencephalogram
uCP	unilateral cerebral palsy
FMA	Fugl-Meyer assessment
AD	Alzheimer's disease
MCI	mild cognitive impairment

Author details

Shoya Fujikawa[1,2], Shun Sawai[1,2], Ryosuke Yamamoto[1,3] and Hideki Nakano[1*]

1 Neurorehabilitation Laboratory, Graduate School of Health Sciences, Kyoto Tachibana University, Kyoto, Japan

2 Department of Rehabilitation, Kyoto Kuno Hospital, Kyoto, Japan

3 Department of Rehabilitation, Tesseikai Neurosurgical Hospital, Osaka, Japan

*Address all correspondence to: nakano-h@tachibana-u.ac.jp

References

[1] Boddington LJ, Reynolds JNJ. Targeting interhemispheric inhibition with neuromodulation to enhance stroke rehabilitation. Brain Stimulation. 2017;**10**(2):214-222. DOI: 10.1016/j.brs.2017.01.006

[2] Mirdamadi JL, Xu J, Arevalo-Alas KM, Kam LK, Borich MR. State-dependent interhemispheric inhibition reveals individual differences in motor behavior in chronic stroke. Clinical Neurophysiology. 2023;**149**:157-167. DOI: 10.1016/j.clinph.2023.02.177

[3] Creutzfeldt OD, Baumgartner G, Schoen L. Reaktionen einzelner Neurone des senso-motorischen Cortex nach elektrischen Reizen. I. Hemmung und Erregung nach direkten und kontralateralen Reizen. Archiv für Psychiatrie und Nervenkrankheiten. 1956;**194**:597-619

[4] Roick H, von Giesen HJ, Benecke R. On the origin of the postexcitatory inhibition seen after transcranial magnetic brain stimulation in awake human subjects. Experimental Brain Research. 1993;**94**(3):489-498. DOI: 10.1007/BF00230207

[5] Fuhr P, Agostino R, Hallett M. Spinal motor neuron excitability during the silent period after cortical stimulation. Electroencephalography and Clinical Neurophysiology. 1991;**81**(4):257-262. DOI: 10.1016/0168-5597(91)90011-l

[6] Day BL, Rothwell JC, Marsden CD. Transmission in the spinal reciprocal Ia inhibitory pathway preceding willed movements of the human wrist. Neuroscience Letters. 1983;**37**(3):245-250. DOI: 10.1016/0304-3940(83)90438-x

[7] Cook ND. Callosal inhibition: The key to the brain code. Behavioral Science. 1984;**29**(2):98-110. DOI: 10.1002/bs.3830290203

[8] Ferbert A, Priori A, Rothwell JC, Day BL, Colebatch JG, Marsden CD. Interhemispheric inhibition of the human motor cortex. The Journal of Physiology. 1992;**453**:525-546. DOI: 10.1113/jphysiol.1992.sp019243

[9] Addamo PK, Farrow M, Bradshaw JL, Moss S, Georgiou-Karistianis N. The effect of attending to motor overflow on its voluntary inhibition in young and older adults. Brain and Cognition. 2010;**74**(3):358-364. DOI: 10.1016/j.bandc.2010.10.001

[10] McGregor KM, Nocera JR, Sudhyadhom A, Patten C, Manini TM, Kleim JA, et al. Effects of aerobic fitness on aging-related changes of interhemispheric inhibition and motor performance. Frontiers in Aging Neuroscience. 2013;**5**:66. DOI: 10.3389/fnagi.2013.00066

[11] Morishita T, Timmermann JE, Schulz R, Hummel FC. Impact of interhemispheric inhibition on bimanual movement control in young and old. Experimental Brain Research. 2022;**240**(2):687-701. DOI: 10.1007/s00221-021-06258-7

[12] Klomjai W, Katz R, Lackmy-Vallée A. Basic principles of transcranial magnetic stimulation (TMS) and repetitive TMS (rTMS). Annals of Physical and Rehabilitation Medicine. 2015;**58**(4):208-213. DOI: 10.1016/j.rehab.2015.05.005

[13] Kesikburun S. Non-invasive brain stimulation in rehabilitation. Turkish Journal of Physical and Medical Rehabilitation. 2022;**68**(1):1-8. DOI: 10.5606/tftrd.2022.10608

[14] Meyer BU, Röricht S, Woiciechowsky C. Topography of fibers in the human corpus callosum mediating interhemispheric inhibition between the motor cortices. Annals of Neurology. 1998;**43**(3):360-369. DOI: 10.1002/ana.410430314

[15] Jin K, Xie L, Sun F, Mao X, Greenberg DA. Corpus callosum and experimental stroke: Studies in callosotomized rats and acallosal mice. Stroke. 2011;**42**(9):2584-2588. DOI: 10.1161/STROKEAHA.111.613349

[16] Fling BW, Benson BL, Seidler RD. Transcallosal sensorimotor fiber tract structure-function relationships. Human Brain Mapping. 2013;**34**(2):384-395. DOI: 10.1002/hbm.21437

[17] Chen JE, Glover GH. Functional magnetic resonance imaging methods. Neuropsychology Review. 2015;**25**(3):289-313. DOI: 10.1007/s11065-015-9294-9

[18] Allison JD, Meador KJ, Loring DW, Figueroa RE, Wright JC. Functional MRI cerebral activation and deactivation during finger movement. Neurology. 2000;**54**(1):135-142. DOI: 10.1212/wnl.54.1.135

[19] Gröschel S, Sohns JM, Schmidt-Samoa C, Baudewig J, Becker L, Dechent P, et al. Effects of age on negative BOLD signal changes in the primary somatosensory cortex. NeuroImage. 2013;**71**:10-18. DOI: 10.1016/j.neuroimage.2012.12.039

[20] Langan J, Peltier SJ, Bo J, Fling BW, Welsh RC, Seidler RD. Functional implications of age differences in motor system connectivity. Frontiers in Systems Neuroscience. 2010;**4**:17. DOI: 10.3389/fnsys.2010.00017

[21] Feyissa AM, Tatum WO. Adult EEG. Handbook of Clinical Neurology. 2019;**160**:103-124. DOI: 10.1016/B978-0-444-64032-1.00007-2

[22] Babiloni C, Barry RJ, Başar E, et al. International Federation of Clinical Neurophysiology (IFCN) – EEG research workgroup: Recommendations on frequency and topographic analysis of resting state EEG rhythms. Part 1: Applications in clinical research studies. Clinical Neurology. 2020;**131**(1):285-307. DOI: 10.1016/j.clinph.2019.06.234

[23] Sauseng P, Gerloff C, Hummel FC. Two brakes are better than one: The neural bases of inhibitory control of motor memory traces. NeuroImage. 2013;**65**:52-58. DOI: 10.1016/j.neuroimage.2012.09.048

[24] Chettouf S, Rueda-Delgado LM, de Vries R, Ritter P, Daffertshofer A. Are unimanual movements bilateral? Neuroscience and Biobehavioral Reviews. 2020;**113**:39-50. DOI: 10.1016/j.neubiorev.2020.03.002

[25] Bönstrup M, Hagemann J, Gerloff C, Sauseng P, Hummel FC. Alpha oscillatory correlates of motor inhibition in the aged brain. Frontiers in Aging Neuroscience. 2015;7:193. DOI: 10.3389/fnagi.2015.00193

[26] Ishibashi K, Ishii D, Yamamoto S, Okamoto Y, Wakatabi M, Kohno Y. Asymmetry of interhemispheric connectivity during rapid movements of right and left hands: A TMS-EEG study. Journal of Motor Behavior. 2022;**54**(2):135-145. DOI: 10.1080/00222895.2021.1930993

[27] Bodwell JA, Mahurin RK, Waddle S, Price R, Cramer SC. Age and features of movement influence motor overflow. Journal of the American Geriatrics Society. 2003;**51**(12):1735-1739. DOI: 10.1046/j.1532-5415.2003.51557.x

[28] Armatas CA, Summers JJ, Bradshaw JL. Mirror movements in normal adult subjects. Journal of Clinical and Experimental Neuropsychology. 1994;**16**:405-413. DOI: 10.1080/01688639408402651

[29] Cernacek J. Contralateral motor irridation—cerebral dominance. Archives of Neurology. 1961;**4**:61-68

[30] Sehm B, Steele CJ, Villringer A, Ragert P. Mirror motor activity during right-hand contractions and its relation to white matter in the posterior Midbody of the *Corpus callosum*. Cerebral Cortex. 2016;**26**(11):4347-4355. DOI: 10.1093/cercor/bhv217

[31] Welniarz Q, Dusart I, Gallea C, Roze E. One hand clapping: Lateralization of motor control. Frontiers in Neuroanatomy. 2015;**9**:75. DOI: 10.3389/fnana.2015.00075

[32] Hoy KE, FitzgeraldP B, Bradshaw JL, Armatas CA, Georgiou-Karistianis N. Investigating the cortical origins of motor overflow. Brain Research Reviews. 2004;**46**(3):315-327. DOI: 10.1016/j.brainresrev.2004.07.013

[33] Luo Y, Chen C, Adamek JH, Crocetti D, Mostofsky SH, Ewen JB. Altered cortical activation associated with mirror overflow driven by non-dominant hand movement in attention-deficit/hyperactivity disorder. Progress in Neuropsychopharmacology and Biology Psychiatry. 2022;**112**:110433. DOI: 10.1016/j.pnpbp.2021.110433

[34] Baliz Y, Armatas C, Farrow M, Hoy KE, Fitzgerald PB, Bradshaw JL, et al. The influence of attention and age on the occurrence of mirror movements. Journal of the International Neuropsychological Society. 2005;**11**(7):855-862. DOI: 10.1017/s1355617705051003

[35] Addamo PK, Farrow M, Hoy KE, Bradshaw JL, Georgiou-Karistianis N. The influence of task characteristics on younger and older adult motor overflow. Quarterly Journal of Experimental Psychology (Hove). 2009;**62**(2):239-247. DOI: 10.1080/17470210802269217

[36] Addamo PK, Farrow M, Hoy KE, Bradshaw JL, Georgiou-Karistianis N. A developmental study of the influence of task characteristics on motor overflow. Brain and Cognition. 2009;**69**(2):413-419. DOI: 10.1016/j.bandc.2008.09.005

[37] Addamo PK, Farrow M, Bradshaw JL, Moss S, Georgiou-Karistianis N. Characterizing the developmental profile of effort-induced motor overflow across a timed trial. The American Journal of Psychology. 2013;**126**(2):227-234. DOI: 10.5406/amerjpsyc.126.2.0227

[38] Simon-Martinez C, Decraene L, Zielinski I, Hoare B, Williams J, Mailleux L, et al. The impact of brain lesion characteristics and the corticospinal tract wiring on mirror movements in unilateral cerebral palsy. Scientific Reports. 2022;**12**(1):16301. DOI: 10.1038/s41598-022-19920-z

[39] Nelles G, Cramer SC, Schaechter JD, Kaplan JD, Finklestein SP. Quantitative assessment of mirror movements after stroke. Stroke. 1998;**29**(6):1182-1187. DOI: 10.1161/01.str.29.6.1182

[40] Dai J, Wu F, Li J, Yu M, Liao C, Shou Y. Surface electromyography analysis of mirror movements under unilateral movement in stroke patients: A retrospective study. Frontiers in Human Neuroscience. 2022;**16**:1079596. DOI: 10.3389/fnhum.2022.1079596

[41] Ejaz N, Xu J, Branscheidt M, Hertler B, Schambra H, Widmer M, et al. Evidence for a subcortical origin

of mirror movements after stroke: A longitudinal study. Brain. 2018;**141**(3):837-847. DOI: 10.1093/brain/awx384

[42] Hinder MR, Fujiyama H, Summers JJ. Premotor-motor interhemispheric inhibition is released during movement initiation in older but not young adults. PLoS One. 2012;7(12):e52573. DOI: 10.1371/journal.pone.0052573

[43] Chettouf S, Triebkorn P, Daffertshofer A, Ritter P. Unimanual sensorimotor learning-a simultaneous EEG-fMRI aging study. Human Brain Mapping. 2022;**43**(7):2348-2364. DOI: 10.1002/hbm.25791

[44] Wang J, Meng HJ, Ji GJ, Jing Y, Wang HX, Deng XP, et al. Finger tapping task activation vs. TMS hotspot: Different locations and networks. Brain Topography. 2020;**33**(1):123-134. DOI: 10.1007/s10548-019-00741-9

[45] Suzumura S, Kanada Y, Osawa A, Sugioka J, Maeda N, Nagahama T, et al. Assessment of finger motor function that reflects the severity of cognitive function. Fujita Medical Journal. 2021;7(4):122-129. DOI: 10.20407/fmj.2020-013

[46] Kandori A, Yokoe M, Sakoda S, Abe K, Miyashita T, Oe H, et al. Quantitative magnetic detection of finger movements in patients with Parkinson's disease. Neuroscience Research. 2004;**49**(2):253-260. DOI: 10.1016/j.neures.2004.03.004

[47] Shima K, Tsuji T, Kan E, Kandori A, Yokoe M, Sakoda S. Measurement and evaluation of finger tapping movements using magnetic sensors. Annual International Conference IEEE Engineering Medical and Biology Society. 2008;**2008**:5628-5631. DOI: 10.1109/IEMBS.2008.4650490

[48] Suzumura S, Osawa A, Nagahama T, Kondo I, Sano Y, Kandori A. Assessment of finger motor skills in individuals with mild cognitive impairment and patients with Alzheimer's disease: Relationship between finger-to-thumb tapping and cognitive function. Japanese Journal of Comprehensive Rehabilitation Science. 2016;7:19-28. DOI: 10.11336/jjcrs.7.19

[49] Sugioka J, Suzumura S, Kawahara Y, Osawa A, Maeda N, Ito M, et al. Assessment of finger movement characteristics in dementia patients using a magnetic sensing finger-tap device. Japanese Journal of Comprehensive Rehabilitation Science. 2020;**14**:91-94. DOI: 10.11336/jjcrs.11.91

[50] Tomita Y, Tanaka S, Takahashi S, Takeuchi N. Detecting cognitive decline in community-dwelling older adults using simple cognitive and motor performance tests. Geriatrics & Gerontology International. 2020;**20**(3):212-217. DOI: 10.1111/ggi.13863

[51] Enokizono T, Ohto T, Tanaka M, Maruo K, Sano Y, Kandori A, et al. Quantitative assessment of fine motor skills in children using magnetic sensors. Brain & Development. 2020;**42**(6):421-430. DOI: 10.1016/j.braindev.2020.03.004

[52] Enokizono T, Ohto T, Tanaka M, Maruo K, Mizuguchi T, Sano Y, et al. Boys with attention-deficit/hyperactivity disorder perform wider and fewer finger tapping than typically developing boys—Peer comparisons and the effects of methylphenidate from an exploratory perspective. Brain & Development. 2022;**44**(3):189-195. DOI: 10.1016/j.braindev.2021.11.002

[53] Sugioka J, Suzumura S, Kuno K, Kizuka S, Sakurai H, Kanada Y, et al. Relationship between finger movement characteristics and brain voxel-based

morphometry. PLoS One. 2022;**17**(10):e0269351. DOI: 10.1371/journal.pone.0269351

[54] Suzumura S, Osawa A, Kanada Y, Keisuke M, Takano E, Sugioka J, et al. Finger tapping test for assessing the risk of mild cognitive impairment. Hong Kong Journal of Occupational Therapy. 2022;**35**(2):137-145. DOI: 10.1177/15691861221109872

[55] Liu B, Chen X, Li Y, Liu H, Guo S, Yu P. Effect of passive finger exercises on grip strength and the ability to perform activities of daily living for older people with dementia: A 12-week randomized controlled trial. Clinical Interventions in Aging. 2018;**13**:2169-2177. DOI: 10.2147/CIA.S174756

[56] Wang J, Xie J, Li M, Ren D, Li Y, He Y, et al. Finger exercise alleviates mild cognitive impairment of older persons: A community-based randomized trial. Geriatric Nursing. 2022;**47**:42-46. DOI: 10.1016/j.gerinurse.2022.06.014

[57] Naito E, Morita T, Hirose S, Kimura N, Okamoto H, Kamimukai C, et al. Bimanual digit training improves right-hand dexterity in older adults by reactivating declined ipsilateral motor-cortical inhibition. Scientific Reports. 2021;**11**(1):22696. DOI: 10.1038/s41598-021-02173-7

Chapter 5

Transcranial Magnetic Stimulation as Neuroplasticity Modulation Tool in Rehabilitation

Marziyya Mammadova

Abstract

Since the study of the neuroplastic processes of the brain, it was understood that these processes could be modulated and used in the neurorehabilitation of patients with brain damage. The optimal method of neuromodulation of plasticity is noninvasive transcranial magnetic stimulation (TMS), which can also be used to induce nerve impulses in the parameters we need. This technique allows for measuring the functional state of the central nervous system (CNS) using neurophysiological methods, measuring the effectiveness of rehabilitation, and predicting the restoration of lost functions. We measured the effectiveness of TMS in modulating neuroplasticity using clinical-neurophysiological data and scores of rating scales in rehabilitation. The main studies were provided on the rehabilitation of stroke, but these data can be used in the rehabilitation of other brain injuries.

Keywords: transcranial magnetic stimulation (TMS), multilevel magnetic stimulation, neuroplasticity modulation, reorganization of the human brain, rehabilitation

1. Introduction

Rehabilitation in the broadest sense of this concept is a set of general measures aimed at returning to life, returning lost functions, improving damaged functions, adapting to lost functions as much as possible, modifying life to improve the quality of life, and reintegration into society.

As you can see, a small and short-term damage may be just sufficient to disrupt the functioning of the brain, and years and quite a lot of work can be spent on recovery.

Rehabilitation methods are increasing with the progress and growth of the world economy, along with a deep study of the brain and its untapped potential. If earlier rehabilitation used only methods for recovery only in specialized institutions and the approaches were standard, now the approaches have become individualized and rehabilitation activities continue at the patient's home, robotics and telemedicine are used, and ideas from science fiction films are being implemented, for example, using a medical avatar for rehabilitation [1].

It is not for nothing that the World Health Organization (WHO) developed the Rehabilitation 2030 initiative, which aims to draw attention to the acute unmet need for rehabilitation worldwide and highlights the importance of strengthening health systems to ensure rehabilitation [2]. This document emphasizes that rehabilitation must be made accessible to all members of society throughout life, and that rehabilitation is a critical component of health care and plays a critical role in ensuring comprehensive health coverage.

2. The role of TMS in brain neuroplasticity

Transcranial magnetic stimulation (TMS) is a noninvasive method of stimulating nerve cells in the brain by applying a pulsed magnetic field to the skull. Now, despite the name transcranial, TMS is also used to stimulate the spinal cord. By influencing brain activity, TMS can influence neuroplasticity, which is the ability of the brain to modulate its structure and function in response to experience and learning.

With the help of TMS, it is possible to induce an increase in the activity of neurons, which can increase the activity of certain areas of the brain, contribute to their strengthening to improve the functions associated with these areas, and stimulate neurogenesis. This property is widely used to enhance the activity of motor cortical areas in the rehabilitation of stroke patients. TMS can affect the balance between excitation and inhibition in the brain, it can increase or decrease synaptic connections depending on stimulation parameters, and this property is used as a treatment for some mental disorders such as depression.

With all this, the TMS method is very convenient for both studying neuroplasticity and modulating neuroplasticity for therapeutic purposes, and TMS equipment is constantly being updated and improved.

Studies show that TMS may have an effect on the stimulation of neurogenesis, which is the formation of new neurons in certain areas of the brain [3, 4].
The effects of TMS may depend on the intensity of the magnetic field, the frequency of stimulation, the duration and frequency of repetition of stimulations, as well as the specific characteristics of brain tissues and their response to stimulation. Thus, it has been shown that high-frequency TMS causes a stimulating effect, and low-frequency TMS, on the contrary, has an inhibitory effect on neuronal connections.

3. How does TMS work?

The TMS method is based on the impact of pulsed magnetic field (MF) using an electromagnetic coil on the brain and the subsequent induction of an electric current in it. The stimulating coil can be located either directly on the scalp or at some distance from the head (for example, at a different angle), depending on which it changes the zone and depth of propagation of the magnetic pulse (MP) and the focus of the stimulus. In modern devices, a magnetic pulse can propagate to a depth of more than 2–6 cm, that is, mainly to the cortical and subcortical structures. An electric current arises in the nerve fibers entering this MP, which leads to depolarization of neurons in the cerebral cortex, and the subsequent propagation of the impulse along nerve structures that are functionally dependent on the area of influence. In this case, either suppression or enhancement of the activity of a number of enzyme and mediator systems occurs. In response to stimulation of the visual cortex, phosphenes appear, and in the motor cortex, movement of the

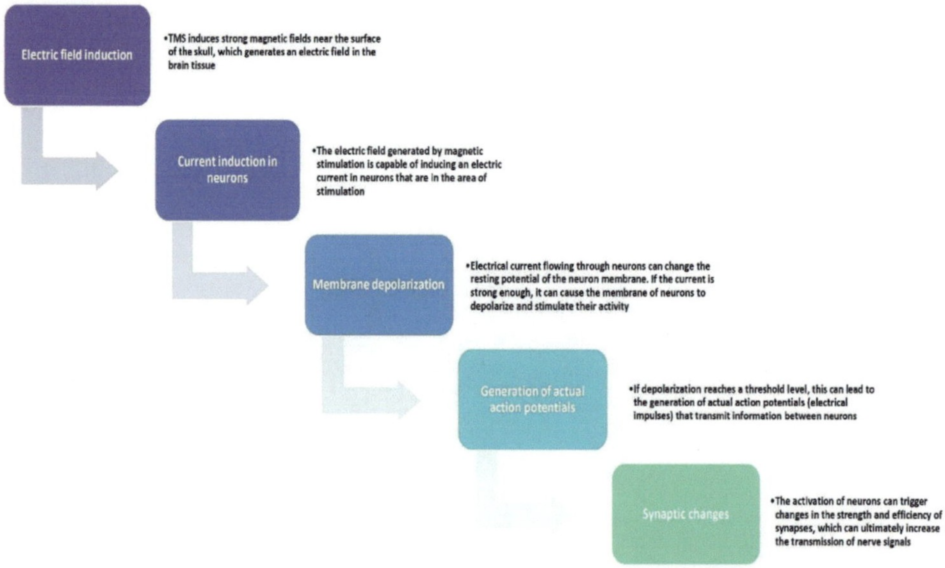

Figure 1.
The steps of TMS's influence processes.

corresponding limbs (according to Penfield's motor "homunculus"), i.e., motor-evoked potential (MEP), takes place.

The effect of TMS on increasing neuronal activity occurs by using magnetic fields to induce electrical currents in the brain, which can excite neurons and help increase their activity. The TMS process can be broken down into the following steps (see **Figure 1**) [5].

Researchers offer several TMS methods to study brain function (see **Figure 2**).

The effects of TMS may depend on various parameters, such as the intensity of the magnetic field, the frequency of stimulation, the duration and repetition rate of stimulation, as well as the specific characteristics of brain tissue and its response to stimulation. Single-pulse TMS involves the delivery of single magnetic pulses to a specific area of the brain; this technique is used to diagnose and study brain reactions. Electroencephalography (EEG) and electromyography (EMG) can record TMS-evoked potentials (TEPs), which provide insight into cortical reactivity [5]. Paired-Pulse TMS are applied one after the next to assess connectivity between cortical areas. The type of effect depends on their intensity and the interval between them. Triple-Pulse combines TMS with electrical stimulation to study the integrity of the corticospinal tract and measures the percentage of excited fibers. Quadripulse is a unique form of repetitive TMS (rTMS) that allows inducing neuroplasticity with short pulse intervals (facilitation) or long ones (depression). Repetitive TMS—A series of pulses are used for prolonged exposure to the cortex. Low-frequency rTMS ($\leq$1 Hz) suppresses cortical activity, while high-frequency rTMS (>1 Hz) increases it and may cause long-term changes. Navigated transcranial magnetic stimulation (nTMS) is designed to map the corresponding stimulated projection areas when TMS is applied to the cerebral cortex [6]. Unlike the alternative to traditional methods, repetitive TMS (rTMS), theta burst stimulation (TBS) has the advantage of faster stimulation. Intermittent TBS (iTBS) has excitatory effects similar to long-term

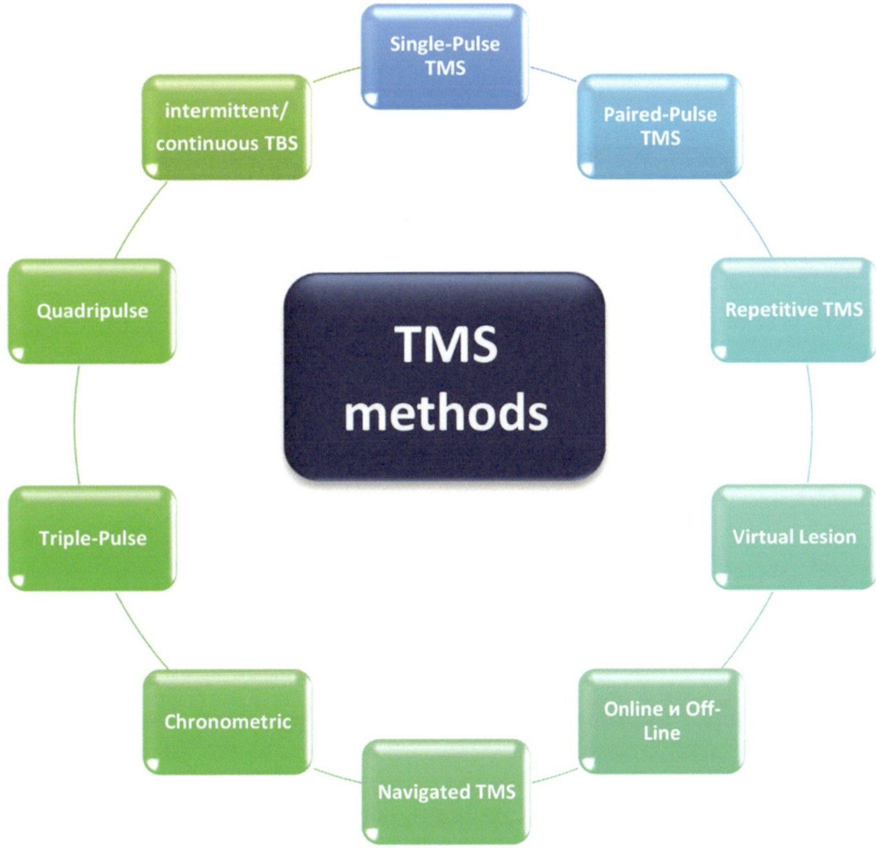

Figure 2.
Transcranial magnetic stimulation methods.

potentiation (LTP), whereas continuous TBS (cTBS) has inhibitory effects similar to long-term depression (LTD) [7].

Transcranial magnetic stimulation can have both short-term and long-term effects on neuronal activity and its use can be employed for therapeutic purposes, in addition, it has local and long-term effects (see **Figure 3**).

Neuroimaging studies have shown that TMS is biologically active both in tissues directly under the coil and in distant areas, probably due to transsynaptic connections. Local changes in brain activity include the appearance of phosphenes and motor effects that occur during TMS as a result of depolarization of neuron membranes in the area of stimulus propagation and the subsequent appearance of an electrical impulse in the cortical axon neurons. Moreover, depending on the parameters of the impulse delivery, stimulation of one hemisphere can inhibit or facilitate the response received from the other hemisphere, which indicates interhemispheric modulatory effects, reflecting the effect of TMS on brain structures remote from the stimulation zone [9]. An example of such an effect is TMS with paired pulses. So, the motor-evoked potential in response to a TMS pulse preceded by a subthreshold "preparing" pulse is weakened when the interstimulus interval is 1 to 4 milliseconds, and strengthened when the interstimulus interval is 1 to 4 milliseconds, but when this interval is between 5 and 30 milliseconds, it reflects intracortical inhibition or facilitation of conduction, respectively [10]. Based on pharmacological

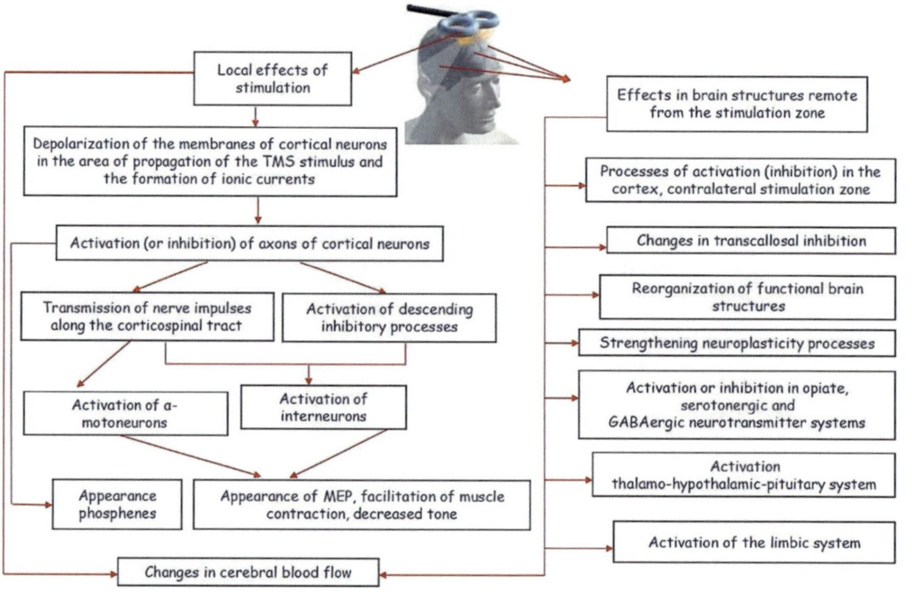

Figure 3.
The effects of TMS directly on the distribution zone and on brain structures remote from the impact zone [8].

effects, it has been shown that activation or inhibition at GABAergic (GABA, gamma-aminobutyric acid) or dopaminergic synapses causes an intracortical inhibitory effect of paired impulses, while the facilitating effect of paired pulses takes place due to excitation in synapses, the mediator of which is N-methyl-D-aspartate, and changes in the motor threshold depend on the conductivity of ion channels. The identified patterns open up new opportunities for studying local damage in neurochemical systems [11].

A number of studies show that during TMS, changes in blood flow occur not only in the zone of impulse propagation but also in brain structures remote from the stimulation zone [10, 12]. Thus, it was shown, for example, that the intensity of rTMS positively correlated with the level of regional cerebral blood flow in the anterior cingulate cortex ipsilaterally, cerebellum, insula contralaterally, primary auditory cortex, and somatosensory cortex (facial projection). According to some authors, rTMS of the left dorsolateral prefrontal cortex (DLPFC) causes changes in blood flow in both the prefrontal cortex and paralimbic structures [13]. According to other authors, exactly the same effect was demonstrated with rTMS of the prefrontal cortex in the blood flow of limbic structures [14]. In human studies, Szuba et al., in subjects with major depression in response to a single session of rTMS of the left DLPFC with a frequency of 10 Hz, compared with sessions of sham rTMS at the same site of action, at the same pulse frequency and session duration, observed an increase in the production of thyroid-stimulating hormone (TSH) [15]. Activation of hypothalamic-pituitary system with this method is similar to the relief of symptoms of depression after a session of electric shock. Finally, normalization of the dexamethasone suppression test with rTMS has been reported [16].

The effect of reducing the excitability of the human brain with low-frequency rTMS is used as therapy for phantom pain in paralyzed patients, as well as for amputations, for inhibition and reorganization of the motor representation of a non-functioning limb. One study showed the inhibitory effects of repetitive transcranial magnetic stimulation (rTMS) on the primary motor cortex (M1) and premotor cortex (PMC) using low-frequency rTMS (0.2–1 Hz) 1200 pulses (20 min) rTMS at 1 Hz and intensity 80-90% of the resting motor threshold and measures of short intracortical inhibition (SICI), intracortical facilitation (ICF) and cortical silent period (CSP), where SICI is a measure of inhibition reflecting intracortical activation of gamma-aminobutyric acid-A receptors (GABA A), ICF is a measure of facilitation, which is mediated by N-methyl-D-aspartate (NMDA) and GABA A receptors, and CSP is a measure of inhibition, reflecting processes mediated by GABA B. This ability to non-invasively induce an inhibitory effect on a specific brain region allows the use of low-frequency rTMS as a therapeutic tool for patients with neurological disorders accompanied by low or excessive cortical inhibition [17].

4. TMS in rehabilitation

Transcranial magnetic stimulation (TMS) has many applications in the field of rehabilitation.

Recovery after a stroke: After a stroke, many patients experience impaired motor and speech functions. TMS can be used to stimulate the brain and promote functional recovery, improving motor skills, coordination, and speech. This helps patients to improve their independence and quality of life. The mechanism of therapeutic action of TMS is based on the restoration of destroyed or creation of new functional systems within the damaged hemisphere, inclusion in the implementation of motor programs of unused neural networks of the damaged hemisphere, activation of uncrossed pyramidal pathways of the intact hemisphere, creation of collateral pathways around damaged structures, and inclusion in already functioning connections of the damaged hemisphere through crossed pathways. In other words, the method of high-intensity rhythmic TMS, being a powerful neuromodulatory factor, includes a mechanism of plastic reorganization of the motor cortex.

Transcranial magnetic stimulation acts directly on the initial segment of the central motor neuron and transsynaptically within the cortex causing an outgoing volley of impulses affecting the spinal cord motoneurons with the subsequent appearance of a motor-evoked potential (MEP). During voluntary muscle contraction, TMS causes a motor-evoked potential (MEP) and after that—a temporary suppression of muscle potentials—a period of silence. The silent period arises mainly due to a synchronous volley of inhibitory postsynaptic potentials produced by an electromagnetic stimulus at the cortical level. These effects of TMS were decisive for the choice as an auxiliary method of rehabilitation of patients with ischemic stroke in the recovery period. Rhythmic TMS is a noninvasive, painless, and safe method for obtaining controlled activation of the human cortex with a potentiation effect. When stimulating the motor areas of the hemisphere with a pulsed magnetic field, not only contralateral but also ipsilateral descending pathways can be activated, since with TMS it is possible to focus the magnetic stimulus and influence the uncrossed pyramidal tract. The activating effect of TMS on the reticular formation and dopaminergic structures of the brain, which contributes to the activation of compensatory and restorative processes in the central nervous system, improvement in cognitive functions, restoration of praxis, and gnosis, has also been shown.

A group of European experts has revised recommendations on the therapeutic effectiveness of repetitive (or rhythmic) TMS (rTMS), previously published in 2014 [18]. These updated recommendations take into account all rTMS publications, including data up to 2014, as well as literature currently reviewed up to the end of 2018. Level A evidence (definite effectiveness) was achieved for low-frequency rTMS (LF-rTMS) contralateral primary motor cerebral cortex (M1) to restore hand motor skills in the subacute stage of stroke. Level B evidence (probably effective) was achieved for: HF-rTMS of ipsilateral M1 to accelerate motor recovery in subacute stroke and LF-rTMS of the right inferior frontal gyrus in chronic motor aphasia after stroke. Level A/B evidence regarding the effectiveness of rTMS for any other conditions has not been achieved. Current recommendations are based on the differences achieved in the therapeutic efficacy of real and sham (sham TMS) rTMS protocols, replicated in a sufficient number of independent studies. An extensive PubMed review identified 213 articles, including 25 original placebo/sham-controlled TMS studies with at least 10 poststroke patients receiving rTMS over multiple daily sessions compared to the affected contra- and/or ipsilateral hemisphere. Among these studies, a number of studies dealt with limb motor rehabilitation in the subacute stage using low-frequency rTMS (LF-rTMS) with contralateral M1 and/or high-frequency rTMS (HF-rTMS) with ipsilateral M1. Some of them dealt with limb motor rehabilitation in the subacute stage with contralateral intermittent theta stimulation-theta burst stimulation (TBS) or ipsilateral intermittent theta burst stimulation (iTBS). Intermittent theta burst stimulation (iTBS) is a more acceptable protocol, administered at lower intensities and shorter intervals, than conventional rTMS protocols. In addition, studies have been conducted on limb motor rehabilitation in the chronic stage, as well as low-frequency rTMS or iTBS of the cerebellum and restoration of swallowing function [19].

We used rTMS according to the method we developed in the rehabilitation program for patients after stroke, which included multilevel magnetic stimulation using a high-intensity pulsed magnetic field (2–2.2 T): Level I – rhythmic TMS of projections of the motor zones of the cortex of the affected hemisphere with a pulse intensity magnetic field of 70–90% of the maximum output of the stimulator, supply frequency stimulus 30–40 Hz, and pulse duration 0.1 ms; Level II – rhythmic TMS of

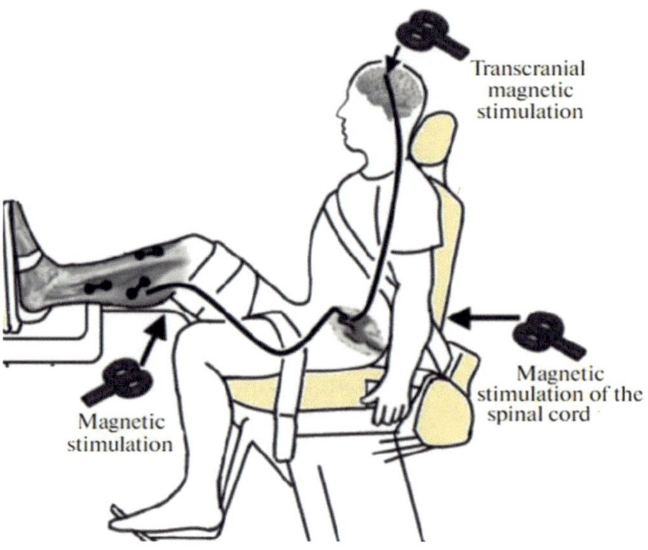

Figure 4.
Multilevel magnetic stimulation technique [20].

segmental reflex zones (cervical and lumbar) with a pulsed magnetic field intensity of 40–60% of the maximum output of the stimulator, supply frequency stimulus 40–50 Hz, and pulse duration 0.1 ms; Level III – rhythmic TMS of the peripheral neuromotor apparatus with a pulse intensity magnetic field of 70–100% of the maximum output of the stimulator, supply frequency stimulus 30–40 Hz, and pulse duration 0.1 ms (see **Figure 4**). The duration of the procedure was 20–25 min (10 procedures per course).

The use of therapeutic techniques of transcranial and multilevel magnetic stimulation in poststroke patients helps to improve the clinical course of the disease and reduce the degree of cognitive impairment—impairment of memory, attention, orientation, speech, reading, reducing maladaptation and thereby helping to increase the level of daily household activity and improve motor functions. Our results allow us to conclude that the effect of transcranial and multilevel magnetic stimulation on brain structures responsible for the cognitive sphere occurs at all stages of recovery after stroke, apparently even residual. Multilevel rhythmic magnetic stimulation is a pathogenetically justified and therapeutically effective method of rehabilitation of poststroke patients, which, acting noninvasively on all levels of the neuromotor apparatus (central, segmental, and peripheral), stimulates afferent and efferent impulses, causes plastic reorganization of the projections of motor zones of paretic limbs in the cortex and, due to a multilevel effect on the activation of fine and gross motor skills, accelerates the restoration of cognitive functions [20].

Transcranial magnetic stimulation can help restore damaged neural connections and improve cognitive function, memory, attention, and learning after traumatic brain injury.

For Parkinson's disease, TMS may help reduce symptoms of movement disorders, and muscle stiffness, and improve motor control.

In the rehabilitation of patients with Alzheimer's disease, TMS can be used to improve cognitive function and slow down the progression of the disease.

For musculoskeletal disorders, paralysis, and spasticity, to relieve pain and speed up the process of physical recovery after surgery or injury, TMS helps to strengthen muscles and improve motor skills, reduce pain and inflammation, and helps to speed up the process of physical and tissue recovery.

The results of a systematic review identified the potential benefits of the combined use of virtual reality (VR) and noninvasive brain stimulation (NIBS) as a new approach to rehabilitation. Most of the studies reviewed in five pathologies: stroke, neuropathic pain, cerebral palsy, phobia, posttraumatic stress disorder, and multiple sclerosis rehabilitation reported positive effects from the use of VR-NIBS, but studies are ongoing [21].

The use of TMS in rehabilitation requires a privatized approach and supervision by qualified neurologists, physiotherapists, and occupational therapists, who must develop treatment plans and adjust stimulation parameters according to the needs of each patient. TMS continues to develop as a noninvasive, effective method of rehabilitation and provides the prerequisites for improving the quality of life of patients.

Acknowledgments

I would like to thank my supervisor Professor, Doctor of Medicine Alishir Musayev (posthumously), my second supervisor Professor, Doctor of Medicine Sadagat Huseynova, and my permanent consultant and reviewer, coauthor of many joint works, Professor, Doctor of Medicine Farkhanda Balakishiyeva, for their great contribution and support in carrying out my work, and for my formation as a scientist and competitor.

Conflict of interest

The author declares no conflict of interest.

Author details

Marziyya Mammadova
Scientific Research İnstitute of Medical Rehabilitation, Baku, Azerbaijan

*Address all correspondence to: mammadovamarziyya@gmail.com

References

[1] Mann J. The medical avatar and its role in neurorehabilitation and neuroplasticity: A review. NeuroRehabilitation. 2020;**46**(4): 467-482. DOI: 10.3233/NRE-203063

[2] World Health Organization. Rehabilitation 2030. 2017. Available from: www.who.int/initiatives/rehabilitation-2030

[3] Muri L et al. Repetitive transcranial magnetic Stimulation activates glial cells and inhibits neurogenesis after pneumococcal meningitis. PLoS One. 2020;**15**(9):e0232863. DOI: 10.1371/journal.pone.0232863

[4] Zhou L, Jin Y, Wu D, Cun Y, Zhang C, Peng Y, et al. Current evidence, clinical applications, and future directions of transcranial magnetic stimulation as a treatment for ischemic stroke. Frontiers in Neuroscience. 2023;**17**:1177283. DOI: 10.3389/fnins.2023.1177283

[5] Rotenberg A et al. Transcranial Magnetic Stimulation: Neuromethods. New York, NY: Springer; 2014

[6] Sandro M, editor. Navigated Transcranial Magnetic Stimulation in Neurosurgery. Krieg Germany: Springer International Publishing; 2017

[7] Stoby KS, Rafique SA, Oeltzschner G, Steeves JKE. Continuous and intermittent theta burst stimulation to the visual cortex do not alter GABA and glutamate concentrations measured by magnetic resonance spectroscopy. Brain Behaviour. 2022;**12**(2):e2478. DOI: 10.1002/brb3.2478

[8] Musaev AV, Nasirova MY. Transcranial magnetic stimulation. Neurophysiological mechanisms, significance in the diagnosis and rehabilitation of patients with diseases of the nervous system. Physiotherapy, Balneology and Rehabilitation. 2008;**2**:3-12

[9] Salerno A, Georgesco M. Interhemispheric facilitation and inhibition studies in man with double magnetic stimulation. Electroencephalography and Clinical Neurophysiology. 1996;**101**:395-403

[10] Kujirai T. Corticocortical inhibition in human motor cortex. The Journal of Physiology (Lond). 1993;**471**:501-519

[11] George MS, Lisanby SH, Sackeim HA. Transcranial magnetic Stimulation (TMS). Achieves in General Psychiatry. 1999;**56**:300-311

[12] Dettmers C, Ridding MC, Stephan KM, et al. Comparison of regional cerebral blood flow with transcranial magnetic stimulation at different forces. Journal of Applied Physiology. 1996;**81**(2):596-603

[13] Teneback CC, Nahas Z, Speer AM, et al. Changes in prefrontal cortex and paralimbic activity in depression following two weeks of daily left prefrontal TMS. The Journal of Neuropsychiatry and Clinical Neurosciences. 1999;**11**(4):426-435

[14] Nahas Z, Lomarev M, Roberts DR, et al. Unilateral left prefrontal transcranial magnetic stimulation (TMS) produces intensity-dependent bilateral effects as measured by interleaved BOLD fMRI. Biological Psychiatry. 2001;**50**(9):712-720

[15] Szuba MP, O'Reardon J, Rai AS, et al. Acute mood and thyroid

stimulating hormone effects of transcranial magnetic stimulation in major depression. Biological Psychiatry. 2001;**50**(1):22-27

[16] Pridmore S. Rapid transcranial magnetic stimulation and normalization of the dexamethasone suppression test. Psychiatry and Clinical Neurosciences. 1999;**53**(1):33-37

[17] Chen M, Deng H, Schmidt RL, Kimberley TJ. Low-frequency repetitive transcranial magnetic stimulation targeted to premotor cortex followed by primary motor cortex modulates excitability differently than premotor cortex or primary motor cortex stimulation alone. Neuromodulation. Dec 2015;**18**(8):678-685. DOI: 10.1111/ner.12337. Epub 2015 Aug 26. PMID: 26307511; PMCID: PMC5154674

[18] Lefaucheur JP, André Obalia N, Antal A, et al. Evidence-based guidelines on the therapeutic use of repetitive transcranial magnetic stimulation (rTMS). Clinical Neurophysiology. 2014;**125**:2150-2206

[19] Lefaucheurab Jean-Pascal, Alemanc André, Baekendef Chris. Evidence-based guidelines on the therapeutic use of repetitive transcranial magnetic stimulation (rTMS): An update (2014-2018). Clinical Neurophysiology. February 2020;**131**(2):474-528

[20] Mamedova MY. Effects of rhythmic transcranial and multilevel magnetic stimulation on cognitive impairments in post-stroke patients. The Bulletin of Contemporary Clinical Medicine. 2021;**14**(3):23-32. DOI: 10.20969/VSKM.2021.14(3).23-32

[21] Cassani R, Novak GS, Falk TH, et al. Virtual reality and non-invasive brain stimulation for rehabilitation applications: A systematic review. Journal of NeuroEngineering Rehabilitation. 2020;**17**:147. DOI: 10.1186/s12984-020-00780-5

Chapter 6

Somatosensory Stimulation (Acupuncture) Modulates Spinal and Supraspinal Motor Neuron Excitability

Akira Nihonmatsu

Abstract

It has been reported that acupuncture is effective in alleviating abnormalities of muscle tone caused by abnormal motor neuron excitability such as spastic paralysis caused by cerebrovascular disorder. However, the underlying mechanism is unclear. Thus, we examined the effect of acupuncture stimulation on long-latency reflexes (LLR) to determine the site of action of acupuncture stimulation in modulating motor reflexes. The amplitude ratio of LLR/M was reduced by the acupuncture stimulation of LI4 (hand). Furthermore, we examined the effect of acupuncture stimulation on blink reflexes. The R2 component of blink reflexes was decreased by the acupuncture stimulation of LI4 (hand). LLR is the motor reflex of the central nervous system via such as cerebral cortex of supraspinal pathways. In addition, blink reflexes are the motor reflex of the central nervous system via such as brain stem. These findings suggest that acupuncture stimulation inhibits motor nerve reflexes via supraspinal modulation systems. Furthermore, we examined the effect of acupuncture stimulation on electromyogram F-wave to determine the effect of acupuncture stimulation on the excitability of spinal motor neurons. The result of this study indicated that acupuncture stimulation may have a greater effect on the excitability of spinal motor neurons.

Keywords: acupuncture stimulation, Li4 acupuncture point, long-latency reflex, blink reflex, F-wave

1. Introduction

It has been reported that acupuncture is effective in alleviating abnormalities of muscle tone caused by abnormal motor neuron excitability such as spastic paralysis caused by cerebrovascular disorder and rigidity in Parkinson's disease [1, 2]. These reports that acupuncture stimulation suppresses motor nerve excitability and may alleviate abnormalities in muscle tone. However, the underlying mechanism is unclear. The next section introduces our research on motor reflexes via the cerebral cortex, brainstem, and spinal cord through acupuncture stimulation.

2. Effect of acupuncture stimulation on the long-latency reflex

2.1 Background and purpose

Many reports have shown the effects of acupuncture stimulation on motor reflexes via the motor cortex using motor-evoked potentials (MEP) [3–7]. There are reports that acupuncture stimulation of the upper and lower limbs suppresses MEPs in the muscles of the upper limbs and reports that MEPs are stimulated, but this has not been determined [3–7]. In this study, we investigated the effects of acupuncture stimulation on long-latency reflexes (LLR), which are motor reflexes that pass through the cerebral cortex.

2.2 Materials and methods

2.2.1 Participants

Sixteen healthy volunteers (mean – standard deviation [SD]:28.9–6.6 years; 10 males and 6 females) with no known neurological dysfunction, and stable appearance of LLR agree to participate in this study. Written informed consent was obtained from all subjects. This study was approved by the Research Ethics Committee at Hokkaido College of Oriental Medicine.

2.2.2 Study design

This study applied the crossover protocol; therefore, each experiment was randomly needled on separate days. The experiments were performed under two conditions: (1) acupuncture stimulation of right LI4, (2) control (no acupuncture stimulation). To prevent a carryover effect, more than 1 week intervals between each acupuncture stimulation were maintained.

2.2.3 Apparatus and condition for the LLR recording

Prior to the experiment, the maximum amount of contraction due to the opposite movement of the thumb and middle finger on the measurement side was measured using a load transducer (Showa Sokki load cell), and 20% of that force was maintained. During continuous muscle contraction in that state, electrical stimulation was performed, and LLR was measured. LLR were recorded and analyzed by using a Neuropack MEB 9204 recorder (Nihon Koden, Tokyo, Japan) with a band-pass filter of 5 Hz to 2 kHz. Thirty-two LLR waves, elicited by electric stimulation of the median nerve to the wrist, were recorded from the opponens pollicis muscle on the right hand of each subject in a resting sitting position. The stimulus intensity used to elicit LLR was more than the 120% that is required to elicit an M-wave response. The electrical stimulus rate and duration were 1 Hz and 0.2 milliseconds, respectively. Electromyographic electrodes were attached firmly over the opponens pollicis muscle, With the anode positioned thumb phalanges. The ground electrode was placed between the stimulating and recording electrodes. The electrode impedance was below 5KΩ. The experiments were performed in a quiet room with a consistent temperature of 23–25°C.

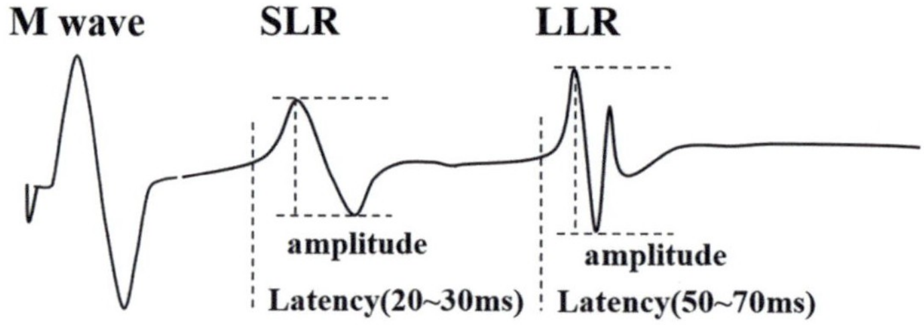

Figure 1.
Analysis of LLR. Median nerve stimulation resulted in well known two component reflex responses in the adductor pollicis muscle. The first component (SLR) is short latency (20–30 msec) responses. In contrast, the second component (LLR) is of longer latency (40–60 msec) responses (reprinted from [8]).

2.2.4 Data analysis for the LLR

Sample images of the LLR and M-wave are shown in **Figure 1**. The LLR was analyzed with respect to three parameters: occurrence, the LLR/M amplitude ratio, and the latency. The sensitivity was set at 5 mV/div for the M-wave and 0.5 mV/div for the LLR. The occurrence was defined as the number of detected LLR responses to 32 electrical stimuli and expressed as percentage (%). The LLR/M amplitude ratio was defined as the peak-to-peak amplitudes of LLR and M-waves were measured, and the amplitude ratio of LLR/M was expressed as the ratio of LLR amplitude and the maximal amplitude of M-wave. LLR latency was defined as the period from the stimulus to the LLR evocation.

2.2.5 Acupuncture stimulation

An acupuncturist applied a needle at the right LI 4 (radial to the midpoint of the second metacarpal bone) (**Figure 2**). Disposable stainless steel needles (diameter, 0.18 mm; length, 40 mm; Seirin Co., Ltd. Shizuoka, Japan) were used. The depth of needle insertion was 10 mm, and the needle was at a right angle to the skin and was maintained in this position (needle retention) for 5 minutes. No manipulation was performed during needle retention.

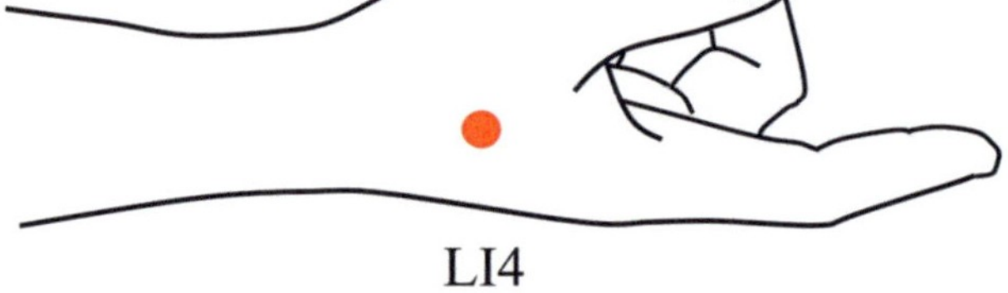

Figure 2.
Acupuncture stimulation site (LI4). An acupuncturist applied a needle at the right LI 4 (radial to the midpoint of the second metacarpal bone). Disposable stainless steel needles (diameter, 0.18 mm; length, 40 mm; Seirin Co., ltd. Shizuoka, Japan) were used. The depth of needle insertion was 10 mm, and the needle was at a right angle to the skin and was maintained in this position (needle retention) for 5 minutes. No manipulation was performed during needle retention.

2.2.6 Experimental setting

M-wave and LLR wave were measured before and after acupuncture (5-minute needle retention). M-wave and LLR wave in the control group were measured at the same timepoints acupuncture.

2.2.7 Statistical analysis

The data are reported as means ± standard deviation (mean ± S.D.). A Wilcoxon signed-rank test was used to compare occurrence, the LLR/M amplitude ratio, and the latency results after acupuncture and before acupuncture. For other statistical analyses, P values <0.05 were considered significant. Statistical analyses were performed using a commercially available statistical package (SPSS, Ver11.0.1, SPSS, Tokyo, Japan).

2.3 Results

2.3.1 Typical electromyogram waveform under before acupuncture stimulation and during acupuncture stimulation

Figure 3 illustrates a sample recording of the LLR wave from a typical subject. LLR wave decreased after acupuncture stimulation (right side), compared with those before acupuncture stimulation. No effect of acupuncture stimulation was observed on the M-wave.

2.3.2 Changes in LLR induced by acupuncture stimulation

The changes in LLR are shown in **Table 1**. The LLR occurrence was significantly reduced by acupuncture stimulation. There was no significant change in the control group. The LLR/M amplitude ratio was significantly reduced by acupuncture stimulation. There was no significant change in the control group. The LLR latency was no significant change in either group.

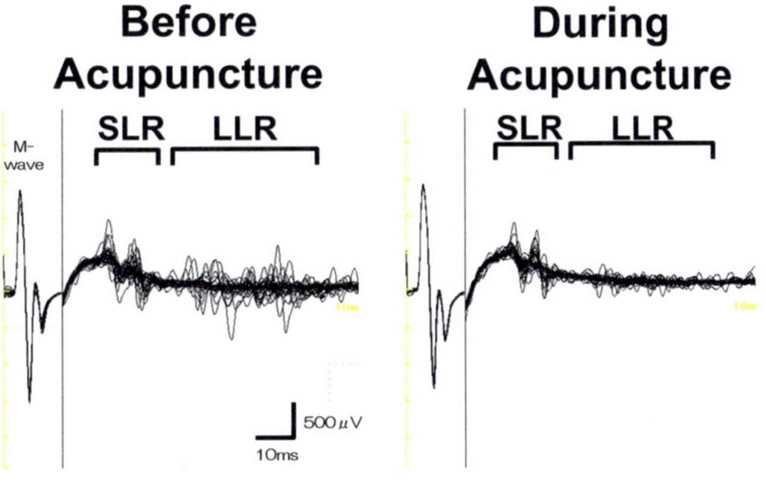

Figure 3.
Typical electromyogram waveform under resting condition (left side) and during acupuncture stimulation (right side). Typical electromyogram waveform under resting condition and during acupuncture stimulation. LLR was decreased during acupuncture stimulation (reprinted from [8]).

	Acupuncture		Control	
	Before	**After**	**Before**	**After**
LLR occurrence (%)	78.7 ± 18.9	62.2 ± 23.7**	87.8 ± 10.0	77.4 ± 11.8
LLR/M ratio (%)	1.95 ± 0.72	1.57 ± 0.72**	1.64 ± 0.32	1.70 ± 0.59
LLR latency (ms)	56.2 ± 3.4	57.6 ± 4.0	56.5 ± 2.3	59.1 ± 2.5

*Mean ± SD. **: P < 0.01 Wilcoxon signed-rank test vs. before acupuncture.*

Table 1.
Changes in LLR induced by acupuncture stimulation.

2.4 Discussion

Sudden mechanical stretch of the wrist flexor muscles gives rise to EMG responses, including both short-latency and long-latency components [9]. Marsden et al. measured electromyograms of the flexor pollicis longus by abruptly extending the thumb. They reported that following a monosynaptic spinal cord reflex with a latency of 25 ms, long-latency reflexes of 55 ms could be measured [10]. In addition, Previous studies have shown that LLR is absent in patients with dorsal column injury [11] and patients with lesions in the corticospinal tract (motor area, internal capsule) [12]. Therefore, LLR is considered to be expressed by a supraspinal mechanism such as the cerebrum. It has been shown that LLR is induced not only by mechanical stimulation but also by electrical stimulation. Previous studies have reported lacking LLR in hemiplegia, posterior spinal cord injury, and pontine hemorrhage [13–15]. Therefore, LLR induced by electrical stimulation is considered to be a reflex that occurs by descending the corticospinal tract via the spinal cord, sensory cortex, and motor cortex. In this study, LLR occurrence and LLR/M amplitude ratio were significantly reduced by acupuncture stimulation. In addition, we reported that acupuncture-induced changes in the LLR/M ratio were associated with changes in SEP N20 amplitude [8]. N20 of SEP is the potential induced when electrical stimulation ascends the dorsal cord of the spinal cord and excites the somatosensory area of the cerebral cortex [16, 17]. In addition, there is evidence that the afferent pathway for the LLR to the cortex is identical to that for the somatosensory evoked cortical potential (SEP) after median nerve stimulation [17]. Therefore, it is thought that changes in the excitability of the somatosensory area of the cerebral cortex are involved in the suppression of LLR occurrence and LLR/M amplitude ratio by acupuncture stimulation. In addition, reflexes via the brainstem such as spino-bulbo-spinal reflex and transcerebellar loop reflex are thought to be involved in LLR [18, 19]. It is also possible that acupuncture stimulation affected this mechanism. However, Previous studies have shown that brainstem-mediated reflexes have faster latencies than LLRs, and cerebellar-mediated reflexes have slower latencies than LLRs [18, 19]. In this study, no significant changes were observed in LLR latency. Therefore, it is thought that the decrease in LLR occurrence and LLR/M amplitude ratio due to acupuncture stimulation is due to an inhibitory mechanism via the cerebral cortex.

2.5 Conclusion

These findings suggest that acupuncture stimulation inhibits motor nerve reflexes via such cerebral cortex modulation systems.

3. Effect of acupuncture stimulation on the blink reflex

3.1 Background and purpose

The blink reflex can be quantitatively measured from the magnitude of the reaction of the muscle action potential of the orbicularis oculi muscle induced when the supraorbital nerve, which is the first branch of the trigeminal nerve, is electrically stimulated. The electromyogram associated with the blink reflex consists of two components called R1 and R2. R1 is a relatively stable early component that appears with a latency of 10 msec and appears only in stimulus measurements. R2 is a late component that appears bilaterally after R1. The R1 component is the potential where electrical stimulation to the supraorbital nerve alters neurons in the facial nucleus at the pons and leads to the orbicularis oculi muscle. Several studies have considered the R2 component of the blink reflex to be evoked through a polysynaptic pathway in the pons and the lateral part of the medulla [20, 21]. In fact, impulses of the R2 component travel along a longer pathway through the medulla up to the thalamus or cerebral cortex [20, 21]. Peripheral facial nerve palsy causes R1 and R2 component suppression, and hemifacial spasm causes an increase in the R2 component [20, 21]. Furthermore, it has been reported that the R2 component reflects the disappearance of Myerson's sign upon administration of L-dopa in patients with Parkinson's disease [22, 23]. Therefore, it is thought that not only the brainstem but also a wide range of central nervous systems, including are involved in the expression of the R2 component of the blink reflex. In this study, we investigated the effects of acupuncture stimulation on BR, which are motor reflexes that pass through the supraspinal modulation systems.

3.2 Materials and methods

3.2.1 Participants

Fifteen healthy volunteers (mean – standard deviation [SD]:30.3–6.2 years; 15 males and 1 female) with no known neurological dysfunction and stable appearance of BR agree to participate in this study. Written informed consent was obtained from all subjects. This study was approved by the Research Ethics Committee at Hokkaido College of Oriental Medicine.

3.2.2 Study design

This study applied the crossover protocol; therefore, each experiment was randomly needled on separate days. The experiments were performed under two conditions: (1) acupuncture stimulation of right LI4 and (2) control (no acupuncture stimulation). To prevent a carryover effect, intervals of more than 1 week between each acupuncture stimulation were maintained.

3.2.3 Experimental setting

BR was measured before and after acupuncture (5-minute needle retention). BR in the control group was measured at the same timepoints acupuncture.

3.2.4 Measurement of BR

BR was recorded and analyzed by using a Neuropack MEB 9204 recorder (Nihon Koden, Tokyo, Japan) with a band-pass filter of 5 Hz to 2 kHz. Five BR waves, elicited by electric stimulation of the supraorbital nerve, were recorded from the orbicularis oculi muscle of each subject. The stimulus intensity was twice the intensity the R2 component responded to. The electrical stimulus rate and duration were 0.1 Hz and 0.2 milliseconds, respectively. Electromyographic electrodes were attached firmly over the orbicularis oculi muscle, With the anode positioned lateral canthus. The ground electrode was placed forehead. The electrode impedance was below 10KΩ. The experiments were performed in a quiet room with a consistent temperature of 23–25°C.

3.2.5 Data analysis for the BR

Analysis was performed on waveforms in which the blink reflex appeared stable (**Figure 4**). The obtained waveforms were analyzed with R1 as the waveform rising at the latency of 10 msec and R2 as the waveform rising at the latency of 30 msec.

3.2.5.1 R1 component

The R1 component was analyzed with respect to two parameters: the R1 latency and R1 amplitude. The R1 latency was defined as the time from the electrical stimulation to the rise of the waveform that appeared around 10 msec was measured. The R1 amplitude ratio was defined as the peak-to-peak amplitudes of R1, An average of waveforms of 60 μV or more was obtained.

3.2.5.2 R2 component

The R1 component was analyzed with respect to three parameters: the R2 latency, R2 amplitude, and R2 duration. The R2 latency was defined as the time from the

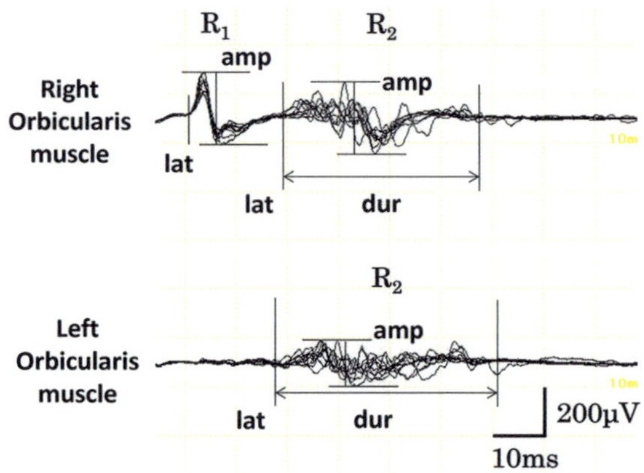

Figure 4.
Analysis of BR. Analysis was performed on waveforms in which the appearance of the blink reflex was stable. The obtained waveforms were analyzed with R1 as the waveform rising at the latency of 10 msec and R2 as the waveform rising at the latency of 30 msec. Lat: Latency, amp: Amuplitude, dur: Duration.

electrical stimulation to the rise of the waveform that appeared around 30 msec was measured. The average of 5 waveforms was obtained. The R2 amplitude ratio was defined as the peak-to-peak amplitudes of R2. The time from the first negative peak of the R2 waveform to the last negative peak of the waveform was measured.

3.2.5.3 Measurement of electrical stimulation pain assessment

The subjective magnitude of electrical stimulation pain was rated by visual analog scale (VAS). It was recorded as no pain at the left end (0 mm) and the maximum pain the participant experienced in the past at the right end (100 mm) on a linear scale of 100 mm.

3.2.6 Acupuncture stimulation

An acupuncturist applied a needle at the right LI 4 (radial to the midpoint of the second metacarpal bone) (**Figure 2**). Disposable stainless steel needles (diameter, 0.18 mm; length, 40 mm; Seirin Co., Ltd. Shizuoka, Japan) were used. The depth of needle insertion was 10 mm, and the needle was at a right angle to the skin and was maintained in this position (needle retention) for 5 minutes. No manipulation was performed during needle retention.

3.2.7 Statistical analysis

The data are reported as means ± standard deviation (mean ± S.D.). A Wilcoxon signed-rank test was used to compare BR results after acupuncture and before acupuncture. For other statistical analyses, P values <0.05 were considered significant. Statistical analyses were performed using a commercially available statistical package (SPSS, Ver11.0.1, SPSS, Tokyo, Japan).

3.3 Results

3.3.1 Typical electromyogram waveform under before acupuncture stimulation and during acupuncture stimulation

Figure 5 illustrates a sample recording of the BR from a typical subject. R2 decreased after acupuncture stimulation (right side). There was no change in the R1 component.

3.3.2 Changes in R1 component induced by acupuncture stimulation

The changes in the R1 component are shown in **Table 2**. The R1 latency and amplitude showed no significant change in both groups.

3.3.3 Changes in R2 component induced by acupuncture stimulation

The changes in the R2 component are shown in **Table 2**. Acupuncture stimulation depressed the latency, amplitude, and duration of the R2 component on both sides. There was no change in the control group.

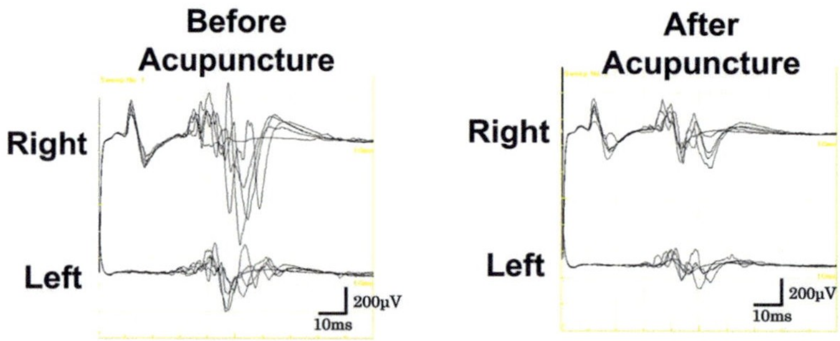

Figure 5.
Typical electromyogram waveform under resting condition (left side) and during acupuncture stimulation (right side). R2 component decreased after acupuncture stimulation. There was no change in the R1 component.

	Acupuncture		Control	
	Before	After	Before	After
Right R1 latency (ms)	10.3 ± 2.0	10.4 ± 1.7	10.3 ± 2.0	10.3 ± 2.0
Right R1 amplitude (%)	281.5 ± 124.2	269.3 ± 106.5	259.5 ± 117.2	254.7 ± 106.5
Right R2 latency (ms)	34.8 ± 3.6	36.0 ± 2.8**	35.4 ± 7.2	36.9 ± 5.1
Right R2 amplitude (%)	287.9 ± 198.5	225.9 ± 154.9**	312.4 ± 281.3	290.4 ± 242.1
Right R2 duration (ms)	28.2 ± 15.9	21.2 ± 10.5**	24.3 ± 9.3	22.3 ± 9.8
Left R2 latency (ms)	37.5 ± 6.7	39.0 ± 6.3**	35.7 ± 11.2	38.5 ± 8.5
Left R2 amplitude (%)	183.8 ± 120.5	152.1 ± 102.5**	219.9 ± 148.7	203.2 ± 136.8
Left R2 duration (ms)	25.9 ± 14.0	20.6 ± 6.9**	27.2 ± 7.9	26.0 ± 11.0

*Mean ± SD. **: P < 0.01 Wilcoxon signed-rank test vs. before acupuncture.*

Table 2.
Changes in BR induced by acupuncture stimulation.

3.3.4 Changes in electrical stimulation pain induced by acupuncture stimulation

The changes in electrical stimulation pain are shown in **Table 3**. The electrical stimulation pain was no significant change in either group.

3.4 Discussion

The blink reflex can be quantitatively measured from the magnitude of the reaction of the muscle action potential of the orbicularis oculi muscle induced when the supraorbital nerve, which is the first branch of the trigeminal nerve,

	Acupuncture	Control
VAS (mm)	29.14 ± 26.33	26.71 ± 23.19

Table 3.
Changes in electrical stimulation pain induced by acupuncture stimulation.

is electrically stimulated. The electromyogram associated with the blink reflex consists of two components called R1 and R2. R1 is a relatively stable early component that appears with a latency of 10 msec and appears only in stimulus measurements. The R1 component is the potential where electrical stimulation to the supraorbital nerve alters neurons in the facial nucleus at the pons and leads to the orbicularis oculi muscle. Several studies have considered the R2 component of the blink reflex to be evoked through a polysynaptic pathway in the pons and the lateral part of the medulla [20, 21]. Peripheral facial nerve palsy causes R1 and R2 component suppression; hemifacial spasm causes an increase in the R2 component [20, 21]. Thalamic hemorrhage and lesions in the sensory cortex have also been reported to cause R2 abnormalities [21]. Furthermore, it has been reported that the R2 component reflects the disappearance of Myerson's sign upon administration of L-dopa in patients with Parkinson's disease [22, 23]. Therefore, it is thought that not only the brainstem but also a wide range of central nervous systems including are involved in the expression of the R2 component of the blink reflex. No significant changes were observed in the latency and amplitude of the R1 component in both control group and acupuncture group. Thus, our results show that the R1 component of the blink reflex was not changed by acupuncture stimulation, suggesting that acupuncture stimulation has no effect on the monosynaptic reflex of the brain stem. Acupuncture stimulation depressed the latency, amplitude, and duration of the R2 component on both sides. It is well known that acupuncture activates various groups of afferent fibers. Kagitani et al. demonstrated that manual acupuncture needle stimulation to the hind limbs activated the single-unit afferents belonging to the group I, II, III, and IV fibers in the spinal dorsal roots [24]. Acupuncture signals are conveyed by afferent fibers to the dorsal horn of the spinal cord. Then, they project to the thalamus via spinothalamic tract (STT) and spinoreticulothalamic tract (SRT). It has been shown to project to various regions such as the lateral reticular formation, central midbrain gray matter, basal ganglia, and sensory cortex [25, 26]. Willer JC et al. reported that electroacupuncture stimulation depresses the R2 component. In addition, they assumed the involvement of endogenous morphine-like systems since the depression of R2 components by electroacupuncture was antagonized by naloxone administration [27]. This study found no effect of acupuncture on electrical pain. Therefore, we suggest that the depression of R2 components by acupuncture is not due to the suppression of pain caused by evoked electrical stimulation. Furthermore, it has been suggested that there is a longer pathway involving the cerebral cortex for the inhibition of R2 components by acupuncture stimulation.

3.5 Conclusion

Acupuncture stimulation may inhibit R2 components via longer pathways involving the cerebral cortex.

DOI: http://dx.doi.org/10.5772/intechopen.1002498

4. Effect of acupuncture stimulation on excitability of spinal motor neurons

4.1 Background and purpose

F-waves are muscle action potentials recorded from muscle fibers of motor units activated by antidromic action potentials ascending in motor axons to the anterior horn cell [28–30]. F-waves are late motor responses observed following supramaximal electrical stimulation of a peripheral nerve causing an antidromic activation of motor neurons [28–30]. Zhao et al. found that the F/M ratio decreased following acupuncture treatment in patients with spastic hypertonia from stroke; this result indicated that the acupuncture treatment could inhibit neuron excitability in patients with spastic hypertonia from stroke [1]. Futhermore, Matsumoto et al. reported that the F/M ratio decreased following acupuncture treatment in patients with Chronic Disorder of Consciousness Following Traumatic Brain Injury [31]. As described above, the effect of acupuncture stimulation on the induced F-wave has been mainly applied to the effect of patients with motor symptoms such as spastic paralysis. In this study, we examined the effects of acupuncture stimulation on the spinal motor neuron in healthy adults, using the electromyographic F-waves of the first dorsal interosseous muscle immediately below the acupuncture stimulation site.

4.2 Materials and methods

4.2.1 Participants

Ten healthy volunteers (mean–standard deviation [SD]:30.3–6.2 years; 15 males and 1 female) with no known neurological dysfunction agree to participate in this study. Written informed consent was obtained from all subjects. This study was approved by the Research Ethics Committee at Hokkaido College of Oriental Medicine.

4.2.2 Study design

This study applied the crossover protocol; therefore, each experiment was randomly needled on separate days. The experiments were performed under two conditions: (1) acupuncture stimulation of right LI4 and (2) control (no acupuncture stimulation). To prevent a carryover effect, more than 1 week intervals between each acupuncture stimulation were maintained.

4.2.3 Experimental setting

M-wave and F-wave were measured before and after acupuncture (5-minute needle retention). M-wave and F-wave in the control group were measured at the same timepoints acupuncture.

4.2.4 Measurement of F-wave

F-waves were recorded and analyzed by using a Neuropack MEB 9204 recorder (Nihon Koden, Tokyo, Japan) with a band-pass filter of 5 Hz to 2 kHz. Thirty-two F-waves, elicited by electric stimulation of the ulnar nerve to the wrist, were recorded from the first dorsal interosseous muscle on the right side of each subject in a resting sitting position. The stimulus intensity used to elicit F-wave was more than the 120% that is required to elicit a maximal M-wave response. The electrical stimulus rate and duration were 1 Hz and 0.2 milliseconds, respectively. Electromyographic electrodes were attached firmly over the first dorsal interosseous muscle, With the anode positioned second phalanges. The ground electrode was placed between the stimulating and recording electrodes. The electrode impedance was below 5KΩ. The experiments were performed in a quiet room with a consistent temperature of 23–25°C.

4.2.5 Data analysis for the F-wave

Sample images of the F-wave and M-wave are shown in **Figure 6**. The F-wave was analyzed with respect to three parameters: occurrence, the F/M amplitude ratio, and the latency. The sensitivity was set at 5 mV/div for the M-wave and 0.5 mV/div for the F-wave. The occurrence was defined as the number of detected F-wave responses to 32 electrical stimuli and expressed as percentage. The F/M amplitude ratio was defined as the peak-to-peak amplitudes of F- and M-waves were measured, and the amplitude ratio of F/M was expressed as the ratio of F amplitude and the maximal amplitude of M-wave. F-wave latency was defined as the period from the stimulus to the F-wave evocation.

4.2.6 Acupuncture stimulation

An acupuncturist applied a needle at the right LI 4 (radial to the midpoint of the second metacarpal bone) (**Figure 2**). Disposable stainless steel needles (diameter, 0.18 mm; length, 40 mm; Seirin Co., Ltd. Shizuoka, Japan) were used. The depth of needle insertion was 10 mm, and the needle was at a right angle to the skin and was maintained in this position (needle retention) for 5 minutes. No manipulation was performed during needle retention.

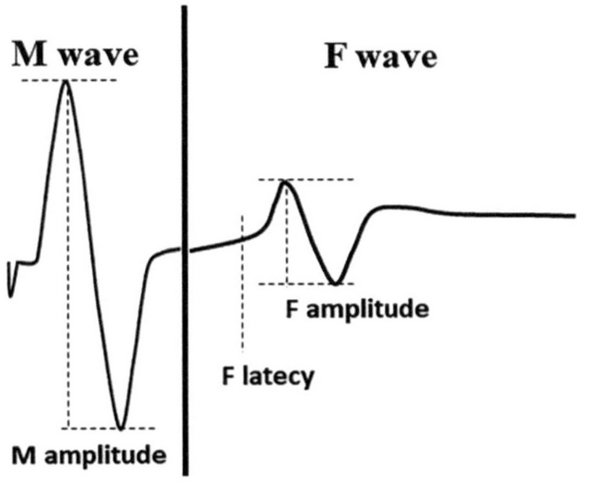

Figure 6.
Analysis of F wave. The F wave was analyzed with respect to three parameters: Occurrence and the F/M amplitude ratio and the latency. The sensitivity was set at 5 mV/div for the M-wave and 0.5 mV/div for the F wave. Occurrence was defined as the number of detected F wave responses to 32 electrical stimuli and expressed as percentage. The F/M amplitude ratio was defined as the peak-to-peak amplitudes of F and M-waves were measured and the amplitude ratio of F/M was expressed as the ratio of F amplitude and the maximal amplitude of M-wave. F-wave latency was defined as the period from the stimulus to the F-wave evocation.

4.2.7 Statistical analysis

The data are reported as means ± standard deviation (mean ± S.D.). A Wilcoxon signed-rank test was used to compare occurrence and the F/M amplitude ratio and the latency results after acupuncture and before acupuncture. For other statistical analyses, P values <0.05 were considered significant. Statistical analyses were performed using a commercially available statistical package (SPSS, Ver11.0.1, SPSS, Tokyo, Japan).

4.3 Results

4.3.1 Typical electromyogram waveform under before acupuncture stimulation and during acupuncture stimulation

Figure 7 illustrates sample recording of the F-wave from a typical subject. F-wave increased after acupuncture stimulation (right side). No effect of acupuncture stimulation was observed on the M-wave.

4.3.2 Changes in F-wave induced by acupuncture stimulation

The changes in the F-wave are shown in **Table 4**. The F-wave occurrence was significantly increased by acupuncture stimulation. There was no significant change in the control group. The F/M amplitude ratio was significantly increased by acupuncture stimulation. There was no significant change in the control group. The F-wave latency was no significant change in either group.

4.4 Discussion

LI4 is located in the area covered by the superficial branch of the radial nerve, and the muscle innervation of the first dorsal interosseus muscle underlying the same skin is supplied by the ulnar nerve. In addition, there are motor points of the first dorsal interosseous muscle around LI4, which may be excited by acupuncture stimulation [32], which may be excited by acupuncture stimulation. Thus, It is

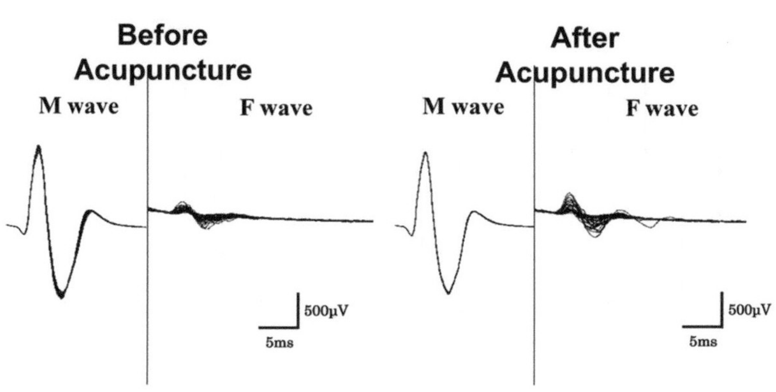

Figure 7.
Typical electromyogram waveform under resting condition (left side) and after acupuncture stimulation (right side). Typical electromyogram waveform under resting condition and during acupuncture stimulation. F wave increased after acupuncture stimulation (right side). No effect of acupuncture stimulation was observed on M wave.

	Acupuncture		Control	
	Before	After	Before	After
F-wave occurrence (%)	40.8 ± 17.2	48.1 ± 19.0**	36.2 ± 25.6	34.3 ± 25.1
F/M ratio (%)	1.73 ± 0.98	2.39 ± 1.56**	1.65 ± 0.63	1.71 ± 0.80
F-wave latency (ms)	29.8 ± 2.6	29.5 ± 2.6	29.5 ± 2.3	29.6 ± 2.3

*Mean ± SD. **: P < 0.01 Wilcoxon signed-rank test vs. before acupuncture.*

Table 4.
Changes in F-wave induced by acupuncture stimulation.

thought that acupuncture stimulation of LI4 excites various sensory receptors in the skin and muscles, spinal motor neuron are thought to undergo various regulations. In this study, F-wave persistence and amplitude F/M ratio increased after acupuncture stimulation. Persistence reflects the number of backfiring spinal anterior horn cells, and the F/M amplitude ratio reflects the synchronization of backfiring spinal anterior horn cells [28–30]. Thus, acupuncture increases the excitability of spinal motor neurons that innervate the muscles immediately below the stimulation site. Previous studies have shown that electrical stimulation of the index finger increases MEP in the first dorsal interosseous muscle [33]. In addition, Previous studies have shown that electrical stimulation of the index finger increases motor unit in the first dorsal interosseous muscle [34]. This suggests that stimulation of the skin may induce facilitation of the spinal motor neuron. Furthermore, It has been reported that pain stimulation to the thumb increases the MEP of the thenar muscle [35]. In addition, groups III and IV muscle afferents facilitated motoneurons and inhibited the motor cortex [36]. This suggests that painful stimuli to the skin and muscles may induce facilitation of the spinal motor neuron. Furthermore, there are motor points of the first dorsal interosseous muscle around LI4, which may be excited by acupuncture stimulation [32]. In addition, it has been reported that the number of Golgi tendon organs in the intrinsic muscle of the hand is maredly small [37]. Koiwa et al. demonstrated that inserted a needle electrode into the muscle motor point of the first dorsal interosseous muscle and measuring the action potential of the ulnar nerve of the elbow, the possibility of activated muscle sensory nerves such as group Ia afferent nerves [38]. Furthermore, we reported that the amplitude F/M ratio increased by acupuncture stimulation was suppressed by vibration stimulation. It is thought that the increase in reflex excitability of spinal motor neurons caused by group Ia afferent nerves excited by acupuncture stimulation is suppressed by presynaptic inhibition caused by the excitation of group Ia afferent nerves by vibration stimulation [39]. Furthermore, we inserted an acupuncture needle into LI4 and applied electrical stimulation to confirm the appearance of F-waves (**Figure 8**). Therefore, it was thought that acupuncture stimulation directly excites the ulnar nerve that innervates the first dorsal interosseous muscle. It may excite various afferent nerves contained within the same nerve trunk. Gracies et al. reported changes in the motor units of each upper extremity muscle by electrical stimulation of the median, ulnar, and radial nerves. They reported that stimulation of homonymous nerves increased the firing of motor units. Furthermore, it is considered that spatial facilitation by skin-afferent nerves and muscle-afferent nerves is involved in this effect [40]. Furthermore, It is well known that acupuncture activates various groups of afferent fibers. Using single-unit nerve recording techniques in rats, Kagitani et al. demonstrated that manual acupuncture needle stimulation to the hind limbs activated the single-unit afferents belonging to groups I–IV fibers in the spinal

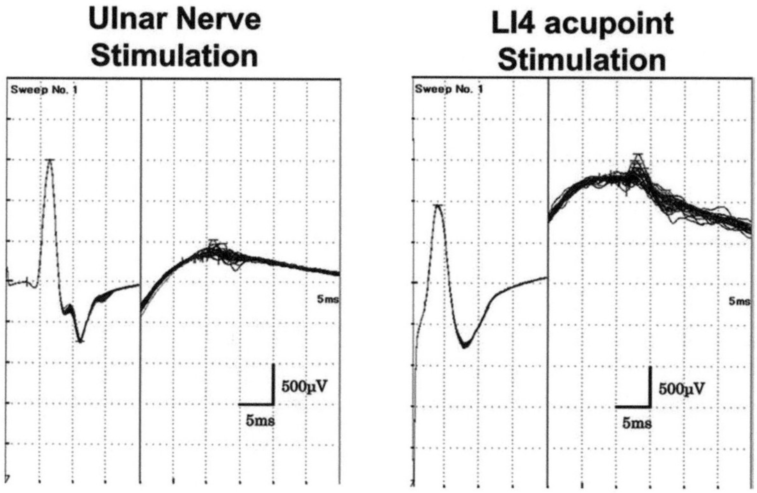

Figure 8.
Electromyograms recorded at the first dorsal interosseous muscle during stimulation of LI4 acupoint (right side) and ulnar nerve trunk (left side) in single subject.

dorsal roots [24]. This suggests that acupuncture stimulated sensory receptors and nerve fibers distributed in the skin and muscles, resulting in increased spinal motor neuron excitability. Furthermore, in our study, subjects cannot avoid paying attention to the acupuncture site during needle insertion. Previous studies have reported that attention causes the facilitation of MEPs [41]. Therefore, acupuncture effect was compensated by facilitation arising from the concentration to the stimulated site. In addition, the F-wave latency, which is an index showing the conduction velocity of motor nerves, was not affected by acupuncture stimulation. Therefore, it is considered that acupuncture stimulation does not affect the conduction velocity of motor nerves.

4.5 Conclusion

The result of this study indicated that acupuncture stimulation may have a greater effect on the excitability of spinal motor neurons.

5. How to use of acupuncture treatment in neurorehabilitation

In our study, acupuncture stimulation caused suppression of LLR occurrence and amplitude LLR/M ratio. Therefore, the results of this study are considered to explain the mechanism of action of acupuncture for Parkinson's disease and multiple sclerosis [42–44]. Therefore, the results of this study are considered to explain the mechanism of action of acupuncture for Parkinson's disease and multiple sclerosis.

Furthermore, we also found that acupuncture stimulation reduced the amplitude, latency, and duration of the BR R2 component. The results of this study suggest that acupuncture can be used for facial spasms and paralysis [45]. Furthermore, it has been reported that the R2 component reflects the disappearance of Myerson's sign upon administration of L-dopa in patients with Parkinson's disease [22, 23]. The results of this study suggest that acupuncture can be used for Parkinson's disease. Furthermore, it has been reported that acupuncture reduces the amplitude ratio in patients with spastic paralysis due to cerebrovascular disease [1]. In addition, acupuncture has been reported to depress the increase in F-wave frequency and amplitude ratio in patients with chronic consciousness disturbance after traumatic brain injury [31]. In addition, there is also a report that acupuncture reduces the incidence of Parkinson's disease [2]. In our study, the F-wave persistence and amplitude F/M ratio before acupuncture stimulation were not high. Therefore, it is possible that changes in spinal motor neurons by acupuncture may have different effects depending on the state before stimulation.

Acknowledgements

Hokkaido College of Oriental Medicine for many helpful discussions on the experiment and the manuscript.

Conflict of interest

The authors declare no conflict of interest.

Author details

Akira Nihonmatsu
Hokkaido College of Oriental Medicine, Hokkaido, Japan

*Address all correspondence to: nihonmatsu@shinkyu.ac.jp

References

[1] Zhao JG, Cao CH, Liu CZ, Han BJ, Zhang J, Li ZG, et al. Effect of acupuncture treatment on spastic states of stroke patients. Journal of the Neurological Sciences. 2009;**276**(1-2): 143-147. DOI: 10.1016/j.jns.2008.09.018

[2] Fukuda S, Egawa M, Namura M. The clinical effects of acupuncture in patients with Parkinson's disease: A randomized controlled trial. The Bulletin of Meiji University of Integrative Medicine. 2012;**6**:21-45 (in japanese)

[3] Maioli C, Falciati L, Marangon M, Perini S, Losio A. Short- and long-term modulation of upper limb motor-evoked potentials induced by acupuncture. The European Journal of Neuroscience. 2006;**23**(7):1931-1938. DOI: 10.1111/j.1460-9568.2006.04698.x

[4] Lo YL, Cui SL. Acupuncture and the modulation of cortical excitability. Neuroreport. 2003;**14**(9):1229-1231. DOI: 10.1097/00001756-200307010-00008

[5] Lo YL, Cui SL, Fook-Chong S. The effect of acupuncture on motor cortex excitability and plasticity. Neuroscience Letters. 2005;**384**(1-2):145-149. DOI: 10.1016/j.neulet.2005.04.083

[6] Yang Y, Eisner I, Chen S, Wang S, Zhang F, Wang L. Neuroplasticity changes on human motor cortex induced by acupuncture therapy: A preliminary study. Neural Plasticity. 2017;**2017**:4716792. DOI: 10.1155/2017/4716792

[7] Sun ZG, Pi YL, Zhang J, Wang M, Zou J, Wu W. Effect of acupuncture at ST36 on motor cortical excitation and inhibition. Brain and Behavior: A Cognitive Neuroscience Perspective. 2019;**9**(9):e01370. DOI: 10.1002/brb3.1370

[8] Nihonmatsu A, Kudo T, Kawanami K, Kasai M. Effect of acupuncture stimulation on the long latency reflex. Japan Acupuncture & Moxibustion. 2020;**70**(1):26-37. DOI: 10.3777/jjsam.70.26 (in japanese)

[9] Hammond PH. The influence of prior instruction to the subject on an apparently involuntary neuro-muscular response. The Journal of Physiology. 1956;**132**:17-19

[10] Marsden CD, Merton PA, Morton HB. Servo action in human voluntary movement. Nature. 1972;**238**(5360):140-143. DOI: 10.1038/238140a0

[11] Marsden CD, Merton PA, Morton HB. Is the human stretch reflex cortical rather than spinal? Lancet. 1973;**1**:759-761. DOI: 10.1016/s0140-6736(73)92141-7

[12] Marsden CD, Merton PA, Morton HB, Adam J. The effect of lesions of the sensorimotor cortex and the capsular pathways on servo responses from the human long thumb flexor. Brain. 1977;**100**:503-526. DOI: 10.1093/brain/100.3.503

[13] Conrad B, Aschoff JC. Effects of voluntary isometric and isotonic activity on late transcortical reflex components in normal subjects and hemiparetic patients. Electroencephalography and Clinical Neurophysiology. 1977;**42**:107-116. DOI: 10.1016/0013-4694(77)90155-9

[14] Jenner JR, Stephens JA. Cutaneous reflex responses and their central nervous pathways studied in man. The Journal of Physiology. 1982;**333**:405-419. DOI: 10.1113/jphysiol.1982.sp014461

[15] Nakajima Y, Nagaoka M, Narabayashi H. Conduction pathways of long latency (V2) reflex. Clinical Electroencephalography. 1983;**25**(9):608-614 (in japanese)

[16] Allison T, McCarthy G, Wood CC, Jones SJ. Potentials evoked in human and monkey cerebral cortex by stimulation of the median nerve. A review of scalp and intracranial recordings. Brain. 1991;**114**(6):2465-2503. DOI: 10.1093/brain/114.6.2465

[17] Deuschl G, Ludolph A, Schenck E, Lücking CH. The relations between long-latency reflexes in hand muscles, somatosensory evoked potentials and transcranial stimulation of motor tracts. Electroencephalography and Clinical Neurophysiology. 1989;**74**(6):425-430

[18] Kuroiwa Y, Mitani H. Long-loop reflexes. Japanese Journal of Clinical Neurophysiology. 2011;**39**(6):521-528 (in japanese)

[19] Shimamura M, Mori S, Matsushima S, Fujimori S. On the spino-bulbo-spinal reflex in dogs, monkeys and man. The Japanese Journal of Physiology. 1964;**15**(14):411-421. DOI: 10.2170/jjphysiol.14.411

[20] Morikawa K. Clinical and electrophysiological study of the blink reflex. Jibi to Rinsyo. 1979;**25**:707-724. DOI: 10.11334/jibi1954.25.2Supplement5_707 (in japanese)

[21] Morimoto K. Blink Reflex (BR). Medical Technology. 2005;**33**(1):69-76 (in japanese)

[22] Kimura J. Disorder of interneurons in parkinsonism. The orbicularis oculi reflex to paired stimuli. Brain. 1973;**96**(1):87-96. DOI: 10.1093/brain/96.1.87

[23] Agostino R, Berardelli A, Cruccu G, Stocchi F, Manfredi M. Corneal and blink reflexes in Parkinson's disease with "on-off" fluctuations. Movement Disorders. 1987;**2**(4):227-235. DOI: 10.1002/mds.870020401

[24] Kagitani F, Uchida S, Hotta H, Aikawa Y. Manual acupuncture needle stimulation of the rat hindlimb activates groups I, II, III and IV single afferent nerve fibers in the dorsal spinal roots. The Japanese Journal of Physiology. 2005;**55**(3):149-155. DOI: 10.2170/jjphysiol.R2120

[25] Kendall DE. A scientific model for acupuncture (part I). American Journal of Acupuncture. 1989;**17**(3):251-268

[26] Kendall DE. A scientific model for acupuncture (part II). American Journal of Acupuncture. 1989;**17**(4):343-360

[27] Willer JC, Roby A, Boulu P, Boureau F. Comparative effects of Electroacupuncture and transcutaneous never stimulation on the human blink reflex. Pain. 1982;**14**:267-278. DOI: 10.1016/0304-3959(82)90133-6

[28] Curt A, Keck ME, Dietz V. Clinical value of F-wave recordings in traumatic cervical spinal cord injury. Electroencephalography and Clinical Neurophysiology. 1997;**105**(3):189-193. DOI: 10.1016/s0924-980x(97)96626-1

[29] Peioglou-Harmoussi S, Fawcett PR, Howel D. Barwick DD:F-responses: A study of frequency, shape and amplitude characteristics in healthy control subjects. Journal of Neurology, Neurosurgery, and Psychiatry. 1985;**48**(11):1159-1164. DOI: 10.1136/jnnp.48.11.1159

[30] Fisher AM. F-waves--physiology and clinical uses. The Scientific World Journal. 2007;7:144-160. DOI: 10.1100/tsw.2007.49

[31] Matsumoto-Miyazaki J, Asano Y, Ikegame Y, Kawasaki T,

Nomura Y, Shinoda J. Acupuncture reduces excitability of spinal motor neurons in patients with spastic muscle Overactivity and chronic disorder of consciousness following traumatic brain injury. Journal of Alternative and Complementary Medicine. 2016;**22**(11):895-902. DOI: 10.1089/acm.2016.0180

[32] Tinazzi M, Rosso T, Zanette G, Fiaschi A, Aglioti SM. Rapid modulation of cortical proprioceptive activity induced by transient cutaneous deafferentation: Neurophysiologicalevidence of short term plasticity across different somatosensory modalities in humans. European Journal of Neuroscience. 2003;**18**:3053-3060. DOI: 10.1111/j.1460-9568.2003.03043.x

[33] Tomaru T. Effects of cutaneous digital nerve electrical stimulation and transcranial magnetic stimulation on the excitability of the motor cortex in humans. The Japanese Journal of Rehabilitation Medicine. 2003;**40**(11):757-765. DOI: 10.2490/jjrm1963.40.757 (in japanese)

[34] Datta AK, Stephens JA. The effects of digital nerve stimulation on the firing of motor units in human first dorsal interosseous muscle. The Journal of Physiology. 1981;**318**:501-510

[35] Martin PG, Weerakkody N, Gandevia SC, Taylor JL. Group III and IV muscle afferents differentially affect the motor cortex and Motoneurones in humans. The Journal of Physiology. 2008;**586**(5):1277-1289. DOI: 10.1113/jphysiol.2007.140426

[36] Fadiga L, Craighero L, Dri G, Facchin P, Destro MF, Porro CA. Corticospinal excitability during painful self-stimulation in humans: A transcranial magnetic stimulation study. Neuroscience Letters. 2004;**361**(1-3):250-253. DOI: 10.1016/j.neulet.2003.12.016

[37] Devanandan MS, Ghosh S, John KT. A quantitative study of muscle spindles and tendon organs in some intrinsic muscles of the hand in the bonnet monkey (Macaca radiata). The Anatomical Record. 1983;**207**(2):263-266. DOI: 10.1002/ar.1092070204

[38] Koiwa N, Asano T, Kusumi T, et al. Middle latency cortical potential elicited by electrical stimulation of muscle afferents in humans. Human Arts and Sciences. 2015;**15**(1):29-39

[39] Nihonmatsu A. Relationship between changes in electromyogram F wave and changes in local oxygen saturation due to acupuncture stimulation. The Autonomic Nervous System. 2022;**59**:96-100 (in japanese)

[40] Gracies JM, Meunier S, Pierrot-Deseilligny E, Simonetta M. Pattern of propriospinal-like excitation to different species of human upper limb motoneurones. The Journal of Physiology. 1991;**434**:151-167. DOI: 10.1113/jphysiol.1991.sp018463

[41] Rosenkranz K, Rothwell JC. The effect of sensory input and attention on the sensorimotor organization of the hand area of the human motor cortex. The Journal of Physiology. 2004;**561**(Pt 1):307-320. DOI: 10.1113/jphysiol.2004.069328

[42] Tatton WG, Lee RG. Evidence for abnormal long loop reflexes in rigid parkinsonian patients. Brain Research. 1975;**100**:671-676. DOI: 10.1016/0006-8993(75)90167-5

[43] Shibasaki H. Long-loop reflexes and somatosensory evoked potentials. Shinkei kenkyu no shinpo. 1988;**32**:45-57. DOI: 10.11477/mf.1431906165 (in japanese)

[44] Kaneshige Y, Matsumoto H, Chiba S, Hashimoto S, Noro H, Yamada Y.

Correlation between somatosensory evoked potentials and long-loop reflexes—Basic investigation and its application for multiple sclerosis. Cranial Nerves. 1989;**41**:997-1003. DOI: 10.11477/mf.1406206405 (in japanese)

[45] Huang JP, Liang ZM, Zou QW, Zhan J, Li WT, Li S, et al. Electroacupuncture on Hemifacial spasm and temporomandibular joint pain Co-morbidity: A case report. Frontiers in Neurology. 2022;**13**:931412. DOI: 10.3389/fneur.2022.931412

Section 3

Physical Therapy Practice

Chapter 7

Motor Imagery in Evidence-Based Physical Therapy

Yoshibumi Bunno, Chieko Onigata and Toshiaki Suzuki

Abstract

Motor imagery allows patients with difficulty in voluntary movements to mentally practice a target motor task. Numerous neurophysiological studies have investigated the mechanisms underlying the benefits of motor imagery, but many aspects remain unclear. Since both central and spinal neural function need to be leveraged to improve various motor functions, we have investigated motor imagery and spinal neural functions. Our previous research demonstrated a facilitation effect of motor imagery on spinal neural function and an immediate effect on muscle strength. Specifically, a mild imagined muscle contraction strength may be sufficient to enhance the excitability of spinal motor neurons. In addition, kinesthetic imagery or combined action observation and motor imagery may substantially enhance the excitability of spinal motor neurons. Also, keeping a position of the upper or lower extremities close to the desired movements leads to greater enhancement of the excitability of spinal motor neurons during motor imagery.

Keywords: motor imagery, action observation, sensory modality, F-waves, spinal neural function, muscle strength

1. Introduction

Motor imagery (MI) is a cognitive process that is realized when an individual imagines that he/she is creating specific motor actions without actually performing the action or contracting muscles [1–3]. MI does not require special equipment and it can be easily performed at any time and location. Therefore, it can be used in a variety of settings, for example, sports medicine or post-operative and post-stroke rehabilitation. A systematic review and meta-analysis of randomized control trials conducted by Zhao et al. [4] revealed that combined MI training and physical therapy is more beneficial for improving the lower limb motor function, gait function (i.e., gait speed, stride length, and cadence), and activities of daily living (ADL) compared to physical therapy alone in post-stroke patients with lower limb motor dysfunction. Similarly, a systematic review and meta-analysis conducted by Li et al. [5] revealed that MI training is effective for improving range of motion, muscle strength, and independence in ADL and to reduce pain in post-operative patients who underwent total knee arthroplasty. In addition, research has demonstrated the effectiveness of MI both on muscle strength for young and old healthy adults [6] and upper limb motor function in post-stroke patients [7]. The number of systematic reviews and meta-analyses on

MI training has grown in the past years. While the clinical use of MI is expected to increase in the future, the evidence of its effects and knowledge about the underlying neurophysiological mechanisms are not yet sufficient. In this chapter, we provide an overview of our previous studies and we discuss MI training in evidence-based physical therapy, with a special focus on benefits related to spinal neural function.

2. Central and spinal neural excitability during MI

Various neurophysiological studies using positron emission tomography, functional magnetic resonance imaging, and near-infrared spectroscopy have revealed mechanisms underlying the effects of MI on the central nervous system. Specifically, research has shown that MI-induced activity in the primary motor cortex (M1), supplementary motor area (SMA), premotor area (PM), prefrontal cortex (PFC), parietal cortex, and subcortical areas such as the basal ganglia and cerebellum [8]. The SMA, PM, basal ganglia, and cerebellum, are key structures in motor control, particularly the planning and preparation stages [9, 10]. Furthermore, these areas are activated during both MI and motor execution (ME). Although numerous previous studies have provided evidence that MI and ME share many common neural networks [8, 11], the activity of M1 during MI is controversial. Some studies found a significant increase in the activity of M1 during MI [12–16] whereas others did not [10, 17–19]. On the other hand, by evaluating the corticospinal excitability using transcranial magnetic stimulation (TMS) with high temporal resolution, a significantly increased amplitude of motor evoked potentials (MEPs) was observed during MI compared with the rest condition, suggesting elevated corticospinal excitability [20–24]. These results indicated that MI can increase corticospinal excitability. However, corticospinal excitability is lower during MI compared to ME [22]. Similarly, the observed M1 activity has been reported to be lower during MI compared to ME (i.e., less than a half) [13]. Although many motor-related brain areas are activated during MI, the role of M1 in MI is still unclear.

In addition, research suggests that it is important to assess spinal neural function during MI. Lower motor neurons of the spinal cord, namely α motor neurons, directly command muscle contraction. Descending pathways comprising upper motor neurons in the motor cortex or brainstem centers such as the reticular formation modulate the spatial and temporal patterns of activation of α motor neurons. Therefore, α motor neurons are the final common pathway for integrating various excitatory and inhibitory commands from upper motor neurons and for transmitting the information to the skeletal muscles [25]. To effectively improve motor function, it is necessary to facilitate both the central nervous system and spinal neural function. Indeed, a significant reduction of corticospinal excitability including spinal motor neurons was observed in post-stroke patients [26–28]. Also, the function of the corticospinal pathway is associated with the acquisition of dexterous motor skills [29, 30]. Therefore, assessing the excitability of spinal motor neurons during MI could help toward a better understanding of the neurophysiological aspects underlying the beneficial effects of MI.

3. Assessing the spinal neural function

The F-wave, H-reflex, and T-reflex are typically used to assess the spinal neural function. In our laboratory, we mainly used the F-wave to assess the excitability of spinal motor neurons during MI under various conditions. The F-wave is defined as compound action potential resulting from the re-excitation ("backfiring") of spinal anterior horn cells by an antidromic impulse following distal electrical stimulation of α motor neurons [31–33]. When electrical stimulation is applied to α motor neurons, compound muscle action potentials orthodromically propagate through α motor neurons and can be recorded from the corresponding muscles (M-wave). In addition to α motor neurons, the H-reflex and T-reflex involve the Ia fiber or muscle spindle in their reflex pathway, but the reflex pathway involved in the F-wave generation consists only of α motor neurons. Therefore, the F-wave can be suitable to assess the spinal motor neurons excitability. The main indexes used to estimate the excitability of spinal motor neurons are *persistence* and *the F-wave/M-wave (F/M) amplitude ratio*. Specifically, persistence (%) is computed as the number of F-wave responses detected divided by the number of electrical stimuli delivered and it reflects the number of backfiring spinal motor neurons [32, 33]. The F/M amplitude ratio (%) is computed as the mean amplitude of the F-wave responses detected divided by the maximum value of M-wave amplitude observed. The F/M amplitude ratio reflects the number, size, and synchronization of backfiring spinal motor neurons [32, 34].

4. Excitability of spinal motor neurons during MI

4.1 Background

The observed effects of MI on the excitability of spinal motor neurons are inconsistent across studies. For example, research has shown that the excitability of spinal motor neurons was significantly decreased after 3 hours intentional relaxation and that it recovered quickly after ME. In addition, when sustained intentional relaxation and MI of thumb abduction were performed simultaneously, the excitability of spinal motor neurons was maintained at pre-relaxation levels [35]. Also, excitability increased during MI of isometric ankle plantar flexion movement [36, 37]. These results indicate that MI may enhance the excitability of spinal motor neurons. However, studies have shown that MI of thumb abduction [21, 38, 39] or palmar flexion [20, 40] did not alter the excitability of spinal motor neurons. Another study on speed skaters performing MI in a competition showed varying responses in participants as both increased and decreased excitability was observed in different participants compared to that at rest [41].

In the following section, we will introduce previous research from our laboratory regarding the excitability of spinal motor neurons during MI under various conditions. The protocols were approved by the Research Ethics Committee at Kansai University of Health Sciences and conducted in accordance with the Declaration of Helsinki. In addition, written informed consent was obtained from all subjects prior to participation.

4.2 Influence of sensory inputs on the excitability of spinal motor neurons during MI

The influence of sensory inputs on the excitability of spinal motor neurons during MI was investigated in a sample of 11 healthy volunteers (8 males, 3 females; mean age, 34.0 years) [42]. Subjects were in a supine position on a bed and were asked to fix their eyes on the display of the pinch meter (Digital Indicator F340A; Unipulse Corp.,

Tokyo Japan). The F-wave was recorded using a Viking Quest electromyography machine ver. 9.0 (Natus Medical Inc., Pleasanton, CA, USA). A pair of silver EEG cup electrodes (10 mm diameter; Natus Medical Inc., Pleasanton, CA, USA) were placed over the thenar muscles and the base of the first dorsal metacarpal bone. The skin was cleaned with an abrasive gel (Neprep® Skin Prep Gel; Weaver and Company, Inc., Aurora, CO, USA). The F-wave was evoked from the left thenar muscles by delivering supramaximal electrical stimulation to the left median nerve at the wrist. Supramaximal stimulus intensity was set at a level 20% higher than the maximal stimulus intensity that could elicit the largest M-wave amplitude.

The baseline excitability of spinal motor neurons was determined by recording the F-wave during 1 minute of relaxation. Then, the holding trial was performed. Specifically, the F-wave was recorded while the participant was holding the pinch meter sensor between the left thumb and index finger. Following the holding trial, participants were instructed to press the pinch meter sensor between the left thumb and index finger with maximal effort for 5 s. Then, for the motor task, subjects were instructed to exert pinch force at their target pinch force [i.e., the pinch force at 50% maximal voluntary contraction (MVC)] for 10 s with visual feedback. In addition, subjects learned isometric left thenar muscle contraction at 50%MVC by performing the motor task for 1 minute. In the MI with sensor trial, subjects performed MI of the isometric left thenar muscle contraction while holding the pinch meter sensor for 1 minute, whereas in the MI without sensor trial, subjects performed the MI without holding the sensor for 1 minute. The F-wave was recorded during MI in both conditions.

Thirty F-waves were recorded in each trial. For the F-wave analysis, the amplifier gain for the M-wave was set at 5 mV per division, 200 μV per division for the F-wave, and a sweep of 5 ms per division. The bandwidth filter ranged from 20 to 3 Hz. The minimum peak-to-peak amplitude of the F-wave was 20 μV [43]. Persistence and F/M amplitude ratio were estimated from the recordings. In addition, we calculated the relative data obtained by dividing persistence and the F/M amplitude ratio during two MI trials with those obtained at rest.

With regard to the MI with sensor condition, the values of persistence during the holding and MI trials were significantly higher than the values obtained at the baseline. The F/M amplitude ratio during the MI trial was significantly higher than that obtained at the baseline. Regarding the MI without sensor condition, the values of persistence observed during the holding and MI trials were significantly higher than that obtained at the baseline. The F/M amplitude ratio during the holding and MI trials was slightly higher than that obtained at the baseline, but the observed differences were not significant. The relative data for persistence and F/M amplitude ratio during MI with the sensor condition were higher than those obtained during MI without the sensor condition.

Overall, the observed changes of F-wave during MI suggest that MI could increase the excitability of spinal motor neurons. In addition, somatosensory inputs, including tactile and proprioceptive, can help increase the effect of MI on the excitability of spinal motor neurons. However, substantial inter-individual variability in excitability was observed and future studies are needed to further elucidate these mechanisms.

4.3 Influence of imagined muscle contraction strength on the excitability of spinal motor neurons during MI

Our first study using MI of isometric thenar muscle activity at 50%MVC showed that MI can enhance the excitability of spinal motor neurons, as measured by the

F-wave. In ME, the excitability increased linearly with the strength of muscle contraction [44]. To test the hypothesis that MI and ME share common neural networks and, thus, that the excitability of spinal motor neurons should increase with the imagined muscle contraction strength, we performed an experiment of MI of isometric thenar muscle activity at varying %MVC level (i.e., 10, 30, 50, and 70%MVC) [45].

Ten healthy volunteers (5 males, 5 females; mean age, 28.7 years) participated in the study. Subjects were in a supine position on a bed and were asked to fix their eyes on the display of the pinch meter (Digital Indicator F340A; Unipulse Corp., Tokyo Japan) throughout the experiment. The recording condition for the F-wave was the same as in [42]. The F-wave recordings were conducted under three trials termed rest, MI, and post. In the rest trial, subjects kept relaxation for 1 minute. Before the MI trial, subjects learned the isometric left thenar muscle contraction while exerting the pinch force at 10%MVC for 1 minute. In the MI trial, subjects were instructed to imagine the isometric left thenar muscle contraction at 10%MVC for 1 minute. After the MI trial, subjects kept relaxed without performing MI for 1 minute again. The above process was defined as the 10% MI condition. This process was also performed under three other conditions (i.e., the 30, 50, and 70% MI conditions, respectively). The four MI conditions were randomized and performed on different days.

Persistence F/M amplitude ratios under the four MI conditions were significantly higher than those at the rest trial. Both persistence and F/M amplitude ratio in the post-trial under the four MI conditions were similar to those observed at rest.

Also, **Figure 1** shows the relative values of persistence and the F/M amplitude ratio measured in the four MI conditions. Results showed that the relative data for persistence and the F/M amplitude ratio were similar among the four MI conditions.

Overall, these results suggested that MI of isometric thenar muscle contraction under various imagined strengths could enhance the excitability of spinal motor neurons and that the imagined strength did not seem to influence the observed effect. Thus, it may be sufficient to perform MI at mild (e.g., 10%MVC) imagined muscle contraction strength to enhance the spinal motor neuron excitability. However, similar to our previous research [42], there was a lot of variability in the excitability of spinal motor neurons during MI and further research is needed.

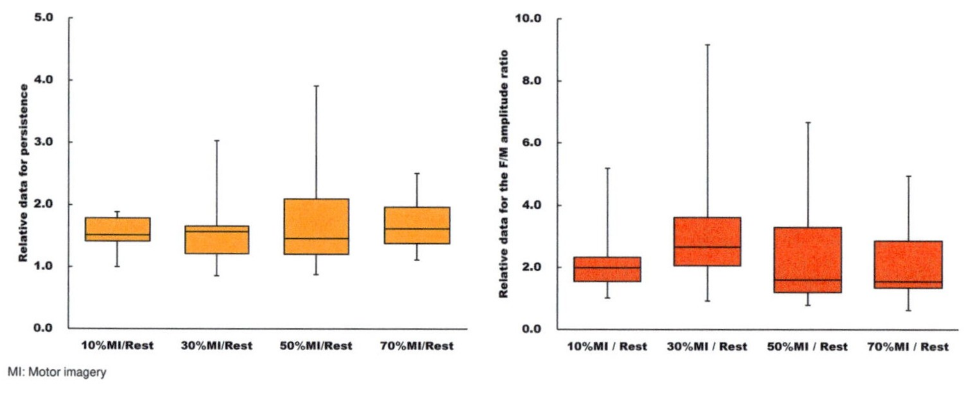

Figure 1.
Relative data for persistence and F/M amplitude ratio under the four MI conditions. There were no differences in relative data for persistence and F/M amplitude ratio among the four MI conditions. (adapted from reference [45]).

4.4 Influence of sensory modality on the excitability of spinal motor neurons during MI

Our previous research [42, 45] revealed that MI of isometric thumb opposition movement enhanced the excitability of spinal motor neurons. However, substantial inter-individual variability was observed. It is hypothesized that this variability could be, at least in part, related to different sensory modalities experienced by the tested subjects.

Sensory experience during MI can be classified into two modalities, specifically kinesthetic and visual. Kinesthetic imagery (KI) is defined as a subject imagining muscle contraction corresponding to actual movements. On the other hand, visual imagery (VI) is defined as a subject imagining movements performed by himself/herself (i.e., internal VI) or performed by another person (i.e., external VI). Previous research has shown that KI can activate motor-related brain regions to a larger extent than VI [46]. In addition, a significantly higher MEPs amplitude (i.e., higher corticospinal excitability) was observed during KI compared to VI [22, 23]. Therefore, we hypothesized that the sensory modality experienced during MI may affect the excitability of spinal motor neurons.

We administered a survey to 85 subjects to investigate the sensory modalities used while performing MI [47]. Results showed that three types of sensory modality were used during MI: kinesthetic, tactile/pressure, and visual, used either alone or combined. In Ref. [48], we investigated the possible influence of the sensory modality of MI on the excitability of spinal motor neurons by using kinesthetic and somatosensory perception.

Fourteen healthy volunteers (10 males, 4 females; mean age, 23.4 years) participated in the study. Subjects were in a supine position on a bed and were asked to fix their eyes on the display of the pinch meter (Digital Indicator F340A; Unipulse Corp., Tokyo Japan) during the experiment. The recording settings for the F-wave were the same as in the above described study and are reported in [42, 45]. The baseline of the excitability was determined in a rest trial by recording the F-wave during relaxation for 1 minute. Next, subjects were instructed to exert isometric left thenar muscle contraction at 50%MVC for 1 minute with visual feedback. Subjects were trained with two sensory modalities: kinesthetic (i.e., thenar muscle contraction while exerting the pinch force at 50%MVC) and somatosensory (i.e., tactile and pressure perception of thumb finger pulp while pressing the pinch meter sensor). Following training, subjects performed a randomized sequence of KI, somatosensory imagery (SI), and combined kinesthetic and somatosensory imagery (SKI), which consisted of imagining kinesthetic and somatosensory perception simultaneously. The F-waves were recorded for 1 minute in each trial. Following the MI trials, subjects were asked how vivid could they imagine the three imagery tasks on a five-point Likert scale ranging from 1 (very hard to image vividly) to 5 (very easy to image vividly).

Persistence and the F/M amplitude ratio were analyzed, as in the above-mentioned studies [42, 45]. Results are summarized in **Figure 2**. Persistence during KI and SI was significantly higher compared to the baseline. The F/M amplitude ratio during KI was significantly higher than that at rest. Both persistence and the F/M amplitude ratio during SKI were higher than that at rest, but the observed differences were not significant. The index of the imagery vividness, as measured using a five-point Likert scale, was significantly lower in the SKI trial than in the KI and SI trials.

Overall, the results of this study indicated that kinesthetic perception may be a more effective sensory modality to enhance the excitability of spinal motor neurons during MI

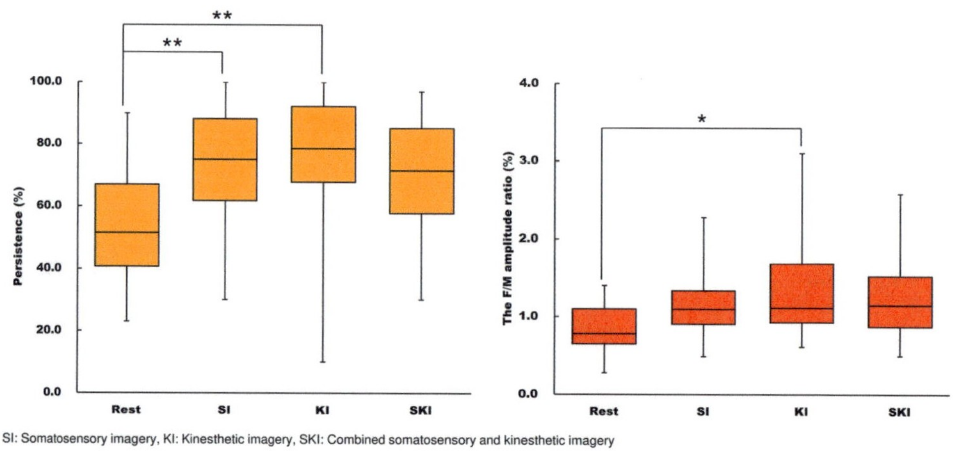

Figure 2.
*Persistence and F/M amplitude ratio during SI, KI, and SKI trials. Persistence was significantly increased during SI and KI compared to rest (**p < 0.01). The F/M amplitude ratio was significantly increased during KI compared to rest (*p < 0.05). (adapted from reference [48]).*

compared to the other sensory modalities investigated. The excitability of spinal motor neurons during SKI was similar to the baseline. This may be, at least in part, related to the relatively low imagery vividness score in the SKI trials, possibly suggesting that subjects could not imagine kinesthetic and somatosensory perceptions simultaneously.

4.5 Influence of combined action observation and MI on the excitability of spinal motor neurons

Previous research [42, 45] has shown inter-individual differences in the spinal motor neurons excitability during MI, which may be influenced by sensory modality during MI or by imagery vividness [48].

Recently, action observation (AO) has received much attention in the fields of sports and neurorehabilitation. AO shares neural substrates with MI and ME, including the PM, parietal cortex, and somatosensory cortices [49]. Numerous TMS studies showed a significant increase in corticospinal excitability during AO [50–53]. In addition, greater enhancement of brain excitability [54] and corticospinal excitability [55–57] were observed during combined AO and MI. AO has also been reported to enable more vivid MI [58]. The study outlined below aimed to investigate whether combined AO and MI can enhance the excitability of spinal motor neurons to a larger extent than AO alone [59].

Thirty-one healthy volunteers (23 males and 8 females; mean age, 23.5 years) participated in this study. Subjects were sitting comfortably in a chair with their left forearm resting on the armrest during the experiment. The left forearm was fully supinated, and the hand was kept open and relaxed with the palm facing upward. Prior to F-wave recording, cyclic left thumb opposition movements at 1 Hz were video-recorded using an iPad (Apple, Inc., Cupertino, CA, USA) for 1 minute. Then, F-wave recordings were performed for three trials, specifically: rest, AO, and combined AO and MI (AO + MI). In the rest trial, the F-wave was recorded during relaxation for 1 minute to determine the baseline. In the AO trial, subjects viewed the video of their own cyclic left thumb opposition movements. To ensure subjects recognized the video as if it was their thumb moving to realize the AO modality, the

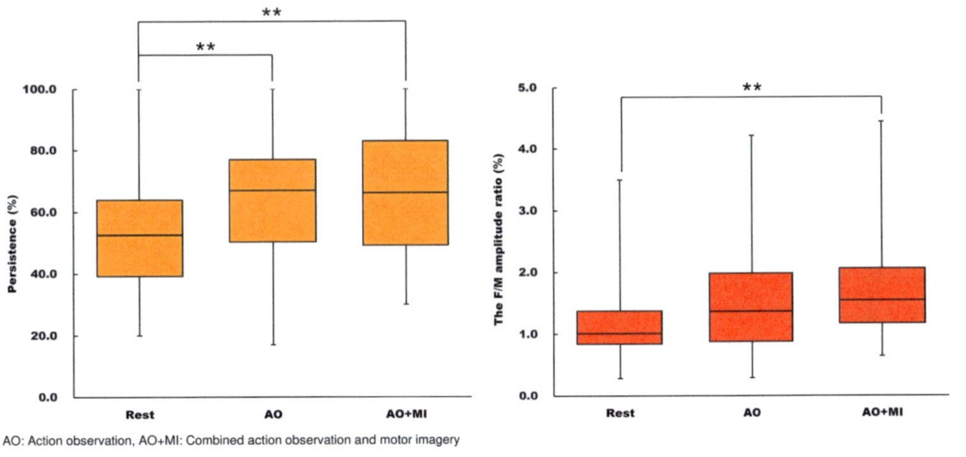

Figure 3.
*Persistence and F/M amplitude ratio during AO and AO + MI trials. Persistence was significantly increased during AO and AO + MI trials compared to rest (**p < 0.01). The F/M amplitude ratio was significantly increased during AO + MI compared to rest (**p < 0.01). (adapted from reference [59]).*

size and position of the hand displayed on the video were adjusted to the size and position of the left hand of the tested subject. For the AO + MI trial, subjects were asked to imagine the left thenar muscle activity while viewing left thumb opposition movements displayed on the iPad for 1 minute. To counterbalance the order effect, 15 subjects performed the tasks in the following order: rest, AO, and AO + MI, whereas the others performed the task in the following order: rest, AO + MI, and AO.

Results are summarized in **Figure 3**. Persistence during AO and during AO + MI was significantly higher than that at rest. The F/M amplitude ratio during AO + MI was significantly higher than that at rest. Overall, these results indicated that AO + MI may facilitate the spinal motor neurons excitability.

5. Immediate effect of MI on muscle strength

In addition to the study of the spinal motor neurons excitability during MI under various imagery conditions outlined in the above sections, we performed a study on the effects of MI on muscle strength [60].

The first study on the effect of MI on muscle strength by Yue & Cole [61] demonstrated a 22% increase in muscle strength following MI training of little finger abduction at MVC for 4 weeks. Similarly, Sidaway et al. [62] demonstrated a 17% increase in muscle strength of ankle dorsiflexion following MI training of ankle dorsiflexion at MVC for 4 weeks. In addition, MI training for 1 week showed a 10% increase in muscle strength of ankle plantar flexion [63]. Overall, these findings suggest that MI training can increase muscle strength in the upper and lower limbs.

It is well known that physical performance improves immediately after MI, and muscle strength may be involved in this process. However, there were no studies demonstrating the immediate effect of MI on muscle strength. In addition, while previous studies [61–64] adopted MI at MVC for MI training, no study investigated the effect of MI at submaximal muscle contraction strength on muscle strength. The study summarized in the following aims to investigate the immediate effect of MI at 50% MVC on muscle strength.

Thirty-six healthy volunteers (20 males, 16 females; mean age, 21.8 years) with no history of orthopedic and neurological disease participated in this study. Subjects were randomly divided into two groups using stratification (i.e., 10 males and 8 females were assigned to each group): MI group (mean age, 22.1 years; mean body weight, 56.7 kg); and control group (mean age, 21.6 years, mean body weight, 59.2 kg). There was no statistical difference in age and body weight between the two groups. The dominant leg of all subjects was the right one. The maximal ankle plantar torque was recorded using a Biodex System 3 dynamometer. Subjects were seated in the adjustable chair of the dynamometer. The right ankle joint was kept in neutral position, and the axis of the dynamometer was aligned with the rotation axis of ankle dorsiflexion/plantar flexion. After warm-up, subjects performed 5 s isometric ankle plantar flexion movement with maximal effort for three times as a pre-intervention trial. Next, all subjects were trained on the isometric right ankle plantar flexion movement at 50%MVC using visual feedback for 1 minute. After training, subjects in the MI group performed MI of isometric right ankle plantar flexion at 50%MVC for 1 minute, whereas subjects in the control group kept relaxed for 1 minute without performing MI. In the post-intervention trial, subjects performed 5 s isometric ankle plantar flexion movement with maximal effort for three times.

Maximal ankle plantar flexion torque (Nm) was determined as the average value of peak ankle plantar flexion torque in the three repeated flexion movements. The maximal ankle plantar flexion torque was normalized to body weight and expressed as Nm/kg. Relative indexes were computed by dividing the normalized maximal ankle plantar flexion torque measured in the post-intervention trial to that obtained in the pre-intervention trial.

In the MI group, the normalized maximal ankle plantar flexion torque at the post-intervention trial was significantly higher than that measured in the pre-intervention trial. In the control group, no significant difference in normalized maximal ankle plantar flexion torque between the pre- and post-intervention trials was observed. The relative index for normalized maximal ankle plantar flexion torque computed in the MI group was significantly higher than that computed in the control group (**Figure 4**).

These results indicated that MI of isometric ankle plantar flexion at 50%MVC could increase maximal ankle plantar torque immediately after MI. However, this

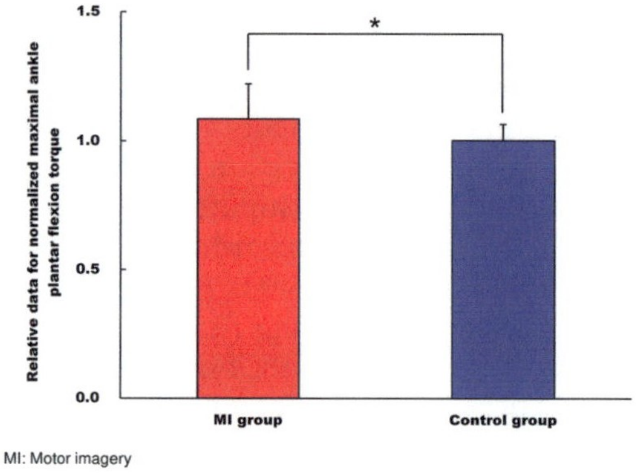

Figure 4.
Relative data for normalized maximal ankle plantar flexion torque during MI and control groups. Relative data for normalized maximal ankle plantar flexion torque in the MI group was significantly higher than that in the control group ($p < 0.05$*). (adapted from reference [60]).*

study did not investigate different imagined muscle contraction strengths, and the effects of MI on muscle strength as a function of the imagined muscle contraction strength need to be investigated in more detail.

6. Application of MI in clinical settings

Our previous findings [42, 45, 48] indicated that MI enhances the excitability of spinal motor neurons and that a mild (e.g., 10%MVC) imagined muscle contraction strength may be sufficient for MI training. However, research also suggested that sensory modality and vividness of MI may influence the excitability of spinal motor neurons during MI.

Different techniques can be introduced to make MI more effective. The first method to enhance the effect of MI is providing sensory inputs, including tactile and proprioceptive perception while performing MI. As discussed above, the excitability of spinal motor neurons during MI while holding the pinch meter sensor was significantly higher than that observed during MI while not holding the sensor [42]. Similarly, Mizuguchi et al. [65] demonstrated that the corticospinal excitability during MI of squeezing a ball while touching the ball was higher than that observed during MI while not touching the ball. Noticeably, no increase in corticospinal excitability was observed while touching the ball with no MI. Accordingly, it is important to perform MI training with the position of the upper or lower extremities close to the actual movements. Secondly, combined AO and MI can be effective. Although, the excitability of spinal motor neurons was increased during AO alone, combined AO and MI increased the excitability to a larger extent than AO alone [59]. These methods may activate motor-related neural function more effectively due to synergistic effects of "MI and sensory inputs" or "MI and AO", and may allow individuals to imagine the movements vividly.

In addition, duration of MI should be considered for MI training. We investigated time-dependent change in the excitability of spinal motor neurons during MI for 5 minutes using the F-wave, and we observed that the excitability of spinal motor neurons at 1-minute and 3-minutes after MI initiation was significantly higher than the baseline, returning to the baseline level after 5 minutes. In addition, subjects could not perform MI vividly for 5 minutes after MI initiation [66]. Mental fatigue caused by repetitive MI of the hand grip movement decreased the corticospinal excitability [67]. These findings indicate that the benefit of MI on the excitability of spinal motor neurons is not necessarily a function of the length of MI. In general, the optimal duration or number of sessions for MI training has not been determined yet, and a detailed investigation is required. In clinical settings, condition of MI training, including sensory inputs, intensity, sensory modalities, the use of AO, and duration, should be set according to the purpose of rehabilitation and individual MI ability.

Finally, the maximal isometric ankle plantar flexion torque was significantly increased immediately after MI at 50%MVC for 1 minute, suggesting that MI at 50%MVC may be beneficial in rehabilitation to improve muscle strength. When utilizing MI in rehabilitation, it is necessary to learn the desired movements in advance, but this may be difficult for specific patients, for example, patients with heart failure who are not able to perform exercise at high intensity. Therefore, MI at 50%MVC may be able to increase the excitability of spinal motor neurons and muscle strength with relatively less physical load than MI at MVC.

7. Conclusion

In this chapter, we presented the influence of MI under various conditions on the excitability of spinal motor neurons and the immediate effect of MI on muscle strength. The F-wave data reported here may provide evidence for elucidating the neurophysiological mechanisms underlying the observed MI effects. Further research is needed to investigate optimal settings for MI in physical therapy and support future, effective application of this technique in clinical settings.

Conflict of interest

The authors declare no conflict of interest.

Author details

Yoshibumi Bunno[1,2]*, Chieko Onigata[2] and Toshiaki Suzuki[1,2]

1 Graduate School of Health Sciences, Graduate School of Kansai University of Health Sciences, Osaka, Japan

2 Faculty of Health Sciences, Clinical Physical Therapy Laboratory, Kansai University of Health Sciences, Osaka, Japan

*Address all correspondence to: bunno@kansai.ac.jp

References

[1] Farah MJ. The neural basis of mental imagery. Trends in Neurosciences. 1989;**12**:395-399. DOI: 10.1016/0166-2236(89)90079-9

[2] Jeannerod M. The representing brain: Neural correlates of motor intention and imagery. The Behavioral and Brain Sciences. 1994;**17**:187-202. DOI: 10.1017/S0140525X00034026

[3] Guillot A, Di Rienzo F, Maclntyre T, Moran A, Collet C. Imagining is not doing but involves specific motor commands: A review of experimental data related to motor inhibition. Frontiers in Human Neuroscience. 2012;**6**:247. DOI: 10.3389/fnhum.2012.00247

[4] Zhao LJ, Jiang LH, Zhang H, Li Y, Sun P, Liu Y, et al. Effects of motor imagery training for lower limb dysfunction in patients with stroke. American Journal of Physical Medicine & Rehabilitation. 2023;**102**:409-418. DOI: 10.1097/FPHM.0000000000002107

[5] Li R, Du J, Yang K, Wang X, Wang W. Effectiveness of motor imagery for improving functional performance after total knee arthroplasty: A systematic review with meta-analysis. Journal of Orthopaedic Surgery and Research. 2022;**17**:65. DOI: 10.1186/s13018-022-02946-4

[6] Liu X, Ge S, Cordova A, Yaghi Z, Jiang BY, Yue GH, et al. Elderly may benefit more from motor imagery training in gaining muscle strength than young adults: A systematic review and meta-analysis. Frontiers in Psychology. 2023;**13**:1052826. DOI: 10.3389/fpsyg.2022.1052826

[7] Villa-Berges E, Laborda Soriano AA, Lucha-López O, Tricas-Moreno JM, Hernández-Secorún M, Gómez-Martínez M, et al. Motor imagery and mental practice in the subacute and chronic phases in upper limb rehabilitation after stroke: A systematic review. Occupational Therapy International. 2023;**2023**:3752889. DOI: 10.1155/2023/3752889

[8] Hanakawa T. Organizing motor imageries. Neuroscience Research. 2016;**104**:56-63. DOI: 10.1016/j.neures.2015.11.003

[9] Lotze M, Halsband U. Motor imagery. Journal of Physiology, Paris. 2006;**99**:386-395. DOI: 10.1016/j.jphysparis.2006.03.012

[10] Hanakawa T, Dimyan MA, Hallett M. Motor planning, imagery, and execution in the distributed motor network: A time-course study with functional MRI. Cerebral Cortex. 2008;**18**:2775-2788. DOI: 10.1093/cercor/bhn036

[11] Mizuguchi N, Nakata H, Uchida Y, Kanosue K. Motor imagery and sport performance. The Journal of Sports Medicine. 2012;**1**:103-111. DOI: 10.7600/jpfsm.1.103

[12] Lotze M, Montoya P, Erb M, Hülsmann E, Flor H, Klose U, et al. Activation of cortical and cerebellar motor areas during executed and imagined hand movements: An fMRI study. Journal of Cognitive Neuroscience. 1999;**11**:491-501. DOI: 10.1162/089892999563553

[13] Porro CA, Francescato MP, Cettolo V, Diamond ME, Baraldi P, Zuiani C, et al. Primary motor and sensory cortex activation during motor performance and motor imagery: A functional magnetic resonance imaging study.

The Journal of Neuroscience. 1996;**16**:7688-7698. DOI: 10.1523/JNEUROSCI.16-23-07688.1996

[14] Ehrsson HH, Geyer S, Naito E. Imagery of voluntary movement of fingers, toes, and tongue activates corresponding body-part-specific motor representations. Journal of Neurophysiology. 2003;**90**:3304-3316. DOI: 10.1152/jn.01113.2002

[15] Kuhtz-Buschbeck JP, Mahnkopf C, Holzknecht C, Siebner H, Ulmer S, Jansen O. Effector-independent representations of simple and complex imagined finger movements: A combined fMRI and TMS study. The European Journal of Neuroscience. 2003;**18**:3375-3387. DOI: 10.1111/j.1460-9568.2003.03066.x

[16] Solodkin A, Hlustik P, Chen EE, Small SL. Fine modulation in network activation during motor execution and motor imagery. Cerebral Cortex. 2004;**14**:1246-1255. DOI: 10.1093/cercor/bhh086

[17] Binkofski F, Amunts K, Stephan KM, Posse S, Schormann T, Freund HJ, et al. Broca's region subserves imagery of motion: A combined cytoarchitectonic and fMRI study. Human Brain Mapping. 2000;**11**:273-285. DOI: 10.1002/1097-0193(200012)11:4%3C273::aid-hbm40%3E3.0.co;2-0

[18] Hanakawa T, Immisch I, Toma K, Dimyan MA, Gelderen PV, Hallett M. Functional properties of brain areas associated with motor execution and imagery. Journal of Neurophysiology. 2003;**89**:989-1002. DOI: 10.1152/jn.00132.2002

[19] Hanakawa T, Parikh S, Bruno MK, Hallett M. Finger and face representations in the ipsilateral precentral motor areas in humans. Journal of Neurophysiology. 2005;**93**:2950-2958. DOI: 10.1152/jn.00784.2004

[20] Kasai T, Kawai S, Kawanishi M, Yahagi S. Evidence for facilitation of motor evoked potentials (MEPs) induced by motor imagery. Brain Research. 1997;**744**:147-150. DOI: 10.1016/S0006-8993(96)01101-8

[21] Stinear CM, Byblow WD. Motor imagery of phasic thumb abduction temporally and spatially modulates corticospinal excitability. Clinical Neurophysiology. 2003;**114**:909-914. DOI: 10.1016/s1388-2457(02)00373-5

[22] Stinear CM, Byblow WD. Modulation of corticospinal excitability and intracortical inhibition during motor imagery is task-dependent. Experimental Brain Research. 2004;**157**:351-358. DOI: 10.1007/s00221-004-1851-z

[23] Fourkas AD, Ionta S, Aglioti SM. Influence of imagined posture and imagery modality on corticospinal excitability. Behavioural Brain Research. 2006;**168**:190-196. DOI: 10.1016/j.bbr.2005.10.015

[24] Mizuguchi N, Umehara I, Nakata H, Kanosue K. Modulation of corticospinal excitability dependent upon imagined force level. Experimental Brain Research. 2013;**230**:243-249. DOI: 10.1007/s00221-013-3649-3

[25] Lemon RN. Descending pathways in motor control. Annual Review of Neuroscience. 2008;**31**:195-218. DOI: 10.1146/annurev.neuro.31.060407.125547

[26] Foltys H, Krings T, Meister IG, Sparing R, Boroojerdi B, Thron A, et al. Motor representation in patients rapidly recovering after stroke: A functional magnetic resonance imaging

and transcranial magnetic stimulation study. Clinical Neurophysiology. 2003;**114**:2404-2015. DOI: 10.1016/S1388-2457(03)00263-3

[27] Fierro B, Raimondo D, Modica A. Analysis of F response in upper motoneurone lesions. Acta Neurologica Scandinavica. 1990;**82**:329-334. DOI: 10.1111/j.1600-0404.1990.tb03311.x

[28] Drory VE, Neufeld MY, Korczyn AD. F-wave characteristics following acute and chronic upper motor neuron lesions. Electromyography and Clinical Neurophysiology. 1993;**33**:441-446

[29] Heffner RS, Masterton RB. The role of the corticospinal tract in the evolution of human digital dexterity. Brain, Behavior and Evolution. 1983;**23**:165-183. DOI: 10.1159/000121494

[30] Lemon RN, Griffiths J. Comparing the function of the corticospinal system in different species: Organization differences for motor specialization? Muscle & Nerve. 2005;**32**:261-279. DOI: 10.1002/mus.20333

[31] Kimura J. F-wave velocity in the central segment of the median and ulnar nerves. A study in normal subjects and in patients with Charcot-Marie-tooth disease. Neurology. 1974;**24**:539-546. DOI: 10.1212/WNL.24.6.539

[32] Mesrati F, Vecchierini MF. F-waves neurophysiology and clinical value. Neurophysiologie Clinique. 2004;**34**:217-243. DOI: 10.1016/j.neucli.2004.09.005

[33] Fisher MA. F-waves-physiology and clinical uses. The Scientific World Journal. 2007;7:144-160. DOI: 10.1100/tsw.2007.49

[34] Peioglou-Harmoussi S, Fawcett PR, Howel D, Barwick DD. F-responses: A study of frequency, shape and amplitude characteristics in healthy control subjects. Journal of Neurology, Neurosurgery, and Psychiatry. 1985;**48**:1159-1164. DOI: 10.1136/jnnp.48.11.1159

[35] Taniguchi S, Kimura J, Yamada T, Ichikawa H, Hara M, Fujisawa R, et al. Effect of motion imagery to counter rest-induced suppression of F-wave as a measure of anterior horn cell excitability. Clinical Neurophysiology. 2008;**119**:1346-1352. DOI: 10.1016/j.clinph.2007.11.179

[36] Bonnet M, Decety J, Jeannerod M, Requina J. Mental simulation of an action modulates the excitability of spinal reflex pathways in man. Cognitive Brain Research. 1997;**5**:221-228. DOI: 10.1016/S0926-6410(96)00072-9

[37] Aoyama T, Kaneko F. The effect of motor imagery on gain modulation of the spinal reflex. Brain Research. 2011;**1372**:41-48. DOI: 10.1016/j.brainres.2010.11.023

[38] Facchini S, Muellbacher W, Battaglia F, Boroojerdi B, Hallett M. Focal enhancement of motor cortex excitability during motor imagery: A transcranial magnetic stimulation study. Acta Neurologica Scandinavica. 2002;**105**:146-151. DOI: 10.1034/j.1600-0404.2002.1o004.x

[39] Stinear CM, Byblow WD, Steyvers M, Levin O, Swinnen SP. Kinesthetic, but not visual, motor imagery modulates corticomotor excitability. Experimental Brain Research. 2006;**168**:157-164. DOI: 10.1007/s00221-005-0078-y

[40] Hashimoto R, Rothwell JC. Dynamic changes in corticospinal excitability during motor imagery. Experimental Brain Research. 1999;**125**:75-81. DOI: 10.1007/s002210050660

[41] Oishi K, Kimura M, Yasukawa M, Yoneda T, Maeshima T. Amplitude reduction of H-reflex during mental movement simulation in elite athletes. Behavioural Brain Research. 1994;**62**:55-61. DOI: 10.1016/0166-4328(94)90037-X

[42] Suzuki T, Bunno Y, Onigata C, Tani M, Uragami S. Excitability of spinal neural function during several motor imagery tasks involving isometric opponens pollicis activity. Neuro Rehabilitation. 2013;**33**:171-176. DOI: 10.3233/NRE-130942

[43] Fisher MA. H reflexes and F waves fundamentals, normal and abnormal patters. Neurologic Clinics of North America. 2002;**20**:339-360. DOI: 10.1016/s0733-8619(01)00004-4

[44] Suzuki T, Fujiwara T, Takeda I. Excitability of the spinal motor neuron pool and F-waves during isometric ipsilateral and contralateral contraction. Physiotherapy Theory and Practice. 1993;**9**:19-24. DOI: 10.3109/09593989309036482

[45] Bunno Y, Onigata C, Suzuki T. The imagined muscle contraction strengths did not affect the changes of spinal motor neurons excitability. The Journal of Novel Physiotherapies. 2016;**S3**:008. DOI: 10.4172/2165-7025.S3-008

[46] Guillot A, Collet C, Nguyen VA, Malouin F, Richards C, Doyon J. Brain activity during visual versus kinesthetic imagery: An fMRI study. Human Brain Mapping. 2009;**30**:2157-2172. DOI: 10.1002/hbm.20658

[47] Todo M, Bunno Y, Yoneda H, Suzuki T. Individual differences in methods of motor imagery. Rigakuryoho Kagaku. 2015;**30**:405-407. (In Japanese). DOI: 10.1589/rika.30.405

[48] Bunno Y. Imagery strategy affects spinal motor neuron excitability - using kinesthetic and somatosensory imagery. Neuroreport. 2019;**30**:463-467. DOI: 10.1097/WNR.0000000000001218

[49] Hardwick RM, Caspers S, Eickhoff SB, Swinnen SP. Neural correlates of action: Comparing meta-analyses of imagery, observation, and execution. Neuroscience and Biobehavioral Reviews. 2018;**94**:31-44. DOI: 10.1016/j.neubiorev.2018.08.003

[50] Fadiga L, Fogassi L, Pavesi G, Rizzolatti G. Motor facilitation during action observation: A magnetic stimulation study. Journal of Neurophysiology. 1995;**73**:2608-2611. DOI: 10.1152/jn.1995.73.6.2608

[51] Strafella AP, Paus T. Modulation of cortical excitability during action observation: A transcranial magnetic stimulation study. Neuroreport. 2000;**11**:2289-2292. DOI: 10.1097/00001756-200007140-00044

[52] Clark S, Tremblay F, Ste-Marie D. Differential modulation of corticospinal excitability during observation, mental imagery and imitation of hand actions. Neurophychologia. 2004;**42**:105-112. DOI: 10.1016/S0028-3932(03)00144-1

[53] Montagna M, Cerri G, Borroni P, Baldissera F. Excitability changes in human corticospinal projections to muscles moving hand and fingers while viewing a reaching and grasping action. The European Journal of Neuroscience. 2005;**22**:1513-1520. DOI: 10.1111/j.1460-9568.2005.04336.x

[54] Berends HI, Wolkorte R, Ijzerman MJ, Van Putten MJAM. Differential cortical activation during observation and observation-and-imagination. Experimental Brain Research. 2013;**229**:337-345. DOI: 10.1007/s00221-013-3571-8

[55] Sakamoto M, Muraoka T, Mizuguchi N, Kanosue K. Combining observation and imagery of an action enhances human corticospinal excitability. Neuroscience Research. 2009;**65**:23-27. DOI: 10.1016/j.neures.2009.05.003

[56] Nojima I, Koganemaru S, Kawamata T, Fukuyama H, Mima T. Action observation with kinesthetic illusion can produce human motor plasticity. The European Journal of Neuroscience. 2015;**41**:1614-1623. DOI: 10.1111/ejn.12921

[57] Wright DJ, Williams J, Holmes PS. Combined action observation and imagery facilitates corticospinal excitability. Frontiers in Human Neuroscience. 2014;**8**:951. DOI: 10.3389/fnhum.2014.00951

[58] Holmes P, Calmels C. A neuroscientific review of imagery and observation use in sport. Journal of Motor Behavior. 2008;**40**:433-445. DOI: 10.3200/JMBR.40.5.433-445

[59] Bunno Y, Suzuki T. Motor imagery while viewing self-finger movements facilitates the excitability of spinal motor neurons. Experimental Brain Research. 2020;**238**:2077-2086. DOI: 10.1007/s00221-020-05870-3

[60] Bunno Y, Kitagawa M, Tsujimura F, Nakatani Y, Nishiura M, Hamamoto H, et al. Motor imagery of ankle plantar flexion at 50% of maximal voluntary contraction increases the maximal torque of ankle plantar flexion. Japanese Journal of Clinical Neurophysiology. 2021;**49**:1-7. (In Japanese). DOI: 10.11422/jscn.49.1

[61] Yue GH, Cole KJ. Strength increases from the motor program: Comparison of training with maximal voluntary and imagined muscle contractions. Journal of Neurophysiology. 1992;**67**:1114-1123. DOI: 10.1152/jn.1992.67.5.1114

[62] Sidaway B, Trzaska AR. Can mental practice increase ankle dorsiflexor torque? Physical Therapy. 2005;**85**:1053-1060. DOI: 10.1093/ptj/85.10.1053

[63] Grosprêtre S, Jacquet T, Lebon F, Papaxanthis C, Martin A. Neural mechanisms of strength increase after one-week motor imagery training. European Journal of Sport Science. 2018;**18**:209-218. DOI: 10.1080/17461391.2017.1415377

[64] Ranganathan VK, Siemionow V, Liu JZ, Sahgal V, Yue GH. From mental power to muscle power-gaining strength by using the mind. Neuropsychologia. 2004;**42**:944-956. DOI: 10.1016/j.neuropsychologia.2003.11.018

[65] Mizuguchi N, Sakamoto M, Muraoka T, Kanosue K. Influence of touching an object on corticospinal excitability during motor imagery. Experimental Brain Research. 2009;**196**:529-535. DOI: 10.1007/s00221-009-1875-5

[66] Bunno Y. Does the duration of motor imagery affect the excitability of spinal anterior horn cells? Somatosensory & Motor Research. 2018;**35**:223-228. DOI: 10.1080/08990220.2018.1538963

[67] Kluger BM, Palmer C, Shattuck JT, Triggs WJ. Motor evoked potential depression following repetitive central motor initiation. Experimental Brain Research. 2012;**216**:585-590. DOI: 10.1007/s00221-011-2962-y

Chapter 8

Motor Imagery-Based Neurofeedback in Physiotherapy Practice

Shun Sawai, Shoya Fujikawa, Ryosuke Yamamoto and Hideki Nakano

Abstract

Neurofeedback (NFB) is a closed-loop technique in which the patient receives feedback on brain activity to encourage voluntary control of brain activity. NFB promotes neuroplasticity and changes the brain functionally and structurally. Motor imagery-based NFB (MI-NFB) can improve motor imagery ability by providing feedback on brain activity during motor imagery, thereby showing effectiveness in performance and motor learning. Furthermore, the effects of MI-NFB are further enhanced when it is combined with noninvasive brain stimulation and motor exercise. Therefore, MI-NFB is used in the physiotherapy of patients with neurological diseases, such as stroke and Parkinson disease, as well as children with attention deficit-hyperactivity disorder and elderly people. This chapter reviews MI-NFB in physiotherapy practice, thus contributing to the development of effective evidence-based physiotherapy.

Keywords: neurofeedback, motor imagery, neurorehabilitation, stroke, Parkinson disease, physiotherapy practice

1. Introduction

Neurofeedback (NFB) is a technique that promotes voluntary control of brain activity by providing feedback on brain activity to the participant [1]. Kamiya found that electroencephalography (EEG) can be used to notice changes in brain states [2] and that it can be controlled spontaneously by feeding back activity in the α-frequency band [3]. These research results were the first step to developing NFB, which has been widely used to treat psychiatric disorders [4], improve cognitive function [5], enhance motor performance [6], and so on. In NFB, brain activity is measured mainly by EEG [7], functional magnetic resonance imaging (fMRI) [8], and functional near-infrared spectroscopy [9], and feedback on the activity in the targeted brain regions is provided to the participant to facilitate self-regulation of the participant's brain activity. The methods used to provide feedback include visual feedback [10], in which brain activity is projected on a monitor, and auditory feedback [11], which uses sound stimuli of different frequencies. These methods are used to encourage participants to voluntarily adjust their brain activity.

Although many neural mechanisms underlying the effects of NFB are still unclear, several potential mechanisms have been proposed [12–14], one of which is the induction of neuroplasticity through NFB. In addition to changing motor performance and brain activity, NFB has also been shown to alter the structure of white matter [15]. For these reasons, neuroplasticity, which causes changes in brain structure, has been proposed to be a mechanism underlying the effects of NFB. The second potential mechanism involves changing the connectivity of the brain. The neural network associated with NFB can be divided into control, learning, and forward-processing networks [16]. The control network is composed of the frontoparietal control network, which consists of the dorsolateral frontal and posterior parietal cortices, with the participation of brain regions related to the processing of feedback stimuli, such as the lateral occipital cortex and thalamus. The dorsolateral frontal and posterior parietal cortices are associated with the execution of imagery and other processes [17] and may be important in the mental processes that control brain activity. The learning network consists of the dorsal striatum, which has been shown to be associated with motor control and learning based on procedural memory [18] and may be involved in learning to coordinate neural activity in NFB. Finally, the reward-processing network consists of the anterior insula, anterior cingulate cortex, and ventral striatum. The anterior insula [19] and anterior cingulate cortex [20] are associated with a conscious perception of reward, whereas the ventral striatum is associated with an unconscious perception of reward [21, 22]. The reward-processing network has been reported to be activated by the NFB [23], which is also known to regulate brain activity. Thus, the knowledge of results (KR) for regulating brain activity conferred by the NFB may be involved in the process of recognizing the accomplishment of the task, and these neural networks have been proposed to be related to NFB.

In addition to the NFB-related networks described above, NFB alters the connectivity of the language network and visual network, which are involved in internal reception [24]. NFB has also been reported to alter connectivity not only within the cerebrum but also between the primary motor cortex and the cerebellum [25], and NFB may produce its effects by altering connectivity between these brain regions. As described above, NFB has been suggested to cause functional and structural changes in the brain. This chapter reviews the NFB to motor imagery frequently used in physiotherapy practice.

2. Motor imagery-based neurofeedback

Recently, the effect of NFB on motor imagery has attracted much attention. This approach is called motor imagery-based NFB (MI-NFB). Motor imagery is a cognitive process of imagining what it is like to exercise without actual movement [26]. Motor imagery can be divided into myosensory first-person imagery and visual third-person imagery, and previous studies have reported individual differences in motor imagery ability [27, 28]. Motor imagery is known to improve performance [29] and has a motor-learning effect [30] even when the participant does not actually exercise. In addition, motor imagery has been supported from a neurological aspect, as there are areas where brain activity similar to that of actual exercise is observed [31], and resting EEG is altered by motor imagery [32]. On the basis of these background characteristics, motor imagery has been used in sports training for athletes [33] and in rehabilitation for stroke patients [34, 35]. However, one limitation of motor imagery is that the participant cannot understand the accuracy of the imagery because the actual movement does not occur [36]. NFB can be used to solve this problem. MI-NFB provides real-time feedback on brain activity during motor imagery to the participant and improves the accuracy of imagery by activating brain regions related to motor imagery [37]. In this section, the mechanism and effects of MI-NFB are explained on the basis of the results of studies conducted in healthy individuals.

MI-NFB has been reported to provide feedback on activity in the primary motor cortex (M1) [38, 39] and supplementary motor area (SMA) [40, 41] in many studies. These areas are activated by motor imagery and have been reported to be related to the accuracy of motor imagery [31]. The blood oxygen-level dependent (BOLD) signal in fMRI [40, 41] and the event-related desynchronization (ERD) of EEG β-rhythms [42] and μ-rhythms [43] are mainly used as feedback stimuli for MI-NFB. In this approach, the ERD reflects a decrease in the EEG signal caused by the occurrence of an event [44]. Control of these parameters related to motor imagery is then encouraged to improve the accuracy of motor imagery and motor performance (**Figure 1**).

MI-NFB has been proposed to facilitate motor learning by providing KR [45]. KR is one of the basic principles underlying motor learning, and if motor learning involves actual exercise, the results are automatically returned as feedback by behavioral indicators and sensory stimuli, and motor learning is based on this information [46]. In contrast, motor imagery does not provide feedback on KR such as behavioral indices and sensory stimuli because it is not accompanied by actual movement. In this context, MI-NFB provides brain activity as KR, and motor learning is facilitated based on this information.

MI-NFB has been shown to alter brain activity and improve motor imagery ability [37]. Hwang et al. tested the effects of MI-NFB with visual stimuli in healthy young individuals [47]. In their study, right- or left-hand movements were used as the imagery task, the μ activity in the sensorimotor area was displayed on a monitor, and the participants received visual feedback regarding brain activity. The findings showed

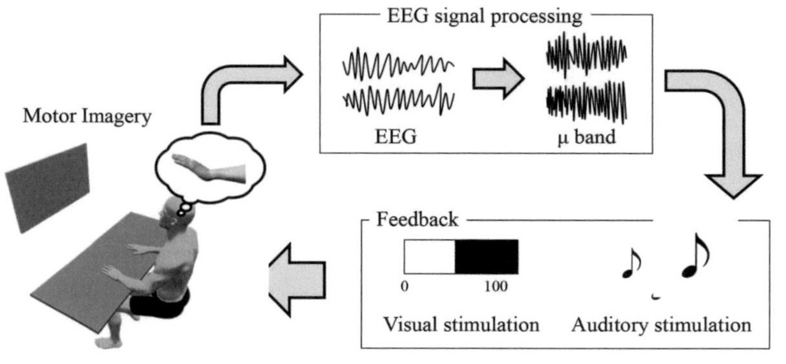

Figure 1.
MI-NFB system using EEG. EEG is measured during motor imagery, and μERD data are used to provide feedback to the patients, including visual feedback using bar graphs or auditory feedback using sound stimuli. This system promotes voluntary control of EEG during motor imagery.

that this system facilitated control of brain activity during motor imagery. Their results indicated that MI-NFB enabled the control of μ activity, potentially indicating an improvement in motor imagery ability. Additionally, Grigorev et al. examined the effects of MI-NFB with vibrotactile stimulation in healthy young individuals [48]. In their study, the imagery task consisted of right- or left-handed movements. Vibration actuators were attached to the bilateral forearms and behind the neck and set to vibrate when μ-rhythmic ERD occurred, providing vibrotactile brain activity feedback (**Figure 2**). Their results showed that MI-NFB produced significantly greater ERD for non-dominant hand motor imagery, but it had no significant difference for dominant hand motor imagery. Since non-dominant hand movements require higher brain activity than dominant hand movements [49], the present results may modulate the brain activity mobilized for these non-dominant hand movements. Although MI-NFB has been suggested to enable the control of brain activity and improve the accuracy of motor imagery, as shown in the above study [48], the effect of MI-NFB varies depending on the conditions. Moreover, the effects of MI-NFB are not consistent in relation to the participant's characteristics [50] and the difficulty of the task [51]. Therefore, improving the accuracy of MI-NFB and evaluating its responsiveness are future research topics.

In this section, the basic mechanisms and effects of MI-NFB are described on the basis of previous studies. MI-NFB provides the participant KR in motor imagery accuracy, encouraging the participant to control brain activity related to motor imagery. This process improves the accuracy of motor imagery. Therefore, MI-NFB may be effective in addressing participants' inability to understand whether their motor imagery is good or poor. However, the effectiveness of MI-NFB varies depending on the difficulty of the task and the participants' characteristics; hence, more accurate MI-NFB is required in the future.

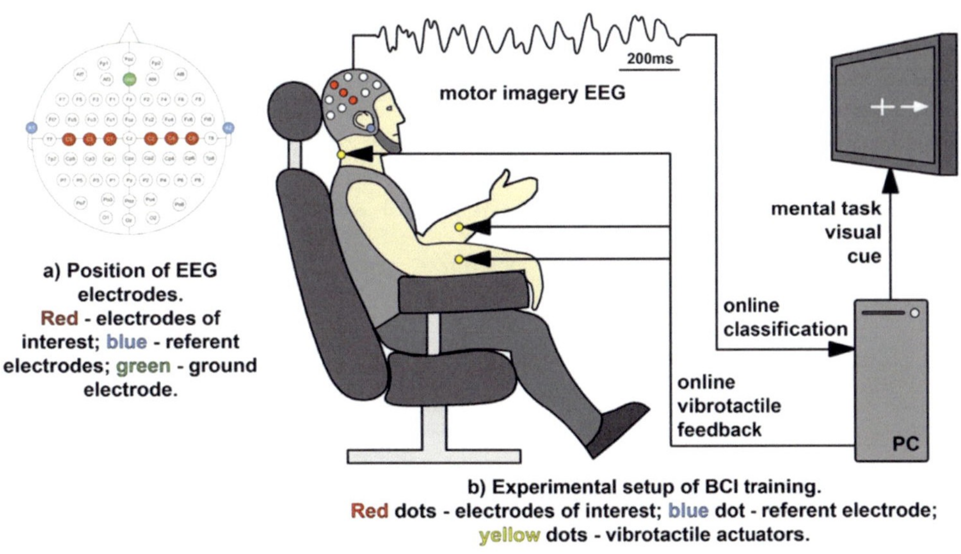

Figure 2.
Experimental setup of MI-NFB using vibrotactile stimulation [48]. EEG was measured during motor imagery, and brain activity was returned as feedback to the participant in real time through a vibration actuator. The participant then had to imagine the hand movement to generate more vibration.

3. Combination of neurofeedback with other techniques

With the evolving usage of stimulators in physiotherapy [52], it is becoming increasingly clear that MI-NFB should not be used alone; rather, it should be used in combination with some other interventions to further amplify its effects. This section describes the use of MI-NFB in combination with other techniques.

3.1 Combination of neurofeedback with transcranial stimulation

Recent studies have begun examining the efficacy of transcranial stimulation combined with MI-NFB. Transcranial stimulation is classified into transcranial direct current stimulation (tDCS), transcranial alternating current stimulation, and transcranial magnetic stimulation [53]. These stimuli are used to promote brain plasticity and alter cognitive and mental functions [54], and their effects have attracted much attention. The effects of transcranial stimulation on motor imagery have been validated, with tDCS [55, 56], transcranial alternating current stimulation [56, 57], and transcranial magnetic stimulation [58] all shown to improve the accuracy of motor imagery. However, the effects of combining transcranial stimulation with MI-NFB are largely unclear.

In a study examining the effects of tDCS on MI-NFB [59], participants were divided into NFB and NFB + tDCS groups, and MI-NFB for left wrist dorsiflexion was performed. For the NFB + tDCS group, tDCS was performed before imaging. During NFB, EEG measurements were obtained, and the ERD of the μ-rhythm in M1 was projected on the monitor (**Figure 3**). In tDCS, the anode was placed on C4 and the cathode on the right upper arm, and anodal stimulation was administered to increase the activity of C4, which corresponds to the sensorimotor area of the left hand (**Figure 4**). The participants performed a motor imagery task without NFB before and after MI-NFB, and the EEG results obtained during the task were compared between the groups. The results showed that the ERD of the μ-rhythm in the

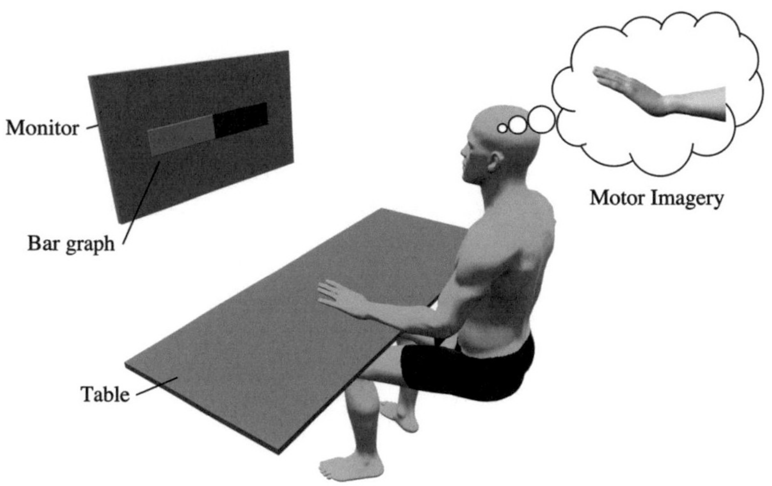

Figure 3.
Experimental setup [59]. The participant sat in a chair and mentally imagined a dorsiflexion movement of the left wrist joint. During the imagery, EEG was measured, and the ERD of the μ-rhythm was represented as a bar graph on the monitor.

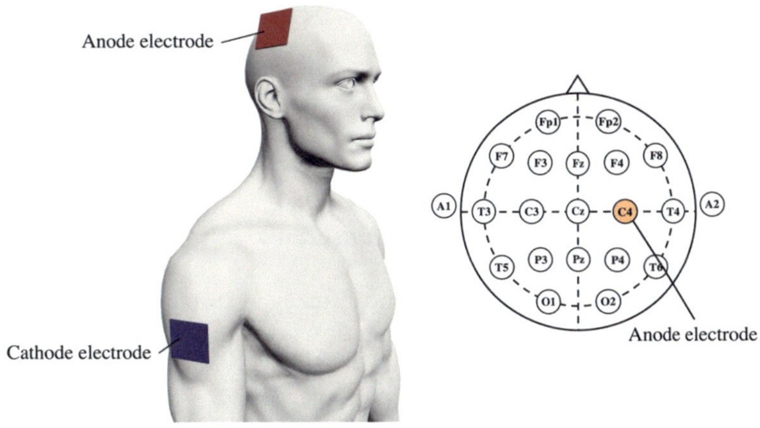

Figure 4.
tDCS setup [59]. A tDCS electrode was placed targeting C4, which corresponds to the sensorimotor area of the left hand. Anodal stimulation was applied to increase activity in this region.

NFB + tDCS group was significantly higher than that in the NFB group. This result indicates that the effect of MI-NFB alone, as well as the combination of MI-NFB and tDCS, can amplify the effect of MI-NFB. Both MI-NFB [37] and tDCS [55, 56] have been shown to improve MI accuracy, but the processes underlying their effects are different. Therefore, the effects of MI-NFB and tDCS do not appear to overlap, indicating the possibility of a synergistic effect.

As shown above, the efficacy of MI-NFB combined with tDCS has been demonstrated. Other electrical and magnetic stimuli also have similar mechanisms of action to tDCS, and their use in combination with MI-NFB may amplify the effects of MI-NFB. Intervention methods that combine such techniques are still in their infancy and require further study. In addition, noninvasive brain stimulation methods such as tDCS are not yet commonly used in physiotherapy practice. With advancements in brain science and engineering, physiotherapy using these devices will become widespread and provide effective rehabilitation.

3.2 Combination of neurofeedback with action observation or motor execution

Action observation and motor execution are often compared with motor imagery, and the accuracy of motor imagery and motor performance are improved when action observation and motor execution are combined with motor imagery [60, 61]. The effects of MI-NFB have also been shown to be improved by combining it with action observation and motor execution.

Action observation is a cognitive process of observing a scene in motion without moving [62]. Action observation and motor imagery have both been used in conjunction with motor execution to support motor learning, but both are different techniques, and it was believed that action observation and motor imagery cannot be used together. However, studies elucidating the neural bases and effects of these techniques have clarified that the combination of motor imagery and action observation improves the accuracy of motor imagery and motor performance [63]. Moreover, the effectiveness of the combination of action observation and MI-NFB has been verified in recent studies. Friesen et al. [64] used a handshake task to examine the effects of MI-NFB in combination with action observation. In their study, participants were divided into two groups: an NFB group, which received EEG feedback during the task, and a sham group, which received false stimulus feedback. The participants were required to watch a video of a complex handshake and simultaneously imagine the action (**Figure 5**). The ERD of μ-rhythms in the sensorimotor area was then measured, and the NFB group received visual feedback of brain activity by changing the saturation of the handshake video. Specifically, a vivid movie was displayed when a sufficient ERD was generated, and a monochrome movie was displayed when the ERD was insufficient (**Figure 6**). A comparison of ERD between groups showed that the NFB group had significantly higher ERD than the sham group, indicating an improvement in the accuracy of motor imagery when NFB is used in combination with action observation and motor imagery. The combination of motor imagery and action observation has been shown to increase cortical excitability [65] and activate motor-related networks [66]. In contrast, the results of this study showed that the

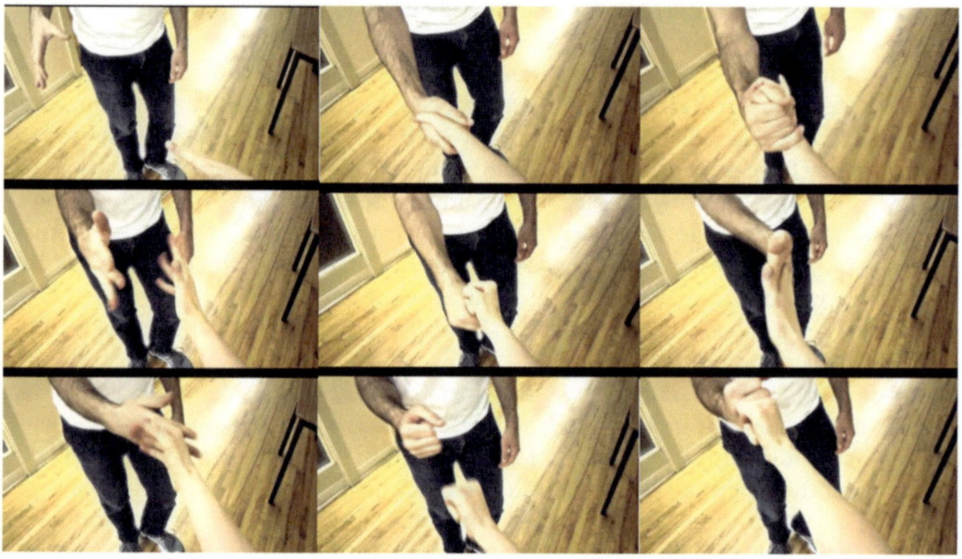

Figure 5.
Action observation of a handshake [64]. The participant was asked to imagine the motion while watching a video of a complex handshake.

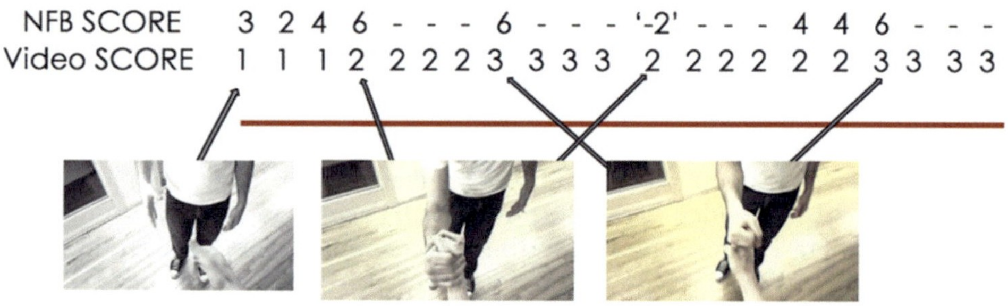

Figure 6.
Providing NFB when action observation and MI-NFB are combined [64]. The participant performed action observation and motor imagery simultaneously, during which EEG measurements were obtained. Then, the handshake video was set to become vivid with the ERD of the μ-rhythm, providing visual feedback on brain activity.

combination of motor imagery and action observation did not have the greatest effect but that the effect was further enhanced when NFB was used in combination.

Ono et al. [67] examined the combined effects of MI-NFB and action observation using proprioceptive NFB. In their study, participants were divided into an NFB group and a control group in which random feedback was provided, and training was conducted using a combination of action observation and motor imagery. A ball-gripping task was used in this study, and participants imagined the motion while watching a video of themselves gripping a ball. An exoskeleton robot was attached to the hand and set to passively generate finger-flexion movements when ERD with a sufficient μ-rhythm was generated during the task. This task was performed six times at 2-week intervals, and the ERD during motor imagery was continuously evaluated. The results showed a significant increase in the ERD in the NFB group in comparison with the control group. These results indicate that the combination of MI-NFB using proprioceptive and behavioral observations can improve the accuracy of motor imagery. Motor imagery and action observation may have activated motor-related areas, which were further modified by NFB. Similar to the findings of the study by Friesen et al. [64], this study showed that the combination of MI-NFB and action observation was effective. Furthermore, since proprioceptive feedback has been reported to be more effective than visual feedback in MI-NFB [68], the feedback system used in this study may have maximized the effects of motor imagery, action observation, and NFB, respectively. As shown in the above studies, the effectiveness of using MI-NFB in combination with action observation is being verified, and more effective methods of motor imagery training are being developed. Action observation is often used in physiotherapy practice, wherein patients observe the actions of physical therapists. Therefore, the results of these studies can be applied to physiotherapy practice to provide effective rehabilitation.

Motor execution generates myosensory and superficial sensory information that does not occur in motor imagery [69], which is thought to support motor imagery as KR [70]. In addition, motor execution has a neural mechanism that is partially similar to motor imagery [31]. For these reasons, the effects of training with motor execution and motor imagery have been examined [71]. The effects of combining MI-NFB and motor execution have been initially verified in recent studies. In one study, the authors examined the effects of combining MI-NFB and motor execution using a standing postural-control task [72]; the participants in this study were divided into the MIME group, which alternated between motor imagery and motor execution, and the MIME + NFB group, in which NFB was added to the motor imagery at that time. The task consisted of an actual exercise, in which the participant stood on an unstable board and kept the board horizontal, and a phase in which the participant imagined the exercise (**Figure** 7). The imagery of the exercise was performed in the resting sitting position, and the participants in the MIME + NFB group received ERD feedback of μ-rhythms in the motor-related regions during the imagery. The feedback method was auditory feedback, wherein higher-frequency sound stimuli were provided as the ERD increased. Performance on the standing postural-control task before and after training was compared between groups. The results showed significantly better standing postural control performance in the MIME + NFB group than in the MIME group. These results indicate that the combination of MI-NFB and motor execution improves the accuracy and performance of motor imagery. NFB provided KR of motor imagery from the neural activity aspect, and motor execution provided KR of motor imagery from the superficial and proprioceptive aspects, and their combined use may have improved the accuracy and

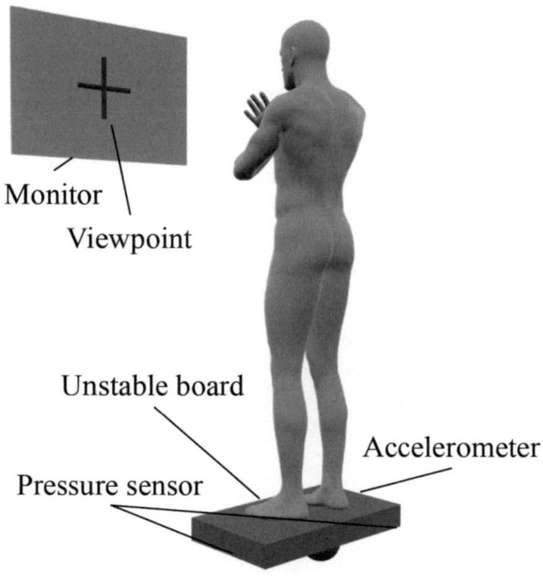

Figure 7.
A standing postural-control task combining MI-NFB and motor execution [72]. The participant stood on an unstable board and maintained the board in horizontal position. In the motor imagery task, the participant was asked to mentally imagine this standing postural-control task in a resting sitting position. Feedback regarding the ERD of the μ-rhythm during motor imagery was provided by auditory stimuli.

effectiveness of motor imagery. Thus, the initial studies on the effects of combining MI-NFB and motor execution have suggested that this approach may improve the accuracy of motor imagery. Since there are many situations in physiotherapy practice where actual exercise and motor imagery are used together, the results of these studies can be applied to clinical treatment.

3.3 Summary

This section described the effects of using MI-NFB in combination with other techniques. The use of noninvasive brain stimulation methods that alter brain states similar to NFB as well as the addition of action observation and motor execution, which are comparable to motor imagery, to MI-NFB can improve its effectiveness. However, further research is needed to provide more effective MI-NFB, since many aspects of this technique remain to be verified, including the effects of the area to be stimulated and the intensity of the stimulation. In physiotherapy practice, motor imagery shows individual differences in its effectiveness [36]. Thus, combining it with the other techniques described above could solve this problem and facilitate effective exercise imagery training for all patients, thereby establishing evidence-based motor imagery and MI-NFB.

4. Neurofeedback in physiotherapy practice

MI-NFB has been validated not only in healthy individuals but also in patients with neurological diseases. This section presents clinical studies of MI-NFB in patients with neurological disorders and describes the physiotherapy practice of MI-NFB.

4.1 Neurofeedback for patients with stroke

The hemiplegia and motor impairment caused by stroke necessitate physical therapy [73]. In particular, stroke patients have reduced motor imagery ability [74, 75], and MI-NFB is used to improve the effectiveness of motor imagery training [76]. Moreover, upper limb function is less likely to recover after stroke than lower limb function [77], and MI-NFB has attracted attention as a new and effective intervention method.

Pichiorri et al. [78] examined the effects of MI-NFB on upper limb movement in patients with subacute stroke. In their study, participants were divided into a control group, which performed motor imagery without NFB, and an MI-NFB group, which performed motor imagery with NFB. EEG measurements were obtained during imaging, and the ERD of the β-rhythm was evaluated. In the MI-NFB group, the virtual hand on the monitor moved to provide visual feedback on brain activity. In this study, participants underwent regular rehabilitation, including physical therapy and occupational therapy for 3 hours a day, and motor imagery training was conducted in addition to these sessions. In a comparison of the control and MI-NFB groups, the MI-NFB group showed a significantly higher ERD of the β-rhythm during imagery, and this phenomenon occurred mainly in the impaired hemisphere. This result suggests that MI-NFB may have enhanced the accuracy of motor imagery by facilitating recruitment of the impaired hemisphere during motor imagery. In addition, an intergroup comparison of the functional connectivity of the resting brain after training showed that the MI-NFB group had significantly increased connectivity between hemispheres in high-frequency bands such as β. The details of this phenomenon are not yet clear, but it is suggested to be related to the compensatory functions of the brain. The injured hemisphere and the unaffected hemisphere may be tightly connected, and bilateral activity may have produced the motor imagery. Interhemispheric connectivity was also observed after imagery training, indicating that it may contribute to brain reorganization. In addition, MI-NFB improved motor function as assessed by the arm section of the Fugl-Meyer Assessment (FMA), the upper limb section of the Medical Research Council scale for muscle strength, and the National Institute of Health Stroke Scale. In particular, the FMA score improved by more than a minimal clinically important difference only in the MI-NFB group. These improvements in brain and motor function indicate that MI-NFB is effective in physiotherapy practice for upper limb function in stroke patients. Zich et al. [79] also examined the effects of frequent MI-NFB on home treatment of chronic stroke patients and presented case reports of three chronic stroke patients more than 6 months after stroke onset, one with mild upper limb paralysis and two with severe upper limb paralysis. In MI-NFB, the participants imagined hand movements and received visual feedback of β-rhythm ERDs assessed from EEG. After 4 weeks of home training with MI-NFB, all participants showed cortical activation in motor-related areas. In addition, upper limb motor function improved in participants who showed mild paralysis. This patient clearly showed functional and structural recovery of the central nervous system after the training. This study did not show motor function or structural brain changes in patients with severe paralysis but showed changes in patients with mild paralysis. These findings indicate that MI-NFB may be effective even in patients with chronic stroke. Future studies should continue to validate MI-NFB in chronic stroke patients, allowing for more widespread use of MI-NFB in physiotherapy practice.

MI-NFB has been examined not only for upper limb function but also for gait function. Mihara et al. [41] performed motor imagery training of gait in patients with gait disorders due to subcortical stroke. During the imagery training, frontal functional near-infrared spectroscopy measurements were obtained to provide visual feedback on blood flow in the SMA associated with the motor imagery. The participants were divided into two groups: the MI-NFB group, which received cerebral blood flow feedback, and the sham group, which received sham feedback. The MI-NFB group showed a significant increase in SMA blood flow in comparison with the sham group. In addition to changes in brain function, the MI-NFB group's score on the Timed Up and Go test, a gait evaluation method, was significantly better after training. The results show that MI-NFB can effectively improve brain and motor function in gait, indicating that MI-NFB can be widely used in physiotherapy practice for stroke patients.

MI-NFB has been shown to improve upper limb and gait functions in stroke patients and may be an effective approach in physiotherapy practice. However, stroke symptoms vary according to the region of injury, and detailed classification of participants and investigation of interventional methods on the basis of the region of injury will contribute to the development of more effective MI-NFB. Conversely, a standard MI-NFB approach for stroke patients could be developed through large-scale studies that are not limited to the region of injury. Further research is needed to establish MI-NFB in physiotherapy practice for stroke patients.

4.2 Neurofeedback for patients with Parkinson disease

Parkinson disease (PD) is a neurological disorder whose main symptoms are resting tremors, muscle stiffness, immobility, and postural dysreflexia [80]. Motor imagery has been shown to be effective in treating these symptoms [81, 82], and MI-NFB is used to improve the effectiveness of motor imagery training. PD patients show decreased motor imagery ability [75, 83], and MI-NFB may contribute to symptom improvement in PD patients.

Subramanian et al. [84] examined the efficacy of MI-NFB in patients with Hoehn and Yahr stage I–III PD. The participants were divided into NFB and control groups and were required to imagine finger-tapping movements of the left hand. fMRI was measured during the imagery, and the BOLD signal of the SMA was returned as feedback to the NFB group. Next, the finger-tapping test and the fMRI BOLD signal during imagery were evaluated before and after training. The finger-tapping test involves tapping the thumb and index finger at maximum speed and reflects the immobility of PD patients [85]. The results showed upregulated SMA brain activity and greater finger-tapping speed in the NFB group in comparison with the control group. The results indicate that MI-NFB modulates brain activity in regions related to PD symptoms and improves immobility. A compensatory network involving the basal ganglia and thalamus is activated in PD as symptoms progress [86]. In addition, SMA projects to the globus pallidus internus of the basal ganglia and thalamus [87, 88], suggesting that MI-NFB may activate the compensatory network. As reported in the above studies, MI-NFB has been shown to be effective in treating motor symptoms in PD patients. Additionally, Subramanian et al. [89] examined the effect of combining exercise therapy and MI-NFB in PD patients. In their study, participants with Hoehn and Yahr stage I–III PD were divided into two groups: the EX group, which received exercise therapy, and the NF group, which received MI-NFB in addition to exercise therapy, and trained for 10 weeks. The EX group performed finger-tapping and postural-control tasks using a virtual reality game device as exercise therapy. In contrast, the NF group performed finger-tapping motor imagery and postural-control tasks.

The motor score of the Movement Disorder Society-sponsored revision of the Unified Parkinson's Disease Rating Scale (MDS-UPDRS) [90] was performed before and after training. The MDS-UPDRS consists of four items: daily motor experiences, daily non-motor experiences, motor tests, and motor complications. In addition, the MDS-UPDRS and other PD symptom scales were assessed before, during, and after the 4-week intervention. The results showed that the motor examination score of MDS-UPDRS significantly improved in the NF group in comparison with the EX group in the unmedicated condition. However, the MDS-UPDRS scores with medication did not show significant group differences for any of the items (**Figure 8**). This result indicates that MI-NFB may contribute to the recovery of basal ganglia function. In the on-medication condition, PD patients are treated with levodopa and other common PD medications that affect the basal ganglia. However, the findings of the study described above showed a difference in motor function with MI-NFB only in the off-medication condition, suggesting that MI-NFB may be an alternative to pharmacotherapy. Thus, MI-NFB has been shown to influence task performance reflecting motor symptoms as well as a general scale assessing the severity of PD. However, MI-NFB did not improve motor function in the on-medication condition. Since most patients with PD are on medication, the clinical usefulness of MI-NFB requires investigation of approaches to improve motor symptoms while on medication.

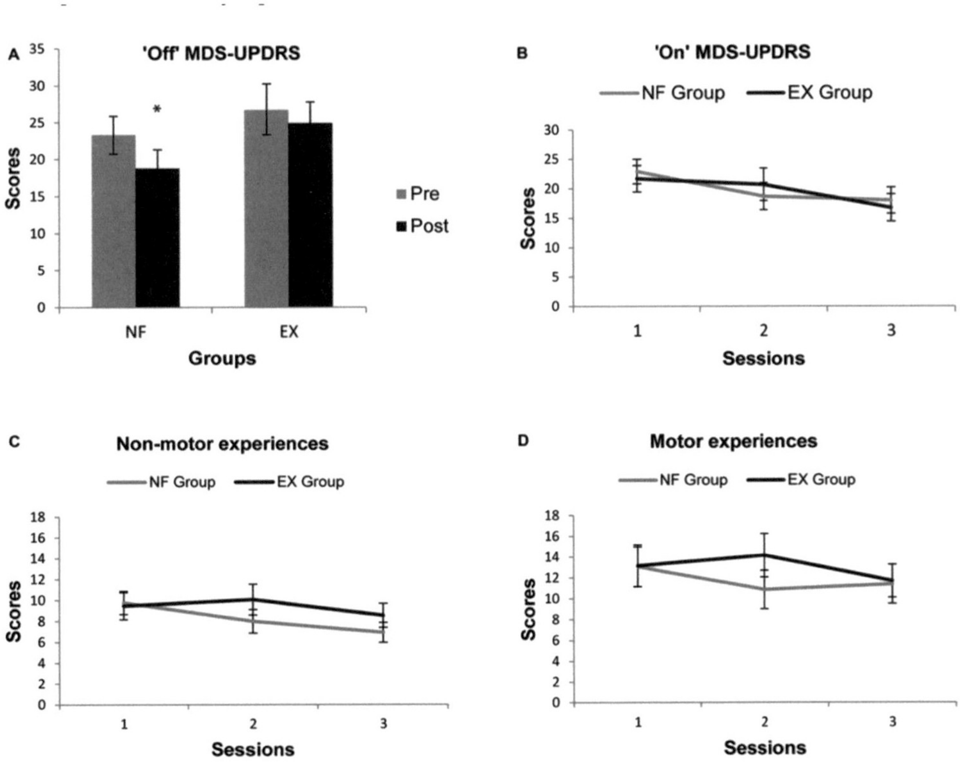

Figure 8.
Effects of MI-NFB combined with exercise therapy in PD patients [89]. (A) The motor examination score of the MDS-UPDRS in the off-medication condition was significantly better in the NF group than in the EX group. (B–D) However, the overall, non-motor experience or motor experience MDS-UPDRS scores with medication showed no significant group differences.

In physiotherapy practice, MI-NFB may be an effective approach to improve motor symptoms such as immobility in PD patients. Since the basal ganglia, which are impaired by PD, are connected to the SMA, which is activated by MI-NFB, MI-NFB can improve symptoms via the SMA. However, the effectiveness of MI-NFB depends on the medication conditions, and further validation is needed to devise an effective MI-NFB protocol. In addition to motor symptoms, PD often presents with non-motor symptoms such as autonomic and psychiatric symptoms. Therefore, the potential effects of non-motor symptoms on the effectiveness of MI-NFB also require consideration.

4.3 Summary

This section presented information regarding the physiotherapy practice of MI-NFB on the basis of its effects on stroke and PD patients; MI-NFB may be effective for stroke and PD caused by brain damage because it encourages the voluntary regulation of brain activity. However, MI-NFB is not always effective for these neurological diseases because their symptoms differ among patients. The findings also indicate the need to develop a method for selecting patients for whom MI-NFB is indicated as well as new MI-NFB protocol that demonstrates a certain level of effectiveness regardless of the characteristics of the patients. With the establishment of additional evidence, MI-NFB may emerge as a standard approach in physiotherapy practice.

5. Conclusion

This chapter described MI-NFB findings from basic studies in healthy individuals and clinical studies in patients with neurological diseases. Many studies have shown that MI-NFB facilitates voluntary control of brain activity and improves motor performance. The use of MI-NFB in combination with other techniques such as transcranial stimulation and action observation has been shown to further enhance its effects. Although clinical studies on patients are still scarce, a certain level of effectiveness has been demonstrated. Therefore, MI-NFB may be an effective approach in the practice of physiotherapy. However, further evidence needs to be developed for the widespread use of MI-NFB; controlling the brain with MI-NFB may raise the level of physiotherapy practice.

Appendices and nomenclature

NFB	neurofeedback
EEG	electroencephalography
fMRI	functional magnetic resonance imaging
MI-NFB	motor imagery-based neurofeedback
M1	primary motor cortex
SMA	supplementary motor area
ERD	event-related desynchronization
KR	knowledge of result
tDCS	transcranial direct current stimulation
ME	motor execution
FMA	Fugl-Meyer assessment

MDS-UPDRS	Movement Disorder Society-sponsored revision of the Unified Parkinson's Disease Rating Scale

Acknowledgements

This work was supported by JSPS KAKENHI (grant number JP23K10417). We would like to thank Editage (www.editage.com) for English language editing.

Conflict of interest

The authors declare no conflict of interest.

Author details

Shun Sawai[1,2], Shoya Fujikawa[1,2], Ryosuke Yamamoto[1,3] and Hideki Nakano[1*]

1 Neurorehabilitation Laboratory, Graduate School of Health Sciences, Kyoto Tachibana University, Kyoto, Japan

2 Department of Rehabilitation, Kyoto Kuno Hospital, Kyoto, Japan

3 Department of Rehabilitation, Tesseikai Neurosurgical Hospital, Osaka, Japan

*Address all correspondence to: nakano-h@tachibana-u.ac.jp

References

[1] Hampson M, Ruiz S, Ushiba J. Neurofeedback. Neuroimage. 2020;**218**:116473. DOI: 10.1016/j.neuroimage.2019.116473

[2] Kamiya J. Operant control of the EEG alpha rhythm and some of its reported effects on consciousness. In: Tart C, editor. Altered States of Consciousness. New York: Wiley; 1969. pp. 507-517

[3] Kamiya J. Conscious control of brain waves. Psychology Today. 1968;**1**:57-60

[4] Arns M, Batail JM, Bioulac S, Congedo M, Daudet C, Drapier D, et al. Neurofeedback: One of today's techniques in psychiatry? Encephale. 2017;**43**:135-145. DOI: 10.1016/j.encep.2016.11.003

[5] Loriette C, Ziane C, Ben HS. Neurofeedback for cognitive enhancement and intervention and brain plasticity. Revue Neurologique (Paris). 2021;**177**:1133-1144. DOI: 10.1016/j.neurol.2021.08.004

[6] Onagawa R, Muraoka Y, Hagura N, Takemi M. An investigation of the effectiveness of neurofeedback training on motor performance in healthy adults: A systematic review and meta-analysis. NeuroImage. 2023;**270**:120000. DOI: 10.1016/j.neuroimage.2023.120000

[7] Batail JM, Bioulac S, Cabestaing F, Daudet C, Drapier D, Fouillen M, et al. EEG neurofeedback research: A fertile ground for psychiatry? Encephale. 2019;**45**:245-255. DOI: 10.1016/j.encep.2019.02.001

[8] Watanabe T, Sasaki Y, Shibata K, Kawato M. Advances in fMRI real-time neurofeedback. Trends in Cognitive Sciences. 2017;**21**:997-1010. DOI: 10.1016/j.tics.2017.09.010

[9] Soekadar SR, Kohl SH, Mihara M, von Lühmann A. Optical brain imaging and its application to neurofeedback. NeuroImage: Clinical. 2021;**30**:102577. DOI: 10.1016/j.nicl.2021.102577

[10] Shabani F, Nisar S, Philamore H, Matsuno F. Haptic vs. visual neurofeedback for brain training: A proof-of-concept study. IEEE Transactions on Haptics. 2021;**14**:297-302. DOI: 10.1109/TOH.2021.3077492

[11] Nakano H, Kodama T, Murata S, Nakamoto T, Fujihara T, Ito Y. Effect of auditory neurofeedback training on upper extremity function and motor imagery ability in a stroke patient: A single case study. International Journal of Clinical Trials. 2018;**3**:126. DOI: 10.15344/2456-8007/2018/126

[12] Marzbani H, Marateb HR, Mansourian M. Neurofeedback: A comprehensive review on system design, methodology and clinical applications. Basic and Clinical Neuroscience. 2016;**7**:143-158. DOI: 10.15412/J.BCN.03070208

[13] Davelaar EJ. Mechanisms of neurofeedback: A computation-theoretic approach. Neuroscience. 2018;**378**:175-188. DOI: 10.1016/j.neuroscience.2017.05.052

[14] Sharon N. Clinical efficacy and potential mechanisms of neurofeedback. Personality & Individual Differences. 2013;**54**:676-686. DOI: 10.1016/j.paid.2012.11.037

[15] Sampaio-Baptista C, Neyedli HF, Sanders ZB, Diosi K, Havard D, Huang Y,

et al. fMRI neurofeedback in the motor system elicits bidirectional changes in activity and in white matter structure in the adult human brain. Cell Reports. 2021;**37**:109890. DOI: 10.1016/j.celrep.2021.109890

[16] Sitaram R, Ros T, Stoeckel L, Haller S, Scharnowski F, Lewis-Peacock J, et al. Closed-loop brain training: The science of neurofeedback. Nature Reviews. Neuroscience. 2017;**18**:86-100. DOI: 10.1038/nrn.2016.164

[17] Seeley WW, Menon V, Schatzberg AF, Keller J, Glover GH, Kenna H, et al. Dissociable intrinsic connectivity networks for salience processing and executive control. The Journal of Neuroscience. 2007;**27**:2349-2356. DOI: 10.1523/JNEUROSCI.5587-06.2007

[18] Kravitz AV, Matikainen-Ankney BA. Motor control: Memory and motor control in the dorsal striatum. Current Biology. 2020;**30**:R1366-R1368. DOI: 10.1016/j.cub.2020.09.018

[19] Billeke P, Ossandon T, Perrone-Bertolotti M, Kahane P, Bastin J, Jerbi K, et al. Human anterior insula encodes performance feedback and relays prediction error to the medial prefrontal cortex. Cerebral Cortex. 2020;**30**:4011-4025. DOI: 10.1093/cercor/bhaa017

[20] Umemoto A, HajiHosseini A, Yates ME, Holroyd CB. Reward-based contextual learning supported by anterior cingulate cortex. Cognitive, Affective, & Behavioral Neuroscience. 2017;**17**:642-651. DOI: 10.3758/s13415-017-0502-3

[21] Ramot M, Grossman S, Friedman D, Malach R. Covert neurofeedback without awareness shapes cortical network spontaneous connectivity. Proceedings of the National Academy of Sciences of the United States of America. 2016;**113**:E2413-E2420. DOI: 10.1073/pnas.1516857113

[22] Daniel R, Pollmann S. A universal role of the ventral striatum in reward-based learning: Evidence from human studies. Neurobiology of Learning and Memory. 2014;**114**:90-100. DOI: 10.1016/j.nlm.2014.05.002

[23] Guler S, Cohen AL, Afacan O, Warfield SK. Matched neurofeedback during fMRI differentially activates reward-related circuits in active and sham groups. Journal of Neuroimaging. 2021;**31**:947-955. DOI: 10.1111/jon.12899

[24] Dobrushina OR, Vlasova RM, Rumshiskaya AD, Litvinova LD, Mershina EA, Sinitsyn VE, et al. Modulation of intrinsic brain connectivity by implicit electroencephalographic neurofeedback. Frontiers in Human Neuroscience. 2020;**14**:192. DOI: 10.3389/fnhum.2020.00192

[25] Vargas P, Sitaram R, Sepúlveda P, Montalba C, Rana M, Torres R, et al. Weighted neurofeedback facilitates greater self-regulation of functional connectivity between the primary motor area and cerebellum. Journal of Neural Engineering. 2021;**18**:056059. DOI: 10.1088/1741-2552/ac2b7e

[26] Olsson CJ, Nyberg L. Motor imagery: If you can't do it, you won't think it. Scandinavian Journal of Medicine & Science in Sports. 2010;**20**:711-715. DOI: 10.1111/j.1600-0838.2010.01101.x

[27] Nakano H, Tachibana M, Fujita N, Sawai S, Fujikawa S, Yamamoto R, et al. Reliability and validity of the Japanese Movement Imagery Questionnaire—Revised Second Version. BMC Research Notes. 2022;**15**:334. DOI: 10.1186/s13104-022-06220-y

[28] Nakano H, Kodama T, Ukai K, Kawahara S, Horikawa S, Murata S. Reliability and validity of the Japanese version of the Kinesthetic and Visual Imagery Questionnaire (KVIQ). Brain Sciences. 2018;**8**:79. DOI: 10.3390/brainsci8050079

[29] MacIntyre TE, Madan CR, Moran AP, Collet C, Guillot A. Motor imagery, performance and motor rehabilitation. Progress in Brain Research. 2018;**240**:141-159. DOI: 10.1016/bs.pbr.2018.09.010

[30] Ruffino C, Papaxanthis C, Lebon F. Neural plasticity during motor learning with motor imagery practice: Review and perspectives. Neuroscience. 2017;**341**:61-78. DOI: 10.1016/j.neuroscience.2016.11.023

[31] Hanakawa T, Dimyan MA, Hallett M. Motor planning, imagery, and execution in the distributed motor network: A time-course study with functional MRI. Cerebral Cortex. 2008;**18**:2775-2788. DOI: 10.1093/cercor/bhn036

[32] Sawai S, Fujikawa S, Ushio R, Tamura K, Ohsumi C, Yamamoto R, et al. Repetitive peripheral magnetic stimulation combined with motor imagery changes resting-state EEG activity: A randomized controlled trial. Brain Sciences. 2022;**12**:1548. DOI: 10.3390/brainsci12111548

[33] Ridderinkhof KR, Brass M. How kinesthetic motor imagery works: A predictive-processing theory of visualization in sports and motor expertise. Journal of Physiology, Paris. 2015;**109**:53-63. DOI: 10.1016/j.jphysparis.2015.02.003

[34] Tong Y, Pendy JT Jr, Li WA, Du H, Zhang T, Geng X, et al. Motor imagery-based rehabilitation: Potential neural correlates and clinical application for functional recovery of motor deficits after stroke. Aging and Disease. 2017;**8**:364-371. DOI: 10.14336/AD.2016.1012

[35] Fujikawa S, Ohsumi C, Ushio R, Tamura K, Sawai S, Yamamoto R, et al. Potential applications of motor imagery for improving standing posture balance in rehabilitation. In: Nakano H, editor. Neurorehabilitation and Physical Therapy. London: IntechOpen; 2022. pp. 27-42. DOI: 10.5772/intechopen.105779

[36] van der Meulen M, Allali G, Rieger SW, Assal F, Vuilleumier P. The influence of individual motor imagery ability on cerebral recruitment during gait imagery. Human Brain Mapping. 2014;**35**:455-470. DOI: 10.1002/hbm.22192

[37] Girges C, Vijiaratnam N, Zrinzo L, Ekanayake J, Foltynie T. Volitional control of brain motor activity and its therapeutic potential. Neuromodulation. 2022;**25**:1187-1196. DOI: 10.1016/j.neurom.2022.01.007

[38] Blefari ML, Sulzer J, Hepp-Reymond MC, Kollias S, Gassert R. Improvement in precision grip force control with self-modulation of primary motor cortex during motor imagery. Frontiers in Behavioral Neuroscience. 2015;**9**:18. DOI: 10.3389/fnbeh.2015.00018

[39] Berman BD, Horovitz SG, Venkataraman G, Hallett M. Self-modulation of primary motor cortex activity with motor and motor imagery tasks using real-time fMRI-based neurofeedback. NeuroImage. 2012;**59**:917-925. DOI: 10.1016/j.neuroimage.2011.07.035

[40] Al-Wasity S, Vogt S, Vuckovic A, Pollick FE. Upregulation of supplementary motor area

activation with fMRI neurofeedback during motor imagery. eNeuro. 2021;**8**:ENEURO.0377-18.2020. DOI: 10.1523/ENEURO.0377-18.2020

[41] Mihara M, Fujimoto H, Hattori N, Otomune H, Kajiyama Y, Konaka K, et al. Effect of neurofeedback facilitation on poststroke gait and balance recovery: A randomized controlled trial. Neurology. 2021;**96**:e2587-e2598. DOI: 10.1212/WNL.0000000000011989

[42] Darvishi S, Gharabaghi A, Boulay CB, Ridding MC, Abbott D, Baumert M. Proprioceptive feedback facilitates motor imagery-related operant learning of sensorimotor β-band modulation. Frontiers in Neuroscience. 2017;**11**:60. DOI: 10.3389/fnins.2017.00060

[43] Pineda JA, Silverman DS, Vankov A, Hestenes J. Learning to control brain rhythms: Making a brain-computer interface possible. IEEE Transactions on Neural Systems and Rehabilitation Engineering. 2003;**11**:181-184. DOI: 10.1109/TNSRE.2003.814445

[44] Pfurtscheller G, Neuper C. Motor imagery and direct brain-computer communication. Proceedings of the IEEE. 2001;**89**:1123-1134. DOI: 10.1109/5.939829

[45] Mihara M, Miyai I, Hattori N, Hatakenaka M, Yagura H, Kawano T, et al. Neurofeedback using real-time near-infrared spectroscopy enhances motor imagery related cortical activation. PLoS One. 2012;7:e32234. DOI: 10.1371/journal.pone.0032234

[46] Winstein CJ. Knowledge of results and motor learning—Implications for physical therapy. Physical Therapy. 1991;**71**:140-149. DOI: 10.1093/ptj/71.2.140

[47] Hwang HJ, Kwon K, Im CH. Neurofeedback-based motor imagery training for brain-computer interface (BCI). Journal of Neuroscience Methods. 2009;**179**:150-156. DOI: 10.1016/j.jneumeth.2009.01.015

[48] Grigorev NA, Savosenkov AO, Lukoyanov MV, Udoratina A, Shusharina NN, Kaplan AY, et al. A BCI-based vibrotactile neurofeedback training improves motor cortical excitability during motor imagery. IEEE Transactions on Neural Systems and Rehabilitation Engineering. 2021;**29**:1583-1592. DOI: 10.1109/TNSRE.2021.3102304

[49] Boe S, Gionfriddo A, Kraeutner S, Tremblay A, Little G, Bardouille T. Laterality of brain activity during motor imagery is modulated by the provision of source level neurofeedback. NeuroImage. 2014;**101**:159-167. DOI: 10.1016/j.neuroimage.2014.06.066

[50] Daeglau M, Zich C, Kranczioch C. The impact of context on EEG motor imagery neurofeedback and related motor domains. Current Behavioral Neuroscience Reports. 2021;**8**:90-101. DOI: 10.1007/s40473-021-00233-w

[51] Bauer R, Vukelić M, Gharabaghi A. What is the optimal task difficulty for reinforcement learning of brain self-regulation? Clinical Neurophysiology. 2016;**127**:3033-3041. DOI: 10.1016/j.clinph.2016.06.016

[52] Ushio R, Tamura K, Fujikawa S, Ohsumi C, Sawai S, Yamamoto R, et al. Clinical application of repetitive peripheral magnetic stimulation in rehabilitation. In: Nakano H, editor. Neurorehabilitation and Physical Therapy. London: IntechOpen; 2022. pp. 43-54. DOI: 10.5772/intechopen.105787

[53] Antal A, Luber B, Brem AK, Bikson M, Brunoni AR, Cohen Kadosh R, et al. Non-invasive brain stimulation and neuroenhancement. Clinical Neurophysiology Practice. 2022;**7**:146-165. DOI: 10.1016/j.cnp.2022.05.002

[54] Yavari F, Jamil A, Mosayebi Samani M, Vidor LP, Nitsche MA. Basic and functional effects of transcranial electrical stimulation (tES)—An introduction. Neuroscience and Biobehavioral Reviews. 2018;**85**:81-92. DOI: 10.1016/j.neubiorev.2017.06.015

[55] Saruco E, Di Rienzo F, Nunez-Nagy S, Rubio-Gonzalez MA, Jackson PL, Collet C, et al. Anodal tDCS over the primary motor cortex improves motor imagery benefits on postural control: A pilot study. Scientific Reports. 2017;**7**:480. DOI: 10.1038/s41598-017-00509-w

[56] Xie J, Peng M, Lu J, Xiao C, Zong X, Wang M, et al. Enhancement of event-related desynchronization in motor imagery based on transcranial electrical stimulation. Frontiers in Human Neuroscience. 2021;**15**:635351. DOI: 10.3389/fnhum.2021.635351

[57] Feurra M, Pasqualetti P, Bianco G, Santarnecchi E, Rossi A, Rossi S. State-dependent effects of transcranial oscillatory currents on the motor system: What you think matters. The Journal of Neuroscience. 2013;**33**:17483-17489. DOI: 10.1523/JNEUROSCI.1414-13.2013

[58] Shu X, Chen S, Chai G, Sheng X, Jia J, Zhu X. Neural modulation by repetitive transcranial magnetic stimulation (rTMS) for BCI enhancement in stroke patients. In: 40th Annual International Conference of the IEEE Engineering in Medicine and Biology Society (EMBC); 18-21 July 2018; Honolulu, HI: IEEE; 2018. pp. 2272-2275. DOI: 10.1109/embc.2018.8512860

[59] Sawai S, Murata S, Fujikawa S, Yamamoto R, Shima K, Nakano H. Effects of neurofeedback training combined with transcranial direct current stimulation on motor imagery: A randomized controlled trial. Frontiers in Neuroscience. 2023;**17**:1148336. DOI: 10.3389/fnins.2023.1148336

[60] McCormick SA, Causer J, Holmes PS. Active vision during action execution, observation and imagery: Evidence for shared motor representations. PLoS One. 2013;**8**:e67761. DOI: 10.1371/journal.pone.0067761

[61] Hardwick RM, Caspers S, Eickhoff SB, Swinnen SP. Neural correlates of action: Comparing meta-analyses of imagery, observation, and execution. Neuroscience and Biobehavioral Reviews. 2018;**94**:31-44. DOI: 10.1016/j.neubiorev.2018.08.003

[62] Jeannerod M. Neural simulation of action: A unifying mechanism for motor cognition. NeuroImage. 2001;**14**:S103-S109. DOI: 10.1006/nimg.2001.0832

[63] Vogt S, Di Rienzo F, Collet C, Collins A, Guillot A. Multiple roles of motor imagery during action observation. Frontiers in Human Neuroscience. 2013;**7**:807. DOI: 10.3389/fnhum.2013.00807

[64] Friesen CL, Bardouille T, Neyedli HF, Boe SG. Combined action observation and motor imagery neurofeedback for modulation of brain activity. Frontiers in Human Neuroscience. 2017;**10**:692. DOI: 10.3389/fnhum.2016.00692

[65] Chye S, Valappil AC, Wright DJ, Frank C, Shearer DA, Tyler CJ, et al. The effects of combined action observation and motor imagery on corticospinal excitability and movement outcomes: Two meta-analyses. Neuroscience and

Biobehavioral Reviews. 2022;**143**:104911. DOI: 10.1016/j.neubiorev.2022.104911

[66] Nedelko V, Hassa T, Hamzei F, Schoenfeld MA, Dettmers C. Action imagery combined with action observation activates more corticomotor regions than action observation alone. Journal of Neurologic Physical Therapy. 2012;**36**:182-188. DOI: 10.1097/NPT.0b013e318272cad1

[67] Ono Y, Wada K, Kurata M, Seki N. Enhancement of motor-imagery ability via combined action observation and motor-imagery training with proprioceptive neurofeedback. Neuropsychologia. 2018;**114**:134-142. DOI: 10.1016/j.neuropsychologia.2018.04.016

[68] Vukelić M, Gharabaghi A. Oscillatory entrainment of the motor cortical network during motor imagery is modulated by the feedback modality. NeuroImage. 2015;**111**:1-11. DOI: 10.1016/j.neuroimage.2015.01.058

[69] Savaki HE, Raos V. Action perception and motor imagery: Mental practice of action. Progress in Neurobiology. 2019;**175**:107-125. DOI: 10.1016/j.pneurobio.2019.01.007

[70] Guillot A, Di Rienzo F, Macintyre T, Moran A, Collet C. Imagining is not doing but involves specific motor commands: A review of experimental data related to motor inhibition. Frontiers in Human Neuroscience. 2012;**6**:247. DOI: 10.3389/fnhum.2012.00247

[71] Wriessnegger SC, Steyrl D, Koschutnig K, Müller-Putz GR. Short time sports exercise boosts motor imagery patterns: Implications of mental practice in rehabilitation programs. Frontiers in Human Neuroscience. 2014;**8**:469. DOI: 10.3389/fnhum.2014.00469

[72] Sawai S, Fujikawa S, Ohsumi C, Ushio R, Tamura K, Yamamoto R, et al. Effects of neurofeedback on standing postural control task with combined imagined and executed movements. Frontiers in Neuroscience. 2023;**17**:1199398. DOI: 10.3389/fnins.2023.1199398

[73] Winstein CJ, Stein J, Arena R, Bates B, Cherney LR, Cramer SC, et al. Guidelines for adult stroke rehabilitation and recovery: A guideline for healthcare professionals from the American Heart Association/American Stroke Association. Stroke. 2016;**47**:e98-e169. DOI: 10.1161/STR.0000000000000098

[74] Braun N, Kranczioch C, Liepert J, Dettmers C, Zich C, Büsching I, et al. Motor imagery impairment in postacute stroke patients. Neural Plasticity. 2017;**2017**:4653256. DOI: 10.1155/2017/4653256

[75] McInnes K, Friesen C, Boe S. Specific brain lesions impair explicit motor imagery ability: A systematic review of the evidence. Archives of Physical Medicine and Rehabilitation. 2016;**97**:478-489.e1. DOI: 10.1016/j.apmr.2015.07.012

[76] Dettmers C, Braun N, Büsching I, Hassa T, Debener S, Liepert J. Neurofeedback-based motor imagery training for rehabilitation after stroke. Der Nervenarzt. 2016;**87**:1074-1081. DOI: 10.1007/s00115-016-0185-y

[77] Liu M, Fujiwara T, Shindo K, Kasashima Y, Otaka Y, Tsuji T, et al. Newer challenges to restore hemiparetic upper extremity after stroke: HANDS therapy and BMI neurorehabilitation. Hong Kong Physiotherapy Journal. 2012;**30**:83-92. DOI: 10.1016/j.hkpj.2012.05.001

[78] Pichiorri F, Morone G, Petti M, Toppi J, Pisotta I, Molinari M, et al.

Brain-computer interface boosts motor imagery practice during stroke recovery. Annals of Neurology. 2015;**77**:851-865. DOI: 10.1002/ana.24390

[79] Zich C, Debener S, Schweinitz C, Sterr A, Meekes J, Kranczioch C. High-intensity chronic stroke motor imagery neurofeedback training at home: Three case reports. Clinical EEG and Neuroscience. 2017;**48**:403-412. DOI: 10.1177/1550059417717398

[80] Tysnes OB, Storstein A. Epidemiology of Parkinson's disease. Journal of Neural Transmission (Vienna). 2017;**124**:901-905. DOI: 10.1007/s00702-017-1686-y

[81] Cuomo G, Maglianella V, Ghanbari Ghooshchy S, Zoccolotti P, Martelli M, Paolucci S, et al. Motor imagery and gait control in Parkinson's disease: Techniques and new perspectives in neurorehabilitation. Expert Review of Neurotherapeutics. 2022;**22**:43-51. DOI: 10.1080/14737175.2022.2018301

[82] Nascimento IAPDS, Santiago LMM, de Souza AA, Pegado CL, Ribeiro TS, Lindquist ARR. Effects of motor imagery training of Parkinson's disease: A protocol for a randomized clinical trial. Trials. 2019;**20**:626. DOI: 10.1186/s13063-019-3694-8

[83] Heremans E, Feys P, Nieuwboer A, Vercruysse S, Vandenberghe W, Sharma N, et al. Motor imagery ability in patients with early- and mid-stage Parkinson disease. Neurorehabilitation and Neural Repair. 2011;**25**:168-177. DOI: 10.1177/1545968310370750

[84] Subramanian L, Hindle JV, Johnston S, Roberts MV, Husain M, Goebel R, et al. Real-time functional magnetic resonance imaging neurofeedback for treatment of Parkinson's disease. The Journal of Neuroscience. 2011;**31**:16309-16317. DOI: 10.1523/JNEUROSCI.3498-11.2011

[85] Picillo M, Vincos GB, Kern DS, Fox SH, Lang AE, Fasano A. Learning more from finger tapping in Parkinson's disease: Up and down from dyskinesia to bradykinesia. Movement Disorders Clinical Practice. 2015;**3**:184-187. DOI: 10.1002/mdc3.12246

[86] Park DC, Reuter-Lorenz P. The adaptive brain: Aging and neurocognitive scaffolding. Annual Review of Psychology. 2009;**60**:173-196. DOI: 10.1146/annurev.psych.59.103006.093656

[87] Ma L, Wang B, Narayana S, Hazeltine E, Chen X, Robin DA, et al. Changes in regional activity are accompanied with changes in inter-regional connectivity during 4 weeks motor learning. Brain Research. 2010;**1318**:64-76. DOI: 10.1016/j.brainres.2009.12.073

[88] Nambu A, Takada M, Inase M, Tokuno H. Dual somatotopical representations in the primate subthalamic nucleus: Evidence for ordered but reversed body-map transformations from the primary motor cortex and the supplementary motor area. The Journal of Neuroscience. 1996;**16**:2671-2683. DOI: 10.1523/JNEUROSCI.16-08-02671.1996

[89] Subramanian L, Morris MB, Brosnan M, Turner DL, Morris HR, Linden DE. Functional magnetic resonance imaging neurofeedback-guided motor imagery training and motor training for Parkinson's disease: Randomized trial. Frontiers in Behavioral Neuroscience. 2016;**10**:111. DOI: 10.3389/fnbeh.2016.00111

[90] Goetz CG, Tilley BC, Shaftman SR, Stebbins GT, Fahn S, Martinez-Martin P, et al. Movement Disorder Society-sponsored revision of the Unified Parkinson's Disease Rating Scale (MDS-UPDRS): Scale presentation and clinimetric testing results. Movement Disorders. 2008;**23**:2129-2170. DOI: 10.1002/mds.22340

Chapter 9

Therapeutic Exercises in Fall Prevention among Older Adults

Olubusola Johnson, Christopher Akosile, Emeka Mong and Ukamaka Mgbeojedo

Abstract

Falls constitute a leading cause of injury-related mortality and morbidity, threatening the independence of older adults. Physical activity levels tend to decrease as the quality of life among older adults with an increasing fear of falls. Exercises of varying types are beneficial in preventing falls among older adults. Despite the assertion that therapeutic exercises are crucial in preventing falls among older adults and promoting their overall health, there is no evidence to favor any exercise type. However, exercise regimens address deficits and needs, plus recommendations exist for regular physical activity. This chapter focuses on falls among older adults. The authors discussed epidemiology, risks, and prevention of falls. Research evidence supports exercises in managing falls with increasing physical activities, quality of life, and reduced fall-related injuries and risks. The chapter highlights the benefits of multifaceted, single-intervention exercises and the Otago Exercise Programme.

Keywords: older adults, fall prevalence, fall risk, fall prevention, exercises

1. Introduction

Falls remain the third leading cause of chronic disability among older adults over 65 [1]. Falls are common in older adults and portend serious problems including physical, injury-related, and psychological health challenges for older adults [2], leading to injury-related morbidity, mortality, and nursing home placement among this population [3]. Aging is associated with increased morbidity, increased fear of falling, and reduced activity, consequently impairing the quality of life of older people. Falls are prevalent among the elderly population. One in three community-dwelling people aged over 65 years falls each year [4, 5]. Burns, Stevens, and Lee [6] reported that one in four people would decrease yearly. Akosile et al. [7] similarly reported a prevalence rate of 27.8% among a sample of older adults in a Nigerian community.

Falls constitute a significant cause of fatal and nonfatal injuries among adults aged ≥65 years [8]. Several factors increase the risks of falls among older adults. Risk factors are intrinsic: related to an individual, and irrelevant: related to the environment. According to Bagiartana and Huriah [9], balance disorders in adults are the primary cause of falls, a significant health concern for older adults. Older people in nursing homes and hospitals also experience falls, which have multifactorial etiology.

Tinetti et al. [10] followed up with a large cohort of older adults. They identified increasing age, female gender, certain medications, history of falls, impaired balance, and lower extremity weakness as significant predictors of falls. In a prospective study of fall risk factors among community-dwelling older adults, muscle weakness, balance impairments, visual impairments, chronic diseases, and cognitive impairment had a significant association with increased risk of falls [11]. Falling is not always reported at hospitals, even though more than one out of four older people falls yearly. Burns, Steven, and Lee [6] said less than half of fall incidents get reported to doctors, and falling once makes you a perpetual faller [12].

In a systematic review, Park [13] reported that falls significantly cause injuries and death in people over 65 [14]. Their systematic review and meta-analysis of observational studies said that risk factors such as previous falls, impaired balance, gait disorders, lower extremity weakness, visual impairments, and polypharmacy were strongly associated with increased fall risk. Rubenstein [15] highlighted factors such as muscle weakness, gait and balance impairments, medications, visual impairment, environmental hazards, chronic conditions, and cognitive decline as significant contributors to fall risk. Falls can result from a combination of risk factors rather than a single cause. Identifying and addressing these risk factors through appropriate interventions, such as exercise programmes, home modifications, medication adjustments, and regular health assessments, can significantly reduce the risk of falls among older adults.

In a study among a community-dwelling sample of older adults, fear of falls was present in nearly one of every four older adults. Distribution is like that among individuals with actual falls [16]. Falls lead to injury and even death in older adults. Fear of falls increases among older adults, and their physical activity levels tend to decrease as age increases, leading to reduced quality of life [2]. According to King and King [2], midlife and older adults represent the most inactive portion of the studied population, and there exists a significant relationship between physical activity, fear of falls, and the quality of life of older adults [17].

Falls among older adults are very costly. Park [13] reported that falls are a significant cause of injury and death in people over 65. In the USA, about $50 billion annually goes to medical costs related to nonfatal fall injuries, and $754 million is spent on fatal fall injuries [18]; this cost will increase as people live longer [19]. Martin et al. [20], in their systematic review of the modified Otago Exercise Programme (OEP), reported that using OEP-modified formats improved balance and functional ability. Kyrdalen et al. [21] asserted that the OEP, with its emphasis on strength and balance exercises, proved to be effective for fall prevention and reducing fall risks. The authors concluded that exercise interventions could reduce fall risks in older adults. Still, the value of different types of exercise activities differs for older adults, as evidence in the literature does not seem to favor any exercise [22].

Therapeutic exercise programmes, specifically for fall prevention, focus on improving strength, balance, flexibility, and coordination. Long-term exercise promotion is recommended for fall prevention. In addition to these physical benefits, therapeutic exercise programmes for fall prevention can positively affect older adults' confidence, self-efficacy, and overall quality of life. Regular participation in these programmes can significantly reduce the risk of falls and their associated consequences. This chapter focuses on falls among older adults, their impacts on aging and vice versa, and the evidence that exercises have been effective in falls, increasing physical activity, and quality of life in this population.

2. Epidemiology of falls

Aging is a critical stage in human life characterized by a series of changes that occur in internal and external organs. These changes help humans adjust to their immediate surroundings. Improving health care and general life services through science and technology has increased the number of older persons. As people age, they experience significant public health concern that results, in most occurrences, in morbidity, cost of health care services, and mortality [23].

Fall is a significant public health concern among older adults, and a faller is someone who has a fall in a stipulated period of 6 months or 1 year [24]. According to Nabavi et al. [25], fall is one of the most common and severe problems among older adults. The World Health Organization sees a fall as an unexpected event where an individual falls to the ground from the same or higher level. It is an event that results in a person coming to rest accidentally on the ground, floor, or other lower level [26]. Older adults are often at risk of falls resulting in severe injuries or even death. Injury from falls in the aging adult population has become widely accepted as a critical health problem [27].

Falls are one of the leading causes of disability and death among older adults or the geriatric population [23, 28]. In a meta-analysis, Salari et al. [29] reported the global percentage of falls among older people from Asia, Europe, Africa, America, and Oceania to be 25.6%. The report showed that the highest prevalence rate of falls in older adults was 34.4% among Oceanians and 27.9% among Americans. Europe's record fall among older adults was 23.4% and the lowest, followed by 25.4 and 25.8% prevalence rates among Africans and Asians, respectively.

Globally, the prevalence of falls in the older adult population in 2022 was 26.5%. In 2012, Japan had a 20.9% prevalence rate of falls, against 15.9% in 2011 [30] and a 28% prevalence rate for Japan in 2018 [31]. Brazil report showed that falls are prevalent, with one in every three older adults experiencing more than one fall in 12 months [32]. In America, falls among adults 65 and older recorded 3 million emergency department visits, causing over 36,000 deaths in 2020 [33]. From Japan's experience, there has been an increase in the number of fallers, which consequently places a more significant burden on care delivery, because of the attendant injuries and morbidity.

Africa also has an aging population, although slower than other world regions. By 2050, the proportion of people aged 60 and older adults in Africa will increase from 5 to 10 percent. The increase in the number of older adults may be dramatic, from 47.4 million in 2005 to two billion by 2050 [34]. In Nigeria, a fall prevalence rate of 23% was reported in 2010, with females experiencing a higher prevalence (24%) of falls compared to males (17.9%) [35, 36]. In 2014, a prevalence rate of 27.8% was reported among older adults (65 years and above) in Nigeria [37]. Older adults in urban areas experience more falls than their counterparts in rural communities. Twenty-five percent (25.3%) of older adults in rural areas reported experiencing a fall within 6 weeks, while a higher percentage of participants (41.3%) in urban communities reported experiencing a fall [37]. In a hospital-based study in Ghana, the prevalence of falls was 40.2% [38]. A study in Malawi reported the prevalence of falls in older adults as 41% [39]. There are very few articles published on the prevalence of falls in Africa. Nevertheless, the increasing adult population is likely a public health concern and a significant reason for emergency department attendance.

Falls are preventable but continue to be a leading cause of mortality, morbidity, and decreased quality of life among older adults already burdened by many other conditions. Globally, the prevalence rate of falls in the aging adult population is at a rate of 1 in 4 or 25.6% prevalence. Oceania has the highest prevalence record of 34.4%, the lowest prevalence rate for Europe at 23.4%, and fall prevalence in Africa is not different from that reported globally.

3. Risk factors for falls

Falls are one of the major causes of injuries, morbidity, and mortality among older adults, impacting older people's quality of life [13] and resulting in social isolation [40]. Identifying the risk factors associated with falls is critical for preventing falls and their consequences [15, 41]. The risk of falls increases with age [42] and the number of risk factors in each person [43]. There are several risk factors for falls in older adults [44]. Risk factors for falls among older adults are multifactorial [26, 44]; and can be classified as extrinsic or intrinsic factors [45, 46] or modifiable and non-modifiable risk factors.

Intrinsic (within-subject) risk factors are those factors related to the individual's specific risk, such as demographic and biological factors, while extrinsic risk factors comprise environmental and behavioral factors [45]. Intrinsic risk factors include previous history of falls, age, gender, living alone, ethnicity, medical conditions and chronic illnesses, impaired mobility and gait, loss of foot sensation, sedentary lifestyle, psychological status, fear of falling, nutritional deficiencies, visual and cognitive impairments. In contrast, extrinsic risk factors include environmental factors (poor lighting, slick floors, slippery bathrooms, rough surfaces), footwear and clothing, and unsuitable walking aids [47, 48].

Modifiable risk factors refer to those risk factors that can be improved or alleviated with an intervention. In contrast, non-modifiable risk factors are those factors that cannot improve with intervention or any treatment [14, 43, 49]. However, most of the associated risk factors for falls and recurrent falls can be modified [42]. According to the American Geriatric Society/British Geriatric Society, modifiable fall risk factors include muscle weakness, imbalance, gait problems, polypharmacy, incontinence, mobility deficits, orthostatic hypotension, and syncope. In contrast, non-modifiable fall risk factors include age, female gender, history of prior falls, and certain chronic health conditions such as dementia, Parkinson's disease, and stroke.

The World Health Organization (WHO) classified risk factors for falls into four categories: biological, behavioral, environmental, and socioeconomic factors [26]. In their systematic review and meta-analysis, Li et al. [50] found depression, history of falls, visual impairment, age, balance disorders, female gender, fear of falling, and dementia as risk factors for falls. Other authors have reported risk factors for falls as a history of previous falls, gait alterations, osteoporosis, loss of functional capacity, fear of future falls, cardiovascular problems, fatigue, and the environment [51, 52]; depression [53, 54]; cognitive impairment [55]; urinary incontinence [54]; polypharmacy (use of ≥ four drugs) [46, 53, 56–58]; visual impairments [54]; use of ambulatory devices [53]; comorbidities [54, 56–58] female gender [42, 54, 59]; diabetes mellitus [42, 59, 60], presence of balance or gait problems or foot abnormalities, and use of antihypertensive [42].

There is an association between diminished balance and reduced physical functioning, plus an increased risk of falling among individuals over 65. Some environmental factors, for example, poor lighting, clutter in and around the house, and improper footwear, are also risks for falls among older persons [43]. Falls often result from a mixture of risk factors rather than a single cause. Identifying and addressing these risk factors through appropriate interventions that include exercise programmes can significantly reduce the risk of falls among older adults. The knowledge, understanding, and exploration of these risk factors would identify areas for improvement and inform targeted interventions that enhance fall prevention which is paramount to improving patient outcomes and reducing the burden of falls.

4. Therapeutic exercises in fall management

Therapeutic exercise is crucial in preventing falls among older adults and promoting their overall health and well-being. Exercise interventions incorporating balance and strength are often components of fall prevention strategies. The effort is usually toward alleviating the numerous debilitating consequences using interventional strategies to prevent falls [61] and improving the overall well-being of older adults. According to [62], prevention of falls can decrease morbidity and mortality among older adults. Sherington et al. [63] reported that interventions that pose an increasing challenge to balance at a higher dose have better fall prevention effects.

Therapeutic exercise programmes for fall prevention focus on improving strength, balance, flexibility, and coordination. Howe et al. [64], in their update of a Cochrane review, concluded that weak evidence supports gait, balance, coordination, and functional tasks, strengthening exercises in managing older adults for balance in 2007. Reduced balance is associated with reduced physical functioning and an increased risk of falling. 3D and multiple exercises were moderately practical immediately post-intervention for balance outcomes in older people [64]. Furthermore, there was insufficient evidence on general physical activity like walking and exercise involving computerized balance programmes or vibration plates [64].

Effective fall prevention strategies are multifactorial interventions targeting specific risk factors and exercises for muscle strengthening with balance training. Weidermann et al. [65], in their meta-analysis on exercise-based reduction of falls, concluded that physical activity and balance exercise are the most effective and rated isolated postural control above multifactorial approaches among community-dwelling older adults.

Research interest in fall prevention intervention began in the 1970s in developed countries. The Center for Disease Control and Prevention (CDC) included information on effective fall prevention interventions in the third edition of the Compendium [66]. Evidence shows that suitably and adequately recommended interventions can prevent falls [1]. Exercise is an evident preference as a fall prevention intervention because defective muscle strength and poor postural control increase fall risks but improve with exercise [64, 67]. Research shows that numerous studies have evaluated different exercise programmes to prevent falls. Exercise is a cost-effective fall prevention strategy [68] and is effective when delivered in a group or individualized setting [69].

The 4th edition of the Centers for Disease Control and Prevention (CDC) Compendium classifies single and multifaceted interventions [70]. Cuevas-Trisan [62] reported the effectiveness of multidimensional intervention strategies for falls. Multifaceted interventions that incorporate exercise have been proven effective in fall prevention. Multifaceted interventions include therapeutic exercise programmes for fall prevention, containing a combination of different forms of exercise to address multiple risk factors simultaneously. These programmes may include education on fall prevention strategies, such as home safety modifications and proper footwear. In their systematic review with meta-analysis, Hopewell et al. [71] reported that exercise is the most common component, including multifaceted interventions for preventing falls in older adults. Individually tailored fall prevention exercise programmes are more common than general programmes.

Multifaceted or multi-component interventions are designed to address multiple fall risk factors by providing participants with two or more individually tailored intervention plans following a pre-executed personalized fall risk assessment. These interventions may include components such as assistive technology, environmental assessment with modifications, quality improvement strategies, and basic fall risk assessments [70, 72]. These strategies had varied combinations of the following interventions: exercise, home/environmental assessment and modification, education, psychological interventions, medication modification/management, vision management, urinary incontinence management, fluid or nutrition therapy including calcium and vitamin D supplementation, sunlight exposure, surgery, referral to appropriate specialists, hip protection. Exercise management of falls is a common denominator often complemented by other interventions to create a comprehensive approach that addresses the broader factors contributing to falls.

A good number of studies with multifaceted intervention strategies have reported significant positive effects on falls [73–75]. Some other studies reported no significant impact of multifaceted interventions on falls [76, 77], while another study found no apparent overall effects of these interventions on falls [78]. A standard, consistent component of multiple interventions significantly associated with reducing the number of fallers and falls rate were exercise, assistive technology, environmental assessment with modifications, quality of life improvement strategies, and basic fall risk assessment. Multifaceted interventions were associated with a reduction in fall rate [RR 0.87; 95% CI 0.80–0.95] but not with a decrease in the number of fallers [RR 0.95; 95% CI 0.89–1.01] [79].

Exercise management of falls is a common denominator often complemented by other interventions to create a comprehensive approach that addresses the broader factors contributing to falls. Single intervention strategies for falls include exercises; cognitive behavioral therapies, environmental or home modification, cognitive-motor interference; manual therapy; virtual reality games; interactive-motor interventions, mind-body interventions involving meditative movements, podiatry, vision intervention, and fall hazard identifications [80–84]. Dautzenberg et al. [79], in a recent meta-analysis with 192 studies, said that single intervention exercises were significantly associated with a reduction in falls rate (RR 0.79; 95% CI 0.73–0.86).

According to the CDC compendium, some single intervention exercises for falls were reported: Simplified Tai Chi, Wolf, et al. [85]; Tai Chi: Moving for Better Balance, Li et al. [86]; The Otago Exercise Programme, Campbell et al. and Robertson et al. [87–89]; Adapted Physical Activity Programme, Kovacs et al. [90]; Freiberger et al. [91]; Falls Management Exercise [FAME] Intervention, Skelton et al. [92]; LiFE (Lifestyle Approach to Reducing Falls Through Exercise), Clemson et al. [93]; Multi-target Stepping Programme, Yamada, et al. [94]; Senior Fitness and Prevention [SEFIP], Kemmler et al. [95]; Stay Safe, Stay Active, Barnett et al. [96]; Strength and Exercise Programme, Kim et al. [97]; PreFalls (Prevent Falls) Programme, Siegrest et al. [98].

The Otago Exercise Programme [OEP] is widespread. It is one of the most tested fall prevention programs by the Centers for Disease Control and Prevention [20, 99]. OEP increases balance and strength, and decreases fall rates, with several other health benefits for older people [100], with a 35% reduction in falls proven [100].

In its original form, the exercise programme comprises individually tailored strength, balance, and endurance exercises plus home-based support, and additional follow-up by telephone over a total exercise period of 1 year. Exercises are performed three times per week, with extra walks twice weekly.

The OEP also positively affected health outcomes when performed two times per week [101]. Dadgari et al. [102] reported that in the experimental group, the mean fall incidence declined from 1.58 to 1.26 from pre- to post-intervention assessment, showing that the Otago exercise programme significantly reduced the incidence of falls. Findings from Kiik et al. [103] showed that the Otago training significantly reduced the risk of falling among the studied older adults ($p = 0.041$). The risk of falls in the intervention group decreased from 14.26 to 12.05 s and increased from 12.94 to 13.26 s in the control group. In their scoping review, Mgbeojedo et al. [104] reported that when the OEP was administered in either group setting or on an individualized basis, it effectively reduced falls. Additionally, balance, strength, mobility, and health-related quality of life within the community and institutionalized older adults were improved.

Regular walking has been suggested as a complement to increase physical activity levels [105]. However, for active and healthy older people with a low fall risk, the OEP's goal to reduce falls may not be sufficiently challenging [106]. This phenomenon highlights the importance of identifying older people who will benefit from fall prevention exercise programmes such as the OEP. The OEP is empirically supported single intervention for fall prevention: a stand-alone programme comprising four home visits over 8 weeks, according to the following schedule: weeks 1, 2, 4, and 8 [107]. It consists of leg muscle strengthening, balance retraining exercises progressing in difficulty, and a walking plan. Each person receives a booklet with instructions for each exercise prescribed and ankle cuff weights (starting at 1 kg) to provide resistance for the strengthening exercises. The OEP programme takes about 30 minutes to complete. To help them adhere to the programme, participants record the days they end it, and the instructor telephones them each month between home visits. Follow-up home visits are conducted every 6 months.

The key components of therapeutic exercise are balance and stability exercises which aim to improve balance and stability by targeting the core muscles, and the lower body. Strengthening exercises for muscle strength are essential for maintaining balance and stability. Stretching exercises help improve and maintain flexibility and range of motion in joints, which enhance mobility, and reduce the risk of falls, progressive challenges, and task-specific training. Task-specific training involves practicing daily activities that older adults commonly encounter, such as stepping over obstacles, reaching for objects, or navigating stairs. These exercises reduce the risk of falls among older adults and have been effective in multifaceted and single programmes with an individual approach.

5. Conclusion

Falls are a significant public health concern. Individualized and multifaceted exercise programmes are essential fall prevention strategies, reducing fall risk and improving the overall well-being of older adults. The current trend in exercise management of falls among older adults focuses on evidence-based and multifaceted approaches that integrate various components to address multiple risk factors tailored to individual needs. Despite the efforts in place, fall prevalence continues to increase globally. One in three older adults falls once a year, one in four are recurrent fallers, and older adults experience fear of falling with or without a history of falling. This trend warrants public health attention globally. Assessing the risks of falls as part of routine health care for older adults is necessary.

Author details

Olubusola Johnson[1*], Christopher Akosile[2], Emeka Mong[3] and Ukamaka Mgbeojedo[4]

1 Obafemi Awolowo University, Nigeria

2 Nnamdi Azikiwe University, Nigeria

3 Ebonyi State University, Nigeria

4 University of Nigeria, Nigeria

*Address all correspondence to: obnik2001@gmail.com

References

[1] Gillespie LD, Robertson MC, Gillespie WJ, et al. Interventions for preventing falls in older people living in the community. Cochrane Database Systematic Review. 2012;(9):Cd007146

[2] King AC, King DK. Physical activity for an aging population. Public Health Review. 2010;**32**:401-426. DOI: 10.1007/BF03391609

[3] Rao SS. Prevention of falls in older patients. American Family Physician. 2005;**72**:81-88

[4] Tinetti MESM, Ginter SF. Risk factors for falls among elderly persons living in the community. New England Journal of Medicine. 1988;**319**:1701-1707

[5] Campbell AJ, Borrie MJ, Spears GF, Jackson SL, Brown JS, Fitzgerald JL. Circumstances, and consequences of falls experienced by a community population 70 years and over during a prospective study. Age and Ageing. 1990;**19**:136-141

[6] Burns ER, Stevens JA, Lee R. The direct costs of fatal and non-fatal falls among older adults — United States. Journal of Safety Research. 2016;**58**:99-103

[7] Akosile CO, Odidika FJ, Okoye EC, Odole AC, Mgbeojedo UG, Fabunmi AA, et al. Physical function, fear of falling, occupational status and falls in a Nigerian older adults sample. Ageing International. 2015;**40**:327-337. DOI: 10.1007/s12126-014-9202-2

[8] Bergen G, Stevens MR, Burns ER. Falls and fall injuries among adults aged ≥65 years - United States, 2014. MMWR Morbidity and Mortality Weekly Report. 2016;**23**(65):993-998. DOI: 10.1007/s12126-014-9202-2

[9] Bagiartana KDA, Huriah TA. Systematic review of the effectiveness of tai chi exercises for improving balance and lower limb muscle strength of the elderly in the community. Open Access Macedonian Journal of Medical Sciences. 2021;**10**:6-12. Available from: https://oamjms.eu/index.php/mjms/article/view/7841

[10] Tinetti ME, Mendes de Leon CF, Doucette JT, Baker DI. Fear of falling and fall-related efficacy in relationship to functioning among community-living elders. Journal of Gerontololgy. 1994;**49**:140-147. DOI: 10.1093/geronj/49.3.m140

[11] Stalenhoef PA, Diederiks JP, Knottnerus JA, Kester AD, Crebolder HF. A risk model for the prediction of recurrent falls in community-dwelling elderly: A prospective cohort study. Journal of Clinical Epidemiology. 2002;**55**:1088-1094. DOI: 10.1016/s0895-4356(02)00502-4

[12] O'Loughlin JL, Robitaille Y, Boivin J, Suissa S. Incidence of and risk factors for falls and injurious falls among the community-dwelling elderly. American Journal of Epidemiology. 1993;**137**:342-354

[13] Park SH. Tools for assessing fall risk in the elderly: A systematic review and meta-analysis. Aging Clinical and Experimental Research. 2018;**30**:1-16. DOI: 10.1007/s40520-017-0749-0

[14] Deandrea S, Lucenteforte E, Bravi F, Foschi R, La Vecchia C, Negri E. Risk factors for falls in community-dwelling older people: A systematic review and meta-analysis. Epidemiology. 2010;**21**:658-668. DOI: 10.1097/EDE.0b013e3181e89905

[15] Rubenstein LZ. Falls in older people: Epidemiology, risk factors and strategies for prevention. Age and Ageing. 2006;**35**:ii37-ii41. DOI: 10.1093/ageing/afl084

[16] Akosile CO, Anukam GO, Johnson OE, Fabunmi AA, Okoye EC, Iheukwumere N, et al. Fear of falling and quality of life of apparently healthy elderly individuals from a Nigerian population. Journal of Cross-Cultural Gerontology. 2014;**29**:201-209. DOI: 10.1007/s10823-014-9228-7

[17] Akosile CO, Igwemmad CK, Okoye EC, et al. Physical activity level, fear of falling and quality of life: A comparison between community-dwelling and assisted-living older adults. BMC Geriatry. 2021;**21**:12. DOI: 10.1186/s12877-020-01982-1

[18] Florence CS, Bergen G, Atherly A, Burns E, Stevens J, Drake C. Medical costs of fatal and nonfatal falls in older adults. Journal of the American Geriatrics Society. 2018;**66**:693-698. DOI: 10.1111/jgs.15304

[19] Sun M, Min L, Xu N, Huang L, Li X. The effect of exercise intervention on reducing the fall risk in older adults: A meta-analysis of randomized controlled trials. International Journal of Environmental Research and Public Health. 2021;**29**(18):12562. DOI: 10.3390/ijerph182312562

[20] Martins AC, Santos C, Silva C, Baltazar D, Moreira J, Tavares N. Does modified Otago exercise program improve balance in older people? A systematic review. Preventive Medicine Reports. 2018;**11**:231-239. DOI: 10.1016/j.pmedr.2018.06.015

[21] Kyrdalen IL, Thingstad P, Sandvik L, Ormstad H. Associations between gait speed and well-known fall risk factors among community-dwelling older adults. Physiotherapy Research International Journal. 2018;**24**:e1743. DOI: 10.1002/pri.1743

[22] Galloza J, Castillo B, Micheo W. Benefits of exercise in the older population. Physical Medicine and Rehabilitation Clinics. 2017;**28**:659-669. DOI: 10.1016/j.pmr.2017.06.001

[23] Del Brutto OH, Mera RM, Peinado CD, Sedler MJ. Prevalence, severity, and risk of future falls in community-dwelling older adults living in a rural community: The Atahualpa project. Journal of Community Health. 2019;**44**:487-491

[24] Masud T, Morris RO. Epidemiology of falls. Age and Ageing. 2001;**30**(S4):3-7. DOI: 10.1093/ageing/30.suppl_4.3

[25] Nabavi SH, Hatami ST, Norouzi F, Gerivani Z, Hatami SE, Monadi Ziarat H, et al. Prevalence of fall and its related factors among older people in Bojnurd in 2015. Salmand Iran Journal of Ageing. 2016;**11**:466-473

[26] World Health Organization. WHO global report on falls prevention in older age: Ageing WHO. Unit LC. 2008

[27] Luang-Ubol T, Thiabrithi S, Glangkarn S, Promasatayaprot V. Prevalence of fall and associated risk factors among older adults in Thailand. Journal of Southwest Jiaotong University. 2021;56:713-720

[28] Dhargave P, Sendhilkumar R. Prevalence of risk factors for falls among older people people living in long-term care homes. Journal of Clinical Gerontology and Geriatrics. 2016;7:99-103

[29] Salari N, Darvishi N, Ahmadipanah M, Shohaimi S,

Mohammadi M. Global prevalence of falls in the older adults: A comprehensive systematic review and meta-analysis. Journal of Orthopaedic Surgery and Research. 2022;**17**:334. DOI: 10.1186/s13018-022-03222-1

[30] Demura S, Yamada T, Kasuga K. Severity of injuries associated with falls in the community dwelling older people are not affected by fall characteristics and physical function level. Archive of Gerontology Geriatrics. 2012;**55**:186-189

[31] Tanaka T, Matsumoto H, Son BK, Imaeda S, Uchiyama E, Taniguchi S, et al. Environmental and physical factors predisposing middle-aged and older Japanese adults to falls and fall-related fractures in the home. Geriatrics and Gerontology International. 2018;**18**:1372-1377

[32] Siqueira FV, Facchini LA, Piccini RX, Tomasi E, Thumé E, Silveira DS, et al. Prevalence of falls and associated factors in the elderly. Revista de Saúde Pública. 2007;**41**:749-756

[33] Center for Disease Control and Prevention. Older adult fall prevention. 2023. Available from: https://www.cdc.gov/falls/index.html

[34] United Nations (UN) (2004). World Population Prospects: The 2004 Revision. New York, USA. Population Ageing in the WHO Global Report on Falls Prevention Older Persons. France: WHO; 2007. p. 3

[35] Bekibele CO, Gureje O. Fall incidence in a population of older people persons in Nigeria. Gerontology. 2010;**56**:278-283. DOI: 10.1159/000236327

[36] Oladele A, Atoyebi OA, Elegbede O, Babatunde OA, Adewoye K, Durowade K, et al. Prevalence and risk factors for falls in urban and rural older adults in Ekiti state, Nigeria. Ghana Medical Journal. 2021;**55**:265-272. DOI: 10.4314/gmj.v55i4.6

[37] Akosile CO, Agu CU, Adegoke BOA, Okoye EC, Okeke IA, Emeahara G. Physical activity, fear of falling, and falls in Nigerian older adults. The International Journal of Aging and Society. 2014;**3**:26-37. DOI: 10.18848/2160-1909/CGP/v03i02/35240

[38] Adanusa M, Pobee SK, Zaabaar E, Mawuko V, Asiedu K, Amuzu SK, et al. Prevalence and risk factors for falls among older adults in a primary care facility in Ghana. Malawi Medical Journal. 2022;**34**:225-230. DOI: 10.4314/mmj.v34i4.1

[39] Allain TJ, Mwambelo M, Mdolo T, Mfune P. Falls and other geriatric syndromes in Blantyre, Malawi: A community survey of older adults. Malawi Medical Journal. 2014;**26**(4):105-108

[40] Thomas SM, Parker A, Fortune J, Mitchell G, Hezam A, Jiang Y, et al. Global evidence on falls and subsequent social isolation in older adults: A scoping review. BMJ Open. 2022;**12**(9):e062124. DOI: 10.1136/bmjopen-2022-062124

[41] Carrasco C, Tomas-Carus P, Bra-vo J, Pereira C, Mendes F. Understanding fall risk factors in community-dwelling older adults: A cross-sectional study. International Journal of Older People Nursing. 2019:1-10. e12294. DOI: 10.1111/opn.12294

[42] Gamage N, Rathnayake N, Alwis G. Prevalence, and associated risk factors of falls among rural community-dwelling older people: A cross-sectional study from southern Sri Lanka. Current Gerontology and Geriatrics Research. 2019;(1). Article ID: 2370796. DOI: 10.1155/2019/2370796

[43] Ambrose AF, Paul G, Hausdorff JM. Risk factors for falls among older persons: A review of the literature. Maturitas. 2013;**75**:51-61. DOI: 10.1016/j.maturitas.2013.02.009

[44] Ooi TC, Singh D, Shahar S, et al. Incidence and multidimensional predictors of occasional and recurrent falls among Malaysian community-dwelling older persons. BMC Geriatrics. 2021;**21**:154. DOI: 10.1186/s12877-021-02103-2

[45] American Geriatrics Society. British geriatrics society and American Academy of orthopaedic surgeons panel on falls prevention. Guideline for the prevention of falls in older persons. Journal of the American Geriatrics Society. 2001;**49**:664-672

[46] Pfortmueller CA, Lindner G, Exadaktylos AK. Reducing fall risk in the elderly: Risk factors and fall prevention, a systematic review. Minerva Medica. 2014;**105**:275-281

[47] Najafi-Ghezeljeh T, Ghasemifard F, Jafari-Oori M. The effects of a multicomponent fall prevention intervention on fall prevalence, depression, and balance among nursing home residents. Nursing and Midwifery Studies. 2019;**8**:78-84

[48] Vu HM, Nguyen LH, Nguyen HLT, Vu GT, Nguyen CT, Hoang TN, et al. Individual and environmental factors associated with recurrent falls in elderly patients hospitalized after falls. International Journal of Environmental Research and Public Health. 2020;**17**:2441

[49] Finlayson ML, Peterson EW. Falls, aging and disability. Physical Medicine and Rehabilitation Clinics. 2010;**21**:357-373

[50] Li Y, Hou L, Zhao H, Xie R, Yi Y, Ding X. Risk factors for falls among community-dwelling older adults: A systematic review and meta-analysis. Frontiers in Medicine. 2023;**9**:1019094. DOI: 10.3389/fmed.2022.1019094

[51] Duarte GP, Santos JLF, Lebrão ML, Duarte YADO. Relationship of falls among the elderly and frailty components. Revista Brasileira de Epidemiologia. 2019;**21**:e180017

[52] Granbom M, Clemson L, Roberts L, Hladek MD, Okoye SM, Liu M, et al. Preventing falls among older fallers: Study protocol for a two-phase pilot study of the multicomponent LIVE LiFE program. Trials. 2019;**20**:2

[53] Pellicer-García B, Antón-Solanas I, Ramón-Arbués E, García-Moyano L, Gea-Caballero V, Juárez-Vela R. Risk of falling and associated factors in older adults with a previous history of falls. International Journal of Environmental Research and Public Health. 2020;**17**:4085. DOI: 10.3390/ijerph17114085

[54] Tsai Y-J, Yang P-Y, Yang Y-C, Lin M-R, Wang Y-W. Prevalence, and risk factors of falls among community-dwelling older people: Results from three consecutive waves of the national health interview survey in Taiwan. BMC Geriatrics. 2020;**20**:529. DOI: 10.1186/s12877-020-01922-z

[55] Blackwood J, Martin A. Screening for cognitive impairment as a part of falls risk assessment in physical therapist practice. Journal of Geriatric Physical Therapy. 2017;**40**:197-203

[56] Ahmadiahangar A, Javadian Y, Babaei M, Heidari B, Hosseini S, Aminzadeh M. The role of quadriceps muscle strength in the development of falls in the elderly people, a cross-sectional study. Chiropractic and Manual Therapies. 2018;**26**:31. DOI: 10.1186/s12998-018-0195-x

[57] Esain I, Rodriguez-Larrad A, Bidaurrazaga-Letona I, Gil SM. Health-related quality of life, handgrip strength and falls during detraining in elderly habitual exercisers. Health and Quality of Life Outcomes. 2017;**15**:226. DOI: 10.1186/s12955-017-0800-z

[58] Gafner SC, Bastiaenen CH, Ferrari S, Gold G, Terrier P, Hilfiker R, et al. Hip muscle and hand-grip strength to differentiate between older fallers and non-fallers: A cross-sectional validity study. Clinical Interventions in Aging. 2017;**13**:1-8. DOI: 10.2147/CIA.S146834

[59] Hsu H, Jhan L. Risk factors of falling among the elderly in Taiwan: A longitudinal study. Taiwan Geriatrics and Gerontology. 2008;**3**:141-154

[60] Paliwal Y, Slattum PW, Ratliff SM. Chronic health conditions as a risk factor for falls among the community-dwelling US older persons: A zero-inflated regres-sion modeling approach. Biomed Research International. 2017;(2):5146378

[61] Okoye EC, Akosile CO, Maruf FA, Onwuakagba IU, Mgbeojedo UG. Falls and fear of falling among older adults in an assisted-living facility: A qualitative and foundational study for intervention development in a developing country. Archives of Gerontology and Geriatrics. 2021;**94**:104375. DOI: 10.1016/j.archger.2021.104375

[62] Cuevas-Trisan R. Balance problems and fall risks in the elderly. Physical Medicine and Rehabilitation Clinics of North America. 2017;**28**:727-737. DOI: 10.1016/j.pmr.2017.06.006

[63] Sherrington C, Michaleff ZA, Fairhall N, Paul SS, Tiedemann A, Whitney J, et al. Exercise to prevent falls in older adults: An updated systematic review and meta-analysis. British Journal of Sports Medicine. 2017;**51**:1750-1758. DOI: 10.1136/bjsports-2016-096547

[64] Howe TE, Rochester L, Neil F, Skelton DA, Ballinger C. Exercise for improving balance in older people. The Cochrane Database of Systematic Reviews. 2011;**9**:CD004963. DOI: 10.1002/14651858.CD004963.pub3

[65] Wiedenmann T, Held S, Rappelt L, Grauduszus M, Spickermann S, Donath L. Exercise based reduction of falls in communitydwelling older adults: A network meta-analysis. European Review of Aging and Physical Activity. 2023;**20**:1. DOI: 10.1186/s11556-023-00311-w

[66] Stevens JA, Burns ER. A CDC Compendium of Effective Fall Interventions: What Works for Community-Dwelling Older Adults. 3rd ed. Vol. 58. Atlanta, GA: Centers for Disease Control and Prevention, National Center for Injury Prevention and Control; 2015. pp. 99-103

[67] Liu CJ, Latham NK. Progressive resistance strength training for improving physical function in older adults. Cochrane Database Systematic Reviews. 2009;**2009**(3):CD002759. DOI: 10.1002/14651858.CD002759.pub2

[68] Davis JC, Robertson MC, Ashe MC, Liu-Ambrose T, Khan KM, Marra CA. Does a home-based strength and balance programme in people aged > or =80 years provide the best value for money to prevent falls? A systematic review of economic evaluations of falls prevention interventions. British Journal of Sports Medicine. 2010;**44**:80-89. DOI: 10.1136/bjsm.2008.060988

[69] Sherrington C, Fairhall N, Wallbank G, Tiedemann A, Michaleff ZA, Howard K, et al. Exercise for preventing falls in older people living

in the community: An abridged Cochrane systematic review. British Journal of Sports Medicine. 2020;**54**:885-891. DOI: 10.1136/bjsports-2019-101512

[70] Burns ER, Kakara R, Moreland B. A CDC Compendium of Effective Fall Interventions: What Works for Community-Dwelling Older Adults. 4th ed. Centers for Disease Control and Prevention, National Center for Injury Prevention and Control: Atlanta, GA; 2022

[71] Hopewell S, Copsey B, Nicolson P, Adedire B, Boniface G, Lamb S. Multifactorial interventions for preventing falls in older people living in the community: A systematic review and meta-analysis of 41 trials and almost 20000 participants. British Journal of Sports Medicine. 2020;**54**:1340-1350. DOI: 10.1136/bjsports-2019-100732

[72] Hopewell S, Adedire O, Copsey BJ, et al. Multifactorial and multiple component interventions for preventing falls in older people living in the community (review). Cochrane Database Systematic Review. 2018;7:1-307. DOI: 10.1002/14651858. CD012221. pub2

[73] Clemson L, Cumming RG, Kendig H, Swann M, Heard R, Taylor K. The effectiveness of a community-based program for reducing the incidence of falls in the elderly: A randomized trial. Journal of American Geriatric Society. 2004;**52**:1487-1494. DOI: 10.1111/j.1532-5415.2004.52411

[74] Palvanen M, Kannus P, Piirtola M, Niemi S, Parkkari J, Järvinen M. Effectiveness of the chaos falls clinic in preventing falls and injuries of home-dwelling older adults: A randomized controlled trial. Injury. 2014;**45**:265-271

[75] Szanton SL, Clemson L, Liu M, Gitlin LN, Hladek MD, LaFave SE, et al. Pilot outcomes of a multicomponent fall risk program integrated into daily lives of community-dwelling older adults. Journal of Applied Gerontology. 2020;**40**:320-327. DOI: 10.1177/0733464820912664

[76] Dillon L, Clemson L, Coxon K, et al. Understanding the implementation and efficacy of a home-based strength and balance fall prevention intervention in people aged 50 years or over with vision impairment: A process evaluation protocol. BMC Health Services Research. 2018;**18**:512. DOI: 10.1186/s12913-018-3304-6

[77] Morello RT, Soh SE, Behm K, Egan A, Ayton D, Hill K, et al. Multifactorial falls prevention programmes for older adults presenting to the emergency department with a fall: Systematic review and meta-analysis. Injury Prevention. 2019;**25**:557-564

[78] Gates S, Fisher JD, Cooke MW, Carter YH, Lamb SE. Multifactorial assessment, and targeted intervention for preventing falls and injuries among older people in community and emergency care settings: Systematic review and meta-analysis. British Medical Journal. 2008;**336**:130. DOI: 10.1136/bmj.39412.525243.BE

[79] Dautzenberg L, Beglinger S, Tsokani S, Zevgiti S, Raijmann RCMA, Rodondi N, et al. Interventions for preventing falls and fall-related fractures in community-dwelling older adults: A systematic review and network meta-analysis. Journal of the American Geriatric Society. 2021;**69**:2973-2984. DOI: 10.1111/jgs.17375

[80] Holt KR, Haavik H, Elley CR. The effects of manual therapy on balance and falls: A systematic review. Journal of Manipulative and Physiological Therapeutics. 2012;**35**:227-234

[81] Schoene D, Valenzuela T, Lord SR, de Bruin ED. The effect of interactive cognitive-motor training in reducing fall risk in older people: A systematic review. BMC Geriatrics. 2014;**14**:1-22

[82] Wang X, Pi Y, Chen P, Liu Y, Wang R, Chan C. Cognitive motor interference for preventing falls in older adults: A systematic review and meta-analysis of randomised controlled trials. Age and Ageing. 2015;**44**:205-212

[83] Wylie G, Torrens C, Campbell P, Frost H, Gordon AL, Menz HB, et al. Podiatry interventions to prevent falls in older people: A systematic review and meta-analysis. Age and Ageing. 2019;**48**:327-336

[84] Weber M, Schnorr T, Morat M, Morat T, Donath L. Effects of mind–body interventions involving meditative movements on quality of life, depressive symptoms, fear of falling and sleep quality in older adults: A systematic review with meta-analysis. International Journal of Environmental Research and Public Health. 2020;**17**:6556

[85] Wolf SL, Barnhart HX, Kutner NG, McNeely E, Coogler C, Xu T. Reducing frailty and falls in older persons: An investigation of tai chi and computerized balance training. Journal of the American Geriatrics Society. 1996;**44**(5):489-497

[86] Li F, Harmer P, Fisher KJ, McAuley E, Chaumeton N, Eckstrom E, et al. Tai chi and fall reductions in older adults: A randomized controlled trial. Journal of Gerontology. 2005;**60A**:187-194

[87] Campbell AJ, Robertson MC, Gardner MM, Norton RN, Tilyard MW, Buchner DM. Randomized controlled trial of a general practice programme of home-based exercise to prevent falls in elderly women. British Medical Journal. 1997;**315**:1065-1069

[88] Campbell AJ, Robertson MC, Gardner MM, Norton RN, Buchner DM. Falls prevention over 2 years: A randomized controlled trial in women 80 years and older. Age and Ageing. 1999;**28**:513-518

[89] Campbell AJ, Robertson MC, La Grow SJ, Kerse NM, Sanderson GF, Jacobs RJ, et al. Randomized controlled trial of prevention of falls in people aged ≥75 with severe visual impairment: The VIP trial. British Medical Journal. 2005;**331**:817-820

[90] Kovács E, Prókai L, Mészáros L, Gondos T. Adapted physical activity is beneficial on balance, functional mobility, quality of life and fall risk in community-dwelling older women: A randomized single-blinded controlled trial. European Journal of Physical and Rehabilitation Medicine. 2013;**49**:301-310

[91] Freiberger E, Menz HB, Abu-Omar K, Rütten A. Preventing falls in physically active community-dwelling older people: A comparison of two intervention techniques. Gerontology. 2007;**53**:298-305

[92] Skelton D, Dinan S, Campbell M, Rutherford O. Tailored group exercise (falls management exercise—FaME) reduces falls in community-dwelling older frequent fallers (an RCT). Age and Ageing. 2005;**34**(6):636-639

[93] Clemson L, Fiatarone Singh MA, Bundy A, Cumming RG, Manollaras K, O'Loughlin P, et al. Integration of balance and strength training into daily life activity to reduce rate of falls in older people (the LiFE study): Randomized parallel trial. British Medical Journal (Clinical Research Ed). 2012;**345**:e4547

[94] Yamada M, Higuchi T, Nishiguchi S, Yoshimura K, Kajiwara Y, Aoyama T. Multi-target

stepping program in combination with a standardized multicomponent exercise program can prevent falls in community-dwelling older adults: A randomized, controlled trial. Journal of the American Geriatrics Society. 2013;**61**:1669-1675

[95] Kemmler W, von Stengel S, Engelke K, Häberle L, Kalender WA. Exercise effects on bone mineral density, falls, coronary risk factors, and health care costs in older women: The randomized controlled senior fitness and prevention (SEFIP) study. Archives of Internal Medicine. 2010;**170**:179-185

[96] Barnett A, Smith B, Lord S, Williams M, Baumand A. Community-based group exercise improves balance and reduces falls in at-risk older people: A randomized controlled trial. Age and Ageing. 2003;**32**:407-414

[97] Kim H, Yoshida H, Suzuki T. Falls, and fractures in participants and excluded non-participants of a fall prevention exercise program for elderly women with a history of falls: 1-year follow-up study. Geriatrics Gerontology International. 2014;**14**:285-292

[98] Siegrist M, Freiberger E, Geilhof B, et al. Fall prevention in a primary care setting: The effects of a targeted complex exercise intervention in a cluster randomized trial. Deutsches Ärzteblatt International. 2016;**113**:365-372

[99] Stevens JA. A CDC Compendium of Effective Fall Interventions: What Works for Community-Dwelling Older Adults. Corporate Authors(s): National Center for Injury Prevention and Control (U.S.). Division of Unin-tentional Injury Prevention. Atlanta, Georgia: Division of Unintentional Injury Prevention National Center for Injury Pre-vention and Control Centers for Disease Control and Prevention (CDC); 2010. Available from: https://stacks.cdc.gov/view/cdc/25333

[100] Robertson MC, Campbell AJ, Gardner MM, Devlin N. Preventing injuries in older people by preventing falls: A meta-analysis of individual-level data. Journal of the American Geriatrics Society. 2002;**50**(5):905-911. DOI: 10.1046/j.1532-5415.2002.50218.x

[101] Thomas S, Mackintosh S, Halbert J. Does the 'Otago exercise programme' reduce mortality and falls in older adults? A systematic review and meta-analysis. Age and Ageing. 2010;**39**(6):681-687. DOI: 10.1093/ageing/afq102

[102] Dadgari A, Aizan Hamid T, Hakim MN, Chaman R, Mousavi SA, Poh Hin L, et al. Randomized control trials on Otago exercise program (OEP) to reduce falls among elderly community dwellers in Shahroud, Iran. Iran Red Crescent Medical Journal. 2016;**18**:e26340. DOI: 10.5812/ircmj.26340

[103] Kiik SM, Vanchapo AR, Elfrida MF, Nuwa MS, Sakinah S. Effectiveness of Otago exercise on health status and risk of fall among elderly with chronic illness. Jurnal Keperawatan Indonesia. 2020;**23**:15-22

[104] Mgbeojedo UG, Akosile CO, Oko-ye EC, Ani KU, Ekechukwu EN, Okezue OC, et al. Effects of Otago exercise program on physical and psychosocial functions among community-dwelling and institutionalized older adults: A scoping review. Inquiry The Journal of Health Care Organization, Provision, and Financing. 2023;**60**:1-16. DOI: 10.1177/00469580231165858

[105] Sherrington C, Tiedemann A, Fairhall N, Close JC, Lord SR. Exercise to prevent falls in older adults: An updated meta-analysis and best practice recommendations. NSW Public Health Bulletin. 2011;**22**:78-83. DOI: 10.1071/NB10056

[106] Gawler S, Skelton DA, Dinan-Young S, Masud T, Morris RW, Griffin M, et al. ProAct65+ team. Reducing falls among older people in general practice: The ProAct65+ exercise intervention trial. Archives of Gerontology and Geriatrics. 2016;**67**:46-54. DOI: 10.1016/j.archger.2016.06.019

[107] Wetherell JL, Johnson K, Chang D, Ward SR, Bower ES, Merz C. Petkus for fear of falling. International Journal of Geriatric Psychiatry. 2016;**31**:791-798. DOI: 10.1002/gps.4393

Chapter 10

Orthopedic Applications: Advancing Physiotherapy in Musculoskeletal Health

Harshavardhan Sai Sadineni

Abstract

Orthopedic physiotherapy is pivotal in musculoskeletal healthcare, addressing diverse musculoskeletal system conditions. This article provides a comprehensive overview of orthopedic physiotherapy, covering historical evolution, evidence-based principles, diagnostic assessments, therapeutic modalities, exercise prescriptions, post-operative considerations, specialized interventions, technological integration, and patient education. It emphasizes the criticality of evidence-based practice, diagnostic precision, and tailored rehabilitation regimens in achieving optimal patient outcomes. Integrating technology, including advanced imaging modalities and wearable devices, enhances diagnostics, treatment planning, and patient engagement. Patient education and self-management strategies empower individuals to participate in their rehabilitation journey actively. This article underscores the evolving landscape of orthopedic physiotherapy, with ongoing collaboration between clinicians, researchers, and technology reshaping musculoskeletal healthcare.

Keywords: orthopedic physiotherapy, musculoskeletal disorders, evidence-based practice, technological integration, patient education

1. Introduction

Orthopedic physiotherapy is a pivotal branch within the broader field of physiotherapeutic practice, focused on assessing, diagnosing, and managing musculoskeletal disorders, involving a comprehensive approach to restoring optimal function, relieving pain, and improving the quality of life for individuals afflicted by a vast array of orthopedic conditions.

Ancient Greece is a foundational period, with luminaries like Hippocrates acknowledging the pivotal role of movement and exercise in joint health. In this era, specific exercises, massage techniques, and hydrotherapy were prescribed to address musculoskeletal issues, such as joint dislocations and fractures. Fast-forward to the nineteenth and early twentieth centuries, and we encounter remarkable pioneers who propelled orthopedic physiotherapy into a formalized medical specialty. Sister Elizabeth Kenny in Australia and Thomas Bertrand in the United States made pioneering contributions. Sister Kenny introduced groundbreaking techniques, particularly for polio treatment [1].

The mid-twentieth century they have marked another key juncture, with influential figures like Dr. James Cyriax in the United Kingdom playing a central role in advancing the field. Dr. Cyriax's work significantly contributed to understanding musculoskeletal conditions and developing specialized manual therapy techniques [2]. These innovations laid a solid foundation for the precise diagnosis and targeted interventions that define orthopedic physiotherapy today.

In recent years, technology has profoundly influenced orthopedic physiotherapy. Tools such as wearable devices, virtual reality simulations, and telehealth platforms have expanded treatment options and patient engagement. In this era of patient-centered care, patient education holds immense importance, comprising proper body mechanics, ergonomics, lifestyle modifications, and strategies to minimize the risk of injury or exacerbation of symptoms.

2. Understanding musculoskeletal disorders

Musculoskeletal disorders (MSDs) represent a broad spectrum of pathological conditions that affect bones, joints, muscles, tendons, ligaments, and connective tissues. The symptoms exhibited by individuals with MSDs are as diverse as the conditions themselves. For instance, Osteoarthritis (OA), the most common form of arthritis, frequently presents with symptoms such as joint pain (arthralgia), crepitus (crackling or grinding sensations within the joint), stiffness, and a gradual loss of joint cartilage, which results in joint space narrowing. As OA advances, patients may also experience joint stiffness after rest periods, often called the "gelling phenomenon," and joint effusion due to synovial inflammation [3].

This condition is further marked by functional impairment, including reduced range of motion and muscle weakness, along with the development of osteophytes (bony outgrowths) at joint margins. In contrast, Rheumatoid Arthritis (RA), an autoimmune MSD, manifests with symptoms such as joint inflammation (synovitis) leading to symmetric polyarthritis (affecting multiple joints on both sides of the body), morning stiffness that lasts for more than 30 minutes, and joint deformities resulting from the erosion of cartilage and bone. Patients with RA may also experience systemic symptoms, including fatigue, fever, and extra-articular manifestations, encompassing rheumatoid nodules, vasculitis, and lung involvement.

Musculoskeletal disorders (MSDs) constitute a substantial global health burden, affecting over 1.3 billion people worldwide and ranking as the leading cause of disability, leading to 121.3 thousand deaths and 138.7 million Disability-adjusted life years (DALYs), according to the World Health Organization (WHO) [4]. The direct and indirect economic costs associated with MSDs were $1.5 and $1.1 billion in 2007 [5]. Moreover, studies have shown that individuals suffering from chronic MSDs experience reduced mobility, increased pain, and diminished overall quality of life.

One of the primary categories of MSDs is degenerative disorders. Among these conditions, osteoarthritis is a highly prevalent musculoskeletal disorder, making it one of the most common joint diseases. Its significance lies in its substantial contribution to pain, disability, and economic costs. Osteoarthritis primarily affects weight-bearing joints such as the hips, knees, and spine. Another degenerative disorder is degenerative disk disease, which affects the intervertebral disks of the spine, causing chronic back pain and potential nerve compression.

Inflammatory disorders, such as rheumatoid arthritis, arise from an autoimmune response targeting the synovial membranes of joints. This results in inflammation, pain, swelling, and joint deformities. Rheumatoid arthritis has systemic effects, impacting multiple organs and systems beyond the joints. Ankylosing spondylitis, another inflammatory disorder, predominantly affects the spine, leading to spinal fusion, reduced mobility, and postural abnormalities, such as an exaggerated forward stoop known as kyphosis and the loss of the normal lumbar curvature (lordosis), which can significantly impact an individual's quality of life and daily functioning.

Acute and chronic traumatic injuries contribute significantly to the spectrum of MSDs. Fractures, dislocations, sprains, and strains can result from accidents, sports injuries, or repetitive overuse. These injuries often require comprehensive management to ensure proper healing, restore function, and prevent long-term complications. Tendonitis and tenosynovitis, characterized by inflammation of tendons and their surrounding structures, encompass various types and examples. Achilles tendonitis, affecting the Achilles tendon at the back of the ankle, and lateral epicondylitis, commonly known as tennis elbow, are well-recognized forms. Additionally, de Quervain's tenosynovitis, impacting the tendons of the thumb, and rotator cuff tendonitis, affecting the shoulder, are among the frequently encountered variations of these chronic overuse injuries.

Alignment and postural disorders are also noteworthy contributors to MSDs. Conditions such as scoliosis, kyphosis, and lordosis involve abnormal spinal curvature, often leading to asymmetry, pain, and compromised respiratory function. Poor posture, frequently exacerbated by prolonged periods of sitting and excessive screen use, can result in muscle imbalances that lead to specific limitations. These limitations often include a decreased range of motion in joints, particularly in the neck, shoulders, and lower back, and compromised spinal alignment, resulting in conditions like forward head posture or increased thoracic kyphosis. Such postural issues can escalate into chronic pain, including neck and back pain, headaches, and shoulder discomfort.

Understanding the pathophysiology of MSDs is essential for effective management. Genetic predisposition, biomechanical factors, systemic inflammation, and environmental influences contribute to the development of these disorders. Inflammation causes the initiation and progression of numerous musculoskeletal disorders. This cascade begins with releasing inflammatory cytokines, such as Tumor necrosis factor-alpha (TNF-α) and Interleukin-1 beta (IL-1β), often triggered by factors like tissue injury or infection. These cytokines serve as signaling molecules, attracting immune cells, primarily neutrophils and macrophages, to the site of injury or inflammation.

Upon arrival, immune cells release enzymes like Matrix metalloproteinases (MMPs) and inflammatory mediators, perpetuating tissue damage by degrading extracellular matrix components like collagen and proteoglycans in joint cartilage. Simultaneously, activated immune cells can initiate an autoimmune response, as observed in conditions like rheumatoid arthritis, where immune cells mistakenly target and attack synovial tissues.

Furthermore, the inflammatory milieu within affected joints amplifies pain signaling. Nociceptive nerve endings become sensitized due to the release of substances like bradykinin and prostaglandins, heightening pain perception. Additionally, the inflammatory process can lead to the formation of pannus, an invasive synovial tissue, which erodes cartilage and bone, altering joint structures and exacerbating functional impairment. These molecular and cellular interactions emphasize the need for targeted anti-inflammatory therapies in their management.

Diagnosing and managing MSDs involves a comprehensive approach, including clinical evaluation, imaging studies, and laboratory tests. Clinical assessments encompass history-taking, physical exams, and functional tests to identify impairments and their impact. Imaging techniques like X-rays, Magnetic resonance imaging (MRI), and ultrasound aid in precise diagnoses. MSD management is multidisciplinary, with orthopedic physiotherapy at its core. Tailored treatment plans include non-pharmacological interventions such as exercise therapy and manual techniques, complemented by medications like Non-steroidal anti-inflammatory drugs (NSAIDs) and Disease-modifying antirheumatic drugs (DMARDs). Surgical interventions may be necessary for joint replacements, followed by post-operative rehabilitation.

3. Principles of evidence-based practice in physiotherapy

Evidence-based practice (EBP) is the cornerstone of modern healthcare, providing a systematic framework for clinical decision-making allowing practitioners to offer optimal care based on research, clinical expertise, and patient preferences. At its core, it emphasizes the integration of three essential components: external clinical evidence, clinical expertise, and patient values.

External clinical evidence is derived from high-quality research studies, including randomized controlled trials, systematic reviews, and meta-analyzes. These studies are designed to rigorously evaluate the efficacy and safety of various interventions, allowing clinicians to make informed decisions about the most appropriate treatment approaches for specific conditions. The critical appraisal of research studies is a skill that physiotherapists must cultivate to determine the reliability and applicability.

Another crucial aspect is clinical expertise gained through years of education, training, and experience. Physiotherapists bring their unique understanding of anatomy, biomechanics, and patient interactions to decision-making, allowing practitioners to adapt interventions based on individual patient needs, comorbidities, and potential contraindications. Incorporating patient values and preferences recognizes that each patient has unique goals, values, and expectations. Practitioners can tailor interventions to various lifestyle and treatment goals by involving patients in decision-making. This enhances patient satisfaction and adherence to treatment plans.

Clinical questions are structured using the Patient, Intervention, Comparison, Outcome (PICO) framework, helping refine the inquiry's focus. Once the question is formulated, a systematic literature search is conducted, and a critical appraisal of these studies follows, evaluating their methodological rigor, validity, and applicability to clinical practice. The synthesis of evidence involves weighing the results of multiple studies to conclude. This synthesis may take the form of systematic reviews or meta-analyzes to provide a comprehensive overview of the available evidence. Based on the evidence synthesis, physiotherapists make informed decisions about treatment approaches, considering each option's benefits, risks, and feasibility.

As new research emerges and treatment guidelines evolve, physiotherapists must stay updated to ensure their practice remains aligned with the latest evidence. Continuing education, attending conferences, and participating in peer discussions are all strategies that facilitate the integration of new knowledge and skills into clinical practice. Through a commitment to ongoing learning and critical appraisal, physiotherapists uphold the highest standards of care, advancing the field and enhancing the well-being of those they serve.

4. Assessment techniques for orthopedic conditions

Accurate and thorough assessment forms the bedrock of effective orthopedic physiotherapy. A diverse array of assessment techniques, ranging from clinical examinations to advanced imaging technologies, helps decipher the intricacies of orthopedic conditions and devise targeted interventions.

Clinical assessments are the initial step, involving comprehensive history-taking and physical examination to establish an understanding of the patient's condition. The patient's medical history, including past injuries, surgeries, and relevant medical conditions, provides context for the current musculoskeletal complaint. The physical examination encompasses evaluating the joint range of motion, muscle strength, and functional movement patterns and identifying areas of pain or discomfort.

Functional movement assessments encompass various specialized tests, each serving a specific purpose. The Functional Movement Screen (FMS), developed by Gray Cook, is a notable example [6]. It evaluates fundamental movement patterns and identifies any imbalances or dysfunctions. By pinpointing areas of weakness or asymmetry, physiotherapists can design exercise regimens tailored to address these vulnerabilities, reducing the risk of future injuries.

Sport-specific functional assessments dive deep into the specific demands of a particular sport, analyzing an athlete's movement patterns and biomechanics about their chosen activity. For instance, in soccer, the FIFA 11+ program is an evidence-based assessment and exercise regimen designed to reduce the risk of soccer-related injuries [7]. By identifying areas of weakness or improper technique that may predispose athletes to injuries, physiotherapists can tailor interventions and exercise programs to enhance performance and significantly reduce the risk of sports-related injuries.

Through comprehensive gait analysis, physiotherapists can detect abnormalities or compensatory movements that may lead to joint stress or pain. For example, 3D motion analysis systems like Vicon provide precise and quantitative data on gait mechanics. Subsequently, physiotherapists can devise personalized interventions and exercise programs to correct gait issues.

Functional assessments have garnered substantial attention due to their capacity to uncover specific movement deficiencies and their direct application in injury prevention and rehabilitation strategies. Researchers like Dr. Phil Plisky have further advanced the understanding of functional assessments' efficacy in reducing injury risk and improving overall musculoskeletal health [8].

By manually palpating muscles, tendons, ligaments, and joints, physiotherapists can identify areas of tenderness, muscle spasms, and tissue abnormalities. It involves a gentle and systematic technique to assess the skin and superficial tissues. Gradually, they delve deeper into the anatomy, evaluating underlying structures meticulously. Bilateral comparison of corresponding structures on both sides of the body helps them uncover disparities in muscle tone, tenderness, or joint mobility. Accurate anatomical landmark identification is integral; for instance, when examining the knee, palpating the patellar tendon insertion at the tibia's tuberosity provides critical insights into its condition and function.

Texture and temperature evaluation are vital. Inflammation, for example, can manifest as warmth in the affected area and may lead to changes in tissue texture, such as swelling or fibrosis. Muscle tone assessment through palpation unveils valuable information about muscle spasms, trigger points, and regions of hypertonicity or hypotonicity. The presence of palpable knots or nodules within a muscle, for instance, may indicate the existence of trigger points, shedding light on potential sources of pain or discomfort.

Furthermore, palpation is instrumental in evaluating joint mobility. Physiotherapists employ this technique to detect restricted joint motion or the presence of crepitus—those telltale crackling or popping sensations that can hint at joint dysfunction, such as osteoarthritis or ligamentous instability. Distinguished figures in physiotherapy, such as Dr. Shirley Sahrmann, have significantly contributed to the refinement and understanding of palpation techniques, particularly in musculoskeletal assessment [9].

A diverse array of specialized tests is meticulously designed to provoke or reproduce symptoms, providing crucial insights for accurate diagnosis and tailored treatment. The Straight Leg Raise Test, a cornerstone in diagnosing nerve root irritation, is often seen in conditions such as herniated disks or sciatica. During the test, the patient lies supine, and the physiotherapist gently raises the patient's straightened leg. If the elevation of the leg elicits radiating pain along the sciatic nerve pathway, it can strongly indicate nerve compression or irritation.

The Apprehension Test is particularly relevant in diagnosing shoulder instability, where the shoulder joint is prone to dislocation. In this test, the physiotherapist gently rotates the patient's arm, placing stress on the anterior shoulder joint. If the patient experiences apprehension or discomfort during this maneuver, it suggests instability, signifying the potential for dislocation.

The McMurray Test is focused on diagnosing meniscal injuries in the knee joint, a crucial assessment tool. During the test, the physiotherapist flexes the patient's knee while externally rotating the leg and applying varus or valgus stress. If the patient experiences a clicking or popping sensation, it may indicate a meniscal tear. The Apley's Compression Test aids in diagnosing meniscal or ligamentous injuries in the knee. The physiotherapist applies downward compression on the patient's knee while rotating the tibia. Pain or discomfort during this maneuver can suggest issues like meniscal tears or ligamentous damage.

The Lachman Test is a central assessment in diagnosing anterior cruciate ligament (ACL) injuries in knee injuries. The physiotherapist stabilizes the patient's femur while applying anterior force to the tibia. Increased anterior tibial translation compared to the uninjured knee can indicate ACL damage. The Phalen's Test is used in diagnosing carpal tunnel syndrome, a common condition affecting the wrist. The physiotherapist flexes the patient's wrists and briefly holds them in a neutral position. Tingling or numbness in the median nerve distribution can indicate carpal tunnel syndrome.

To assess biceps tendon pathology in the shoulder, the Speed's Test requires the patient to flex their shoulder against resistance actively. Pain or discomfort in the bicipital groove may suggest issues like tendinitis or biceps tendon tears. Prominent researchers and practitioners like Dr. James Andrews and Dr. Stuart McGill have contributed significantly to the understanding and refining of these specialized tests, further enhancing their utility in orthopedic physiotherapy.

Advanced imaging modalities offer deeper insights into orthopedic conditions. X-rays provide detailed views of bone structures, aiding in diagnosing fractures, joint degeneration, and alignment abnormalities. Magnetic resonance imaging (MRI) offers high-resolution images of soft tissues, enabling the visualization of ligaments, tendons, cartilage, and internal joint structures. Ultrasound is another valuable tool for visualizing soft tissues in real-time, assisting in assessing muscle injuries, tendonitis, and bursitis.

Objective measurement tools, such as goniometers and inclinometers, enhance the precision of orthopedic assessments. Isokinetic dynamometers measure muscle strength across various joint movements, identifying muscular imbalances and guiding the design of targeted strength training regimens. Three-dimensional motion analysis systems, exemplified by technologies like Vicon, offer a comprehensive view of joint movements in three dimensions. Whether it's assessing the intricate mechanics of a runner's stride or the intricacies of a baseball pitcher's throw, these systems enable detailed and medically specific evaluations.

Electromyography (EMG), like the Noraxon EMG system, allows for the real-time measurement of muscle activity, empowering physiotherapists to pinpoint areas of dysfunction, identify muscle imbalances, and design interventions that precisely target optimal muscle activation [10]. Whether analyzing the firing patterns of muscles in patients with neuromuscular disorders or optimizing the rehabilitation of athletes recovering from injuries, EMG offers medically specific data that inform tailored treatment plans.

Psychosocial assessments recognize the interplay between psychological factors and musculoskeletal health. Pain perception, fear avoidance behaviors, and psychological distress can significantly influence the experience and progression of orthopedic conditions.

Functional outcome measures are often facilitated through questionnaires and standardized scales that span a spectrum of parameters, encompassing pain intensity, functional limitations, and overall quality of life. One widely employed outcome measure is the Visual Analog Scale (VAS), which quantifies pain intensity on a scale from 0 to 10, thereby serving as a vital baseline for treatment planning and progression monitoring.

The Western Ontario and McMaster Universities Osteoarthritis Index (WOMAC) is specifically tailored to assess hip and knee osteoarthritis; this questionnaire delves into pain, stiffness, and physical function [11]. The Disabilities of the Arm, Shoulder, and Hand (DASH) questionnaire is instrumental in evaluating upper extremity musculoskeletal disorders and exploring the impact of these conditions on an individual's ability to perform various activities aids in devising targeted interventions. The Lower Extremity Functional Scale (LEFS) is used for patients with lower limb injuries or disorders. It assesses functional limitations in individuals with conditions affecting the lower extremities, aiding in formulating rehabilitation plans tailored to each patient's unique needs.

Moreover, in spinal conditions, the Oswestry Disability Index (ODI) is invaluable. Specifically designed for individuals with low back pain, it quantifies the impact of pain on various aspects of daily life, from walking to sleeping. From clinical evaluations and functional movement assessments to advanced imaging technologies and objective measurement tools, the information guides the development of individualized treatment plans that address each patient's needs and optimize musculoskeletal health outcomes.

5. Therapeutic modalities and techniques in orthopedic physiotherapy

Orthopedic physiotherapy encompasses therapeutic modalities and techniques to alleviate pain, improve function, and enhance the musculoskeletal health of individuals with various orthopedic conditions. This diverse array of interventions draws upon traditional and innovative approaches.

A hands-on approach, manual involves skilled techniques applied to joints, soft tissues, and other structures to restore mobility, alleviate pain, and enhance tissue healing. Joint mobilizations and manipulations, for instance, are employed to improve joint range of motion, reduce stiffness, and promote synovial fluid circulation. Soft tissue mobilizations, such as myofascial release and trigger point therapy, target muscle tension and adhesions, facilitating tissue relaxation and enhancing blood flow.

Customized exercise programs address muscle imbalances, enhance joint stability, and improve functional capacity. Strengthening exercises target specific muscle groups to address weakness and restore muscular balance around joints. Incorporating proprioceptive and neuromuscular retraining exercises into a rehabilitation program can be instrumental in restoring coordination, balance, and motor control, all essential for functional movements and injury prevention.

Functional movement assessments guide the selection of therapeutic exercises by identifying movement dysfunctions and compensatory patterns. Moreover, progressive loading and resistance adjustments are made as the patient's condition improves, facilitating muscle strengthening, joint stability, and overall functional enhancement. Manual therapy and exercise interventions often synergize with pain management strategies. Manual traction and neural mobilizations target nerve-related pain by relieving nerve compression and promoting glide. Pain modulation strategies, including heat, cold, or electrical stimulation, contribute to pain relief and tissue healing.

Telehealth platforms, like Telerehab, have emerged as powerful tools, enabling remote consultations that transcend geographical constraints. These platforms allow Patients to access expert guidance, exercise regimens, and real-time progress tracking. Wearable devices and sensors, such as the Myo armband and gait analysis systems like the Gait real-time analysis interactive lab (GRAIL), have revolutionized orthopedic physiotherapy by enabling real-time monitoring of movement patterns and biomechanics [12]. These technologies offer quantitative insights into patients' physical activities and aid in the early identification of aberrant movement patterns. Patients engage in therapeutic exercises within virtual environments, like the Oculus Rift, enhancing motivation and significantly improving adherence to prescribed regimens. This gamified approach to rehabilitation holds great potential.

Hydrotherapy, or aquatic therapy, offers a unique therapeutic environment for orthopedic rehabilitation. The buoyancy of water reduces joint loading, allowing patients to perform exercises with less impact on injured or painful areas. Water resistance adds a strengthening component to exercises, contributing to muscle activation and cardiovascular fitness. Hydrotherapy is particularly beneficial for conditions involving weight-bearing joints, such as the spine, hips, knees, and ankles.

Orthopedic physiotherapists harness a variety of manual techniques to address specific conditions. Mulligan's concept of mobilizations with movement (MWM) combines passive joint mobilization with active, pain-free movements, promoting immediate improvements in joint mechanics and functional outcomes [13]. The McKenzie method focuses on patient-specific mechanical assessment and exercise prescription to manage spinal conditions and address radicular symptoms.

Instrument-assisted soft tissue mobilization (IASTM) utilizes specialized tools to target adhesions and scar tissue within soft tissues. This technique improves tissue flexibility, reduces pain, and enhances movement [14]. Similarly, kinesio-taping involves the application of elastic tape to muscles and joints to provide support, enhance proprioception, and facilitate lymphatic drainage.

By harnessing the power of these various modalities, practitioners empower individuals to overcome orthopedic challenges, optimize functional outcomes, and ultimately enhance their overall quality of life.

6. Exercise prescription for musculoskeletal rehabilitation

Exercise prescription guides recovery, strength enhancement, and functional improvement. Tailoring exercise regimens to individuals' unique needs, goals, and pathologies requires a deep understanding of anatomy, biomechanics, and the principles of exercise science. Exercise selection is based on specificity, overload, progression, and individualization. Specificity dictates that exercises should target the muscles, joints, and movement patterns directly relevant to the individual's condition. Overload involves progressively challenging the body's capacities to induce physiological adaptations. Progression ensures that exercises evolve as the patient's strength, endurance, and mobility improve. Individualization tailors exercise to the patient's physical capabilities, ensuring that the prescribed regimen is neither too strenuous nor too easy.

Therapeutic exercise regimens often include three primary categories of exercises: flexibility, strength, and neuromuscular control. Flexibility exercises enhance joint range of motion and tissue extensibility, preventing stiffness and promoting overall joint health. Stretching techniques, including static, dynamic, and proprioceptive neuromuscular facilitation (PNF) stretching, play a role in maintaining or improving flexibility.

Strength exercises form a core component of musculoskeletal rehabilitation. Strengthening weak muscles and addressing muscular imbalances is essential to enhance joint stability and prevent future injuries. Resistance training, involving free weights, machines, resistance bands, or body weight, challenges muscles to generate force against resistance. Eccentric training, focusing on the lengthening phase of muscle contraction, is often employed to manage tendinopathies and enhance tendon health.

Neuromuscular control exercises enhance proprioception, coordination, and motor control. Balance training, functional movements, and proprioceptive exercises challenge the body's ability to maintain equilibrium and control movement. Volume refers to the total amount of exercise performed, encompassing sets, repetitions, and duration. Intensity involves the effort expended during exercises and can be adjusted through factors like resistance, load, or difficulty. Frequency determines how often exercise sessions are performed, considering recovery and adaptational capacities.

Progression within exercise prescription is essential for continuous improvement. Incremental adjustments are made to exercise variables to ensure ongoing adaptation. Gradually increasing resistance, repetitions, or exercise complexity challenges the body and fosters strength gains. Progression is guided by the patient's response to exercise and ability to tolerate increased loads.

Periodization strategies organize exercise programs into distinct phases to optimize long-term progress. These phases often include preparatory, strength-building, and maintenance phases. Periodization allows for systematic progression, recovery, and avoidance of plateaus, ensuring sustained improvements in musculoskeletal health.

Physiotherapists educate patients on proper exercise technique, form, and alignment to minimize the risk of injury and enhance exercise effectiveness. Teaching patients to self-monitor their exertion levels and recognize overexertion signs ensure safe and successful exercise sessions. Motivation and adherence are often seen when patients find their exercise programs enjoyable and aligned with their aspirations. Engaging patients in shared decision-making empowers them to take ownership of their rehabilitation journey and fosters collaboration between the patient and the physiotherapist.

7. Post-operative rehabilitation: orthopedic considerations

Post-operative rehabilitation is crucial in optimizing outcomes and restoring function. The surgical techniques, tissue healing, and rehabilitation strategies all together shape the recovery trajectory. Understanding each procedure is essential for formulating rehabilitation protocols. In the immediate post-operative phase, rehabilitation often focuses on pain management, edema control, and early mobilization. Gentle range of motion exercises and controlled loading are initiated to prevent joint stiffness and muscle atrophy.

In joint replacement surgeries, such as total hip or knee replacements, rehabilitation is critical in restoring joint function and mobility. Initial exercises concentrate on regaining joint range of motion and preventing joint capsule adhesions. Gradual weight-bearing progression and muscle-strengthening exercises are introduced to restore joint stability and enhance functional capacity. A balance between early mobilization and cautious progression is struck to ensure optimal healing and implant longevity. Orthopedic surgeries involving ligament repairs, such as anterior cruciate ligament (ACL) reconstruction, demand meticulous rehabilitation protocols. Progressive strengthening exercises, neuromuscular control drills, and proprioceptive training are crucial to restore joint stability and prevent re-injury.

Spinal surgeries, including spinal fusion or discectomy, require careful consideration of biomechanics and tissue healing. Early mobilization emphasizing proper body mechanics is essential to prevent complications and promote spinal alignment. Strengthening exercises that target the core muscles help in maintaining spinal stability and reducing the risk of post-operative back pain. Fracture fixation surgeries necessitate graded loading and progressive weight-bearing strategies. Rehabilitation begins with gentle range of motion exercises to prevent joint stiffness and promote bone healing. Resistance exercises and functional tasks are integrated as healing progresses to restore bone strength and joint function.

Regular communication between orthopedic surgeons, physiotherapists, and other healthcare providers enables adjustments to the rehabilitation plan based on the patient's progress, complications, and individual needs. This collaborative approach ensures the rehabilitation plan remains dynamic and responsive to the patient's evolving condition. Patient education help gain insight into self-care techniques, precautionary measures, and signs of potential complications, empowering them to participate in their recovery journey actively.

8. Integrating technology in orthopedic physiotherapy

Technology integration into orthopedic physiotherapy has personalized patient care from diagnostics and treatment planning to monitor progress and enhance patient engagement. Imaging modalities such as magnetic resonance imaging (MRI), computed tomography (CT), and ultrasound offer detailed insights into musculoskeletal structures, aiding in identifying pathologies and guiding treatment decisions. Three-dimensional imaging and advanced visualization techniques allow clinicians to assess complex joint and spinal conditions accurately.

Robot-assisted rehabilitation devices have emerged as pioneering tools, catalyzing the recovery process for patients facing severe impairments. One example of robot-assisted rehabilitation is the robotic exoskeletons, such as the Ekso GT, in spinal cord injury rehabilitation. These exoskeletons are meticulously designed to provide individuals with paraplegia or tetraplegia the opportunity to regain mobility. Through a complex system of sensors and actuators, the Ekso GT assists patients in achieving controlled, weight-bearing steps, thus promoting muscle activation and enhancing lower extremity strength [15].

Devices like the ArmeoSpring support and guide the arm through a series of customized exercises. These exercises target specific muscle groups and movement patterns, facilitating neuroplasticity and motor skill recovery. For patients with post-stroke hemiparesis, the ArmeoSpring offers a lifeline toward regaining fine motor control, enhancing activities of daily living, and ultimately, improving overall quality of life [16].

Moreover, robot-assisted rehabilitation is instrumental in addressing knee osteoarthritis through devices like the Lokomat, a robotic gait training system. It also provides objective feedback to physiotherapists, allowing for data-driven adjustments to therapy regimens. Researchers and clinicians, including Dr. Helen Dawes, Dr. Paolo Bonato, and Dr. Michelle Johnson, continue to push the boundaries of this field, ensuring that patients with orthopedic challenges receive the highest standard of care.

Technology-driven biofeedback systems enhance proprioception, coordination, and motor control, making them particularly effective for stroke, spinal cord injuries, and neurological disorders. By promoting neuroplasticity, biofeedback technology aids in restoring functional independence.

Digital platforms and mobile applications deliver personalized exercise programs directly to patients' devices, empower patients with knowledge, enhance adherence, and foster engagement through instructional videos, progress tracking, and interactive reminders. Physitrack is used in the management of chronic musculoskeletal conditions such as osteoarthritis. Patients receive explicit, step-by-step instructional videos directly on their smartphones or tablets, ensuring that exercises are performed correctly. The app offers progress tracking functionalities, allowing patients to monitor their improvement over time and share this data with their physiotherapists for informed adjustments to treatment plans.

Similarly, with MyRehabPro, physiotherapists can prescribe comprehensive exercise programs via the platform after procedures like joint replacements or arthroscopic surgeries. Patients receive detailed video demonstrations and customizable reminders to ensure consistent adherence to their prescribed regimen [17]. Furthermore, applications like PhysioU provide a wealth of clinical resources and tools. Clinicians can access a library of evidence-based exercises, tests, and assessments to create highly personalized treatment plans [18]. The application facilitates real-time documentation, ensuring accurate and comprehensive record-keeping.

Esteemed researchers and experts in the field, such as Dr. Karen Ginn, Dr. Karin Grävare Silbernagel, and Dr. Ann Cools, continue to champion the integration of technology in orthopedic physiotherapy, ensuring that patients receive the highest caliber of care and support throughout their recovery journeys [19].

9. Patient education and self-management strategies

Patient education and self-management strategies are pivotal to imparting knowledge and equipping patients with the skills to actively engage in their recovery process. Clinicians recognize the individuality of each patient, adapting their communication style, content, and pace to match the patient's comprehension level and cultural context. This personalized approach establishes a rapport that encourages open dialog and promotes active participation in decision-making.

Patients gain insights into the underlying anatomy, the factors contributing to their condition, and the implications for their overall well-being. By employing visual aids and straightforward language, clinicians facilitate a clear understanding of complex concepts, fostering a sense of ownership over their health.

The rationale behind treatment interventions is to enhance patient engagement, compliance, and treatment adherence. Pain education is critical, mainly when pain is a significant factor. Patients learn about pain mechanisms, the role of inflammation, and strategies for managing pain. By differentiating between acute and chronic pain and providing techniques for pain relief, clinicians enable patients to participate actively.

Self-management includes teaching techniques for self-mobilization, maintaining proper body mechanics, and being mindful of posture. Functional rehabilitation strategies extend the principles learned in the clinic to real-world scenarios. Patients receive guidance on adapting their daily activities and work tasks to align with their condition. Functional exercises mimic activities patients encounter in their everyday lives, enabling a seamless transition from therapeutic exercises to functional movements.

Setting realistic goals enhances motivation and commitment. Patients gain a clear sense of purpose and direction, understanding how their efforts contribute to their overall progress. Regularly revisiting and adjusting goals ensures patients remain engaged and motivated throughout their rehabilitation. Recognizing the psychosocial dimensions of rehabilitation, clinicians address the emotional challenges that patients may encounter. Patients are provided with coping strategies, resources, and referrals to mental health professionals when needed.

Incorporating diverse learning modalities ensures that patients receive information in ways that resonate with them. Visual aids, written materials, online resources, and interactive tools accommodate various preferences, enhancing understanding and retention of information.

10. Conclusion

Orthopedic physiotherapy is a fundamental pillar in musculoskeletal healthcare, addressing a vast spectrum of conditions affecting bones, joints, muscles, tendons, ligaments, and connective tissues. In this comprehensive exploration, we have gone through the field of orthopedic physiotherapy, traversing its historical evolution, evidence-based foundations, diagnostic capabilities, therapeutic modalities, exercise prescription, post-operative considerations, specialized interventions, technological integration, and patient education.

Orthopedic physiotherapy is vital in musculoskeletal healthcare, underscoring its fundamental contribution to evidence-based practice. A diverse spectrum of conditions, musculoskeletal disorders (MSDs), encompass ailments such as osteoarthritis, ankylosing spondylitis, tendonitis, and tenosynovitis. Each disorder manifests with distinctive clinical presentations, imposing a significant global health burden.

The underlying principles of evidence-based practice emphasize the criticality of empirical data, clinical expertise, and research in molding practical therapeutic approaches. Subsequently, an extensive examination of diagnostic assessment techniques transpired, encompassing clinical evaluation, physical examination, and advanced imaging modalities, including X-rays, magnetic resonance imaging (MRI), and ultrasound. These diagnostic tools serve as indispensable instruments in precisely identifying orthopedic conditions and evaluating their impact on patients' daily lives.

The therapeutic modalities and techniques that constitute the core of this field were highlighted. Exercise therapy assumes a central role within this sphere, targeting muscle strength, joint stability, and mobility enhancement. Manual therapy techniques, including joint and soft tissue mobilizations, were unveiled as valuable assets in pain alleviation, muscle tension reduction, and joint mobility restoration. Furthermore, the chapter delved into the intricacies of exercise prescription for musculoskeletal rehabilitation, emphasizing its critical role in enhancing functional capacity and reducing the risk of future injuries. The meticulous tailoring of exercise regimens to individual patient needs and conditions emerged as a cornerstone, facilitating a personalized approach to rehabilitation.

In the post-operative arena, orthopedic considerations took center stage, shedding light on the importance of post-surgical rehabilitation under the guidance of orthopedic physiotherapists. Surgical interventions, spanning joint replacements, arthroscopic procedures, and spinal surgeries, were subjected to comprehensive examination, highlighting the pivotal role of rehabilitation in optimizing post-operative outcomes, minimizing complications, and restoring function.

Specialized approaches tailored to specific joint and spinal conditions further expanded our horizon, introducing advanced techniques and innovative interventions that provide tailored solutions to orthopedic challenges. Technology integration was unveiled as a driving force in reshaping orthopedic physiotherapy. Imaging modalities, wearable devices, telehealth, virtual reality (VR), augmented reality (AR), robot-assisted rehabilitation, biofeedback systems, digital platforms, and mobile applications were scrutinized for their potential to enhance diagnostics, treatment planning, monitoring, and patient engagement. Patient education and self-management strategies emerged as critical components in empowering individuals to participate in their rehabilitation journey actively. These strategies enhance understanding, adherence, and the long-term management of musculoskeletal conditions.

In this dynamic and ever-evolving field, the collaboration between clinicians, researchers, and technology continues to shape the future of musculoskeletal healthcare. It ensures that patients receive the highest standard of care and support in their journey to recovery. Orthopedic physiotherapy remains at the forefront, poised to further advance musculoskeletal health through its commitment to evidence-based practice, innovative interventions, and patient-centered care.

Author details

Harshavardhan Sai Sadineni
Kasturba Medical College Manipal, Manipal Academy of Higher Education, Manipal, Karnataka, India

*Address all correspondence to: hsadineni1110@gmail.com

References

[1] Navin M. Values and Vaccine Refusal: Hard Questions in Ethics, Epistemology, and Health Care. 1st ed. England, United Kingdom: Routledge; 2015. p. 241

[2] A history of manipulative therapy. Journal of Manual & Manipulative Therapy;**15**(3). Available from: https://www.tandfonline.com/doi/abs/10.1179/106698107790819873 [cited: September 17, 2023]

[3] Duruöz MT, Öz N, Gürsoy DE, Hande GH. Clinical aspects and outcomes in osteoarthritis. Best Practice & Research Clinical Rheumatology. 2023;**36**:101855

[4] Safiri S, Kolahi AA, Cross M, Hill C, Smith E, Carson-Chahhoud K, et al. Prevalence, deaths, and disability-adjusted life years due to musculoskeletal disorders for 195 countries and territories 1990-2017. Arthritis & Rhematology. 2021;**73**(4):702-714

[5] Bhattacharya A. Costs of occupational musculoskeletal disorders (MSDs) in the United States. International Journal of Industrial Ergonomics. 2014;**44**(3):448-454

[6] Jenkins MT, Gustitus R, Iosia M, Kicklighter T, Sasaki Y. Correlation between the functional movement screen and hip mobility in NCAA division II athletes. International Journal of Exercise Science. 1 Oct 2017;**10**(4):541-549

[7] Sadigursky D, Braid JA, De Lira DNL, Machado BAB, Carneiro RJF, Colavolpe PO. The FIFA 11+ injury prevention program for soccer players: A systematic review. BMC Sports Science, Medicine and Rehabilitation. 28 Nov 2017;**9**(1):18

[8] Teyhen DS, Riebel MA, McArthur DR, Savini M, Jones MJ, Goffar SL, et al. Normative data and the influence of age and gender on power, balance, flexibility, and functional movement in healthy service members. Military Medicine. Apr 2014;**179**(4):413-420. DOI: 10.7205/MILMED-D-13-00362

[9] Sahrmann S, Azevedo DC, Dillen LV. Diagnosis and treatment of movement system impairment syndromes. Brazilian Journal of Physical Therapy. 2017;**21**(6):391-399

[10] Weir RF, Troyk PR, DeMichele GA, Kerns DA, Schorsch JF, Maas H. Implantable myoelectric sensors (IMESs) for intramuscular electromyogram recording. IEEE Transactions on Biomedical Engineering. 2009;**56**(1):159-171

[11] Ackerman I. Western Ontario and McMaster universities osteoarthritis index (WOMAC). The Australian Journal of Physiotherapy. 2009;**55**(3):213

[12] Liu WY, Meijer K, Delbressine JM, Willems PJ, Franssen FM, Wouters EF, et al. Reproducibility and validity of the 6-minute walk test using the gait real-time analysis interactive lab in patients with COPD and healthy elderly. PLoS One. 8 Sep 2016;**11**(9):e0162444. DOI: 10.1371/journal.pone.0162444

[13] Vicenzino B, Paungmali A, Teys P. Mulligan's mobilization-with-movement, positional faults and pain relief: Current concepts from a critical review of literature. Manual Therapy. 2007;**12**(2):98-108

[14] Osailan A, Jamaan A, Talha K, Alhndi M. Instrument assisted soft tissue mobilization (IASTM) versus stretching: A comparison in effectiveness on hip active range of motion, muscle torque

and power in people with hamstring tightness. Journal of Bodywork and Movement Therapies. 2021;**27**:200-206

[15] Duddy D, Doherty R, Connolly J, Loughrey J, Condell J, Hassan D, et al. The cardiorespiratory demands of treadmill walking with and without the use of Ekso GT™ within able-bodied participants: A feasibility study. International Journal of Environmental Research and Public Health. 19 May 2022;**19**(10):6176. DOI: 10.3390/ijerph19106176

[16] Gijbels D, Lamers I, Kerkhofs L, Alders G, Knippenberg E, Feys P. The Armeo Spring as training tool to improve upper limb functionality in multiple sclerosis: A pilot study. Journal of NeuroEngineering and Rehabilitation. 24 Jan 2011;**8**:5. DOI: 10.1186/1743-0003-8-5

[17] Fernandez A, Agujar C. PadayonTa: A physical therapy telerehabilitation application for stroke patients. 2022. DOI: 10.13140/RG.2.2.16168.24323

[18] Nash B, MItchell AW, Jones J, Etheridge J. Student self-efficacy levels for performing clinical skills learned virtually during a pandemic. Journal of Occupational Therapy Education. 2022;**6**(3). DOI: 10.26681/jote.2022.060309

[19] Trevithick BA, Ginn KA, Halaki M, Balnave R. Shoulder muscle recruitment patterns during a kayak stroke performed on a paddling ergometer. Journal of Electromyography and Kinesiology. 2007;**17**(1):74-79

Chapter 11

Growth and Regeneration of Intervertebral Discs by Electrophysiological Potential Therapy: Impedance Therapy

Pavol Kostka, Elena Ziakova, Marek Janitor, Nina Sladekova, Martin Janitor, Daniel Vrabel and Paulina Chripkova

Abstract

Impedance therapy (IT) is an electrophysiological potential therapy where specific electrical impulses (SEI) stimulate the human body's skin surface to cause a regenerative cascade in people diagnosed with degenerative disc disease (DDD). An observational retrospective cohort study sought to monitor the effect of IT, as an innovative nonpharmacological therapy that improves the health of DDD patients. The outcome was objectified by magnetic resonance imaging (MRI) of the spine, a neurological examination, patients' own subjective feelings before and after electrotherapy, and confirmation of "disc grow-up" (DGU). The cohort was composed of 161 patients with an ICD diagnosis of G54.0,1,2,4 and/or M54.2,4,5,12,16,17, of whom 66 were women with a mean age of 54.7 years, and 95 were men with a mean age of 50.2 years. The cohort either had undergone or was undergoing IT rehabilitation with specific electrical impulses (SEI). A retrospective analysis of the data from patients who underwent IT rehabilitation in 2019 demonstrated a statistically significant 19% increase in intervertebral disc volume in cm^3, $p < 0.001$ CI 95%, a reduction in pain perception after IT of 75%, $p < 0.001$ 95% CI, and positive changes in tendon-periosteal reflexes (TPR), $p < 0.01$ CI 95%. IT offers new approaches to treating DDD with objective control of structural/degenerative/regenerative changes.

Keywords: IT-electrophysiological potential therapy—impedance therapy, SEI—specific electrical impulse, DGU phenomenon—disc grow-up, DDD—degenerative disc disease, CRF—case report form

1. Introduction

DDD includes spondylotic, arthritic and degenerative disc disease of the spine, either with or without compression of nerve structures, or spinal instability [1, 2]. The main symptoms are axial pain, neck pain, back pain, upper/lower limb pain or a combination of any of them. An acute attack is expressed by the body's inability to tolerate ongoing degeneration, localized in the spine structure. DDD-associated difficulties start with a metabolic imbalance developing at the cellular level in the connective tissue. It dominates in the largest avascular tissue found in humans, the intervertebral disc. The result is a degenerative cascade, according to Kirkaldy-Willisa [3]. The discs desiccate and lose height, volume, shape, elasticity and their optimal position to the adjacent vertebrae. The body becomes increasingly burdened with painful conditions, which are compensated by incorrect posture and positioning, reduced mobility and unevenly balanced loading of individual muscles and tendons. Fatigue sets in at a critical stage due to the lack or impossibility of movement and sleep, which significantly affects and limits a patient's activities and possibilities. IT stimulates the skin surface with specific electrical impulses (SEI), which induce and restore the body's own regeneration of soft tissue. This increases volume and adjusts the body to a physiologically more optimal shape, herniations recede, perforations heal and the intervertebral disc's structure is restored. A secondary outcome is a reduction or significant resolution of the painful conditions DDD manifests. The method has been used in medical practice ever conclusions were drawn from a randomized clinical trial – impedance therapy in rehabilitation of degenerative disc disease and in accordance with them [4].

2. Degenerative disc disease diagnosis

When a patient has degenerative disc disease, it is important to identify where it hurts in good time, assess the severity and dynamics of developing concomitant medical symptoms, and provide him or her with the most effective therapy. Therefore, diagnosis and treatment require a multidisciplinary or team approach involving a general practitioner, neurologist, radiologist, neurosurgeon or spinal surgeon, algesiologist, orthopedic surgeon and physiotherapist. It is also critical to identify the source of vertebrogenic pain early, likewise assess the severity and dynamics of developing concomitant medical symptoms, and provide patients with the most effective treatment for the disease. Radiological findings (native X-ray, CT or MRI) have confirmed that degenerative lumbar spine disease (DLSD) is going to affect 100% of the population over 40 years of age, and a severe degree will have an impact on 60% of the population over 70 [1, 5]. However, the correlation between the degrees of degenerative changes confirmed by imaging and subjective or objective clinical symptoms is low, and so many patients with radiological findings remain free of difficulties [6, 7]. In symptomatic patients, degenerative changes in the discs and facet joints, degenerative spondylosis, soft tissue changes of the spine and compression of nerve structures and roots in the lumbar spinal canal and/or exiting neuroforamina contribute significantly to discomfort. However, discrepancies between the structural changes detected by a CT scan or MRI and clinical findings often impede accurate identification of the source of pain, for example, in surgical procedures, or in minimally invasive or endoscopic surgery. Indeed, the structural changes depicted may frequently not be causally related to clinical symptomatology. Therefore, a misleading diagnosis is not rare and can lead to failure of conservative or surgical treatment and sometimes even to disability [8, 9]. A specific condition requiring urgent neurosurgical attention is acute cauda equina syndrome. It is caused by compression of the cauda equina and is associated with a large medial herniation of the lumbar disc.

Based on conclusions drawn from medical observations, we confirm that the onset of back pain, as a consequence of DDD, takes place predominantly when there is a pattern of peripheral sensitization [10]. The following has been observed in such cases:

- Painful conditions arising without stimulus;
- Damage (mechanically by compression or inflammation) of the sensory nerves leading to nociceptive afferent C unmyelinated fibers;
- Lactic acid accumulating in the degenerated disc with the subsequent acidosis stimulating the nociceptors;
- Production of cytokines – nociceptive molecules;
- Susceptibility of spinal nerve roots to compressive damage because a well-developed blood-nerve barrier is missing;
- In the acute stage, abnormal accumulation of sodium channels in the nociceptors and ganglia of the posterior horns of the spinal cord, with a consequent decrease in the depolarization threshold;
- Increased number of adrenergic receptors and circulating catecholamines;
- Sprouting of neurons and new nerve fiber outgrowth at the site of nerve fiber severance during a period of regeneration. Increased irritability is visible due to the increased concentration of sodium and calcium channels.

These changes raise the sensitivity of nociceptors to various, even painless stimuli and peripheral sensitization and lead to the development of spontaneous ectopic activity in the damaged nerves.

The four sources of pain recognized In DDD are discogenic and facet pain, pain from spinal stenosis and radicular pain [11]. Discogenic pain is associated with pathological neovascularization and axonogenesis of the intervertebral disc. Nerve fibers,, accompanied by blood vessels, grow into the cracks that appear in degenerate discs. In addition, vascularized granulation tissue and extensive innervations form and extend from the outer layer of the annulus fibrosus to the nucleus pulposus. The rate of unmyelinated C-fiber and micro-vessel growing in the intervertebral disc to the depth of the nucleus pulposus of the spine [11] is directly proportional to the rate of degenerative changes associated with discogenic pain. Nociceptive discogenic pain is caused by stimulation of sensory nerve endings (peptidergic substance P [SP], CGRP-calcitonin gene-related peptides [CRGP] and vasoactive intestinal polypeptides [VIP]) in the outer layers of the annulus fibrosus. Another source of discogenic pain is structural failure of the intervertebral disc. When it is burdened, so-called "peripheral sensitization" can cause the usually innocuous mechanical stimuli of nociceptors in the annulus fibrosus to amplify nociceptive stimulation. In degenerated joints, facet pain comes from the ingrowth of blood vessels and unmyelinated C-fibers and radiates from the subchondral bone into the interior of the damaged articular cartilage. The inflammatory cytokines IL-1b and TNFα sensitize nerve fibers, increasing pain transmission and hyperalgesia [2]. Patients with severe facet joint degeneration feel a burning pain. Pain from spinal stenosis develops from hypertrophy of the bony and ligamentous structures, combined with disc bulging in the spinal canal and around the neuroforamina, compressing the nerve roots and making them dysfunctional. The presence of the inflammatory cytokines IL-1b, TNFα, and IL-6 in the facet joints contributes toward the development of pain [12]. Cytokine levels are higher in patients with lumbar spinal stenosis (LSS) than those with herniated discs.

Nociceptive radicular pain, with no concomitant neurological nerve root damage, is felt when the nociceptors in the perineurium of the nerve root are stimulated. It is caused by ectopic discharges from damaged posterior roots or their ganglia. A diagnosis of "definite" neuropathic radicular pain requires the presence of objective sensory symptoms (hyperalgesia, dysesthesia, hypesthesia and allodynia) either with or without motor signs of radiculopathy, while the presence of isolated motor symptoms of radiculopathy is enough for a diagnosis of "probable" neuropathic radicular pain. Conservative treatment of DDD with gabapentin has been ineffective because, in this type of pain, it acts on central sensitization and not on the onset of the painful condition itself [12].

3. Impedance therapy

The key building block in impedance therapy (IT) is the specific electrical impulse (SEI). Alternating SEIs from a current or voltage generator stimulates the body via electrodes placed on a patient's skin. Output current up to 3 mA is used, with consumption up to 5VA. Applying an SEI elicits a sympathetic skin response [11, 13]. This is confirmed by a change in skin conductance due to the changed conductivity of the sweat produced by it. Repeatedly pooled therapeutic procedures provide adequate data to confirm correlation dependencies for SEI frequency and amplitude; stable and dynamic portions of the SEI; electrode surface, size and insulation resistance; and other parameters for defining the baseline SEI stimulation sequence and determining the dynamic SEI [11]. The SEI structure most capable of effectively increasing skin conductance is one that can induce a harmonic change in skin resistance. In IT, the slowed response to regenerative induction highlights the body's inability to react to a harmonic change, so the therapy takes advantage of the feedback response in the patient's body. Therefore, stimulation comes from the body's previous response. It is evaluated in real-time by an information system with a knowledge base. Unless there is an active feedback loop in the internal information system, the SEI's full regenerative effect on the body cannot be ensured. Under the influence of IT, nonphysiological, unmyelinated C-fibers are effectively reduced, eliminating discogenic pain. Follow-up DICOM images from MRI scans confirm reparative changes in the intervertebral disc after completion of the first block of planned long-term rehabilitation. The observed changes are predominantly at the level of reducing intervertebral disc fissures, which are visible on MR images as desiccated changes. Impedance therapy's effectiveness and success are therefore evident in healed cracks and perforations, reduction of the hernia and increased elasticity. Yet these regenerative/reparative processes are dependent on the degree of DDD and the dynamics of degenerative structural changes. A patient can be cured of this disease of civilization (DDD) after having completed a long-term IT rehabilitation plan. Since impedance therapy has been around for over 20 years, information systems have been keeping medical records of all successfully treated patients who have enrolled in a long-term rehabilitation plan.

Timeline of medical practice established concepts and procedures in electrophysiological potential therapy:

- 2000 - Electrophysiological regenerative potential therapy, later called electrophysiological potential therapy
- or impedance therapy (2005).

2009 - Disc grow-up (DGU). The term refers to confirmed growth in intervertebral disc volume after the completion of a long-term IT rehabilitation plan involving SEIs. It confirms not just the gradual elimination of painful conditions but also the change in the disc's structure, a reduction in perforations and disc herniation, and so the elimination of degenerative changes in the spine. Ongoing follow-up measurements of patients who have undergone not just impedance therapy confirm that the regenerated intervertebral disc keeps its condition even several years after long-term rehabilitation ends, at a time when a patient is no longer receiving IT. On the other hand, patients treated with standard nonsurgical procedures only had intervals of slowed progression of degenerative changes recorded. These alternated with intervals of re-accelerated degeneration. Clinical practice consistently confirmed the validity of the unidirectional degenerative cascade mentioned by Kirkalda-Willis [5] until the patient's body received SEIs.

2014 – Initial blood screening introduced with impedance therapy patients receiving detailed blood analysis. Among other things, changes in plasma blood lactate levels from capillary blood and VZV, CMV, HSV and EBV IgG levels were monitored.

2016 – Correlational evaluation of blood screening. The first dependence was recorded on the size of intervertebral disc growth on IgG-VZV, CMV, HSV and EBV IgG levels, with concordant harmonization of blood lactate levels at rest and later during exercise. Continuing medical observations and initial correlational analyses of sample data have empirically demonstrated and continue to demonstrate a dependence between the magnitude of increased intervertebral disc volume and the magnitude of higher plasma VZV, CMV, HSV and EBV immunoglobulin levels in the first block of a long-term rehabilitation plan with IT.

2016–2018 – "Impedance therapy in rehabilitation of degenerative disc disease," a clinical study that confirmed the DGU phenomenon [4].

4. Retrospective cohort study

An observational retrospective cohort study sought to monitor the effect of IT at the level of an innovative nonpharmacological therapy that improves the health of patients with DDD. It was objectified by magnetic resonance imaging (MRI) of the spine, 3D visualization of DICOM images from MRI scans together with an assessment of the DUG phenomenon, a neurological examination and patients' own subjective feeling before and after electrotherapy.

4.1 Participants

Retrospective data processing covered 161 patients (**Table 1**) with an ICD-10 diagnosis of G54.0,1,2,4 and/or M54.2,4,5,12,16,17 who had undergone impedance therapy. There were 66 (41%) women and 95 (59%) men with a mean age of 50 (11)

Participants	Male	Female
Age (years) Mean (SD)	50.3 (11.3)	54.7 (12.6)
N	95 (59%)	66 (21%)

Table 1.
Characteristics of participants.

and 55 (13) years, respectively. Data from all patients who had cervical and lumbar disc volumes evaluated from January 2019 to December 2019 were included. For retrospective analysis, the criteria below were used in the processing of data on patients who had undergone IT. Consent was given by all patients whose data had been retrospectively processed to the therapy, and they were informed of the possibility to opt out of participation in the monitoring of treatment and its effects at any time. Written consents to the anonymous use of data were archived. In order to analyze the 2019 retrospective study and confirm the effects of impedance therapy, every patient's informed consent was kept according to his or her long-term rehabilitation plan after each medical procedure over the time impedance therapy was applied. Design and flow of participants through the trial All administrative processes complied with the guidelines set out in the Declaration of Helsinki [6].

4.2 Methods

A clinical retrospective trial sought to monitor the effect of IT at the level of an innovative nonpharmacological therapy that improves the health of patients with DDD. It was objectified by magnetic resonance imaging (MRI) of the spine, 3D visualization of DICOM images from MRI scans together with an assessment of the DUG phenomenon, a neurological examination and patients' own subjective feeling before and after electrotherapy. A study was conducted with a retrospective analysis of data from the medical records of patients who had undergone rehabilitation at the optimal duration of 5–7 months and completed the first block of their planned rehabilitation between January and December 2019. All of the data processed in the retrospective analysis from the application of electrophysiological potential therapy on patients consisted of anonymized case report forms (CRF) on patients from the outpatient information system.

4.3 Intervention – Rehabilitation

It consists of three blocks of therapies and their associated phases:

Block I focused on reducing pain. It involved the application of standard physiotherapy procedures in combination with impedance therapy.

Phase 1 - Classification.

Phase 2 - Reverse transcription (RT) symptoms.

Phase 3 - Enrollment in kinesiotherapy.

Block II focused on stress testing to increase physical performance in feedback control.

Phase 4 - Enrollment in training sessions.

Phase 5 - Analysis of metabolism.

Phase 6 - Fixation of regeneration.

Block III focused on maintaining proper exercise frequencies and correct weight. Muscle load measurements with a defined blood lactate level.

Patients whose data had been processed in the retrospective study underwent rehabilitation three times every 2 weeks for a total of 29–48 therapy sessions that each lasted between 90 and 120 minutes. The length of each planned rehabilitation was always dependent on the patient's DDD condition, with the patient's comorbidities being an important factor.

Every patient whose data was processed had undergone the following during therapy:

1. Examination of tendon-periosteal reflexes before and after therapy

2. Electrophysiological potential therapy (IT) with a physiotherapy muscle stimulator (PSS)

3. Heat and light therapy (TDP® lamp, Biolamp, Biolaser L1)

4. Dry needling

5. Manual therapy by a physiotherapist

6. Measurement of capillary blood lactate levels [4].

4.3.1 Methods for monitoring safety and accuracy

1. Adverse event monitoring was used to observe each patient's local and systemic tolerance to medical treatment and procedures. Patients were under the direct control of medical staff during every impedance therapy session.

2. During electrophysiological potential therapy, every patient was exposed to physical loads at output currents up to 3 mA, with consumption up to 5VA. Prior to each SEI application to a patient's body, an artificial resistive load with a dynamic waveform was used for control purposes to measure current and voltage from the alternating electrical pulse generator.

3. The trifilar winding at the generator cores was measured at the beginning of each day of therapy. Throughout SEI application, the generators exhibited tolerances within 0.05% of the measured electrical parameters.

4. No notes were made during IT of either electrical inaccuracies or generator failure in patient records that were processed for retrospective analysis.

5. Comparisons made of the outcomes in individual patients were based on anonymized patient data, which was also subordinated to the composition of the final CRF.

6. Intervertebral disc volume was assessed with a DICOM image converter [14].and a magnetic resonance imaging scan, which has a negligible error rate.

7. The precision of MRI equipment was defined from a sample calibration volume that was measured in each MRI scanner. In the retrospective cohort study, a bias of up to 0.9% was accepted. All patients also carried on them a foreign object with a well-defined calibration value to measure the precision of the MRI scan while.

4.3.2 Outcome measures

Primary outcome: Data recorded for each patient over a period before impedance therapy and after a series of therapies were retrospectively evaluated [4]:

1. Pain perception. Pain is assessed on a scale of 1–10 (1 = no pain, 10 = unbearable pain) [4].

2. Magnetic resonance (MR) imaging. MR images were used to visualize the discs in 3D, with the findings evaluated in DICOM files in order to assess and compare the effect of the therapy. The DICOM images were processed by InVesallius a DICOM data converter program (Paulo 2014). DGU was subsequently confirmed by visions of images of regenerated intervertebral discs that had healed and grown. A Siemens 1.5 T MRI scanner provided the MR images. They were produced in the following sequences:

    a. transversal T2 weighted images,

    b. sagittal T2 weighted images and 3D data. The sequences were always at the same level, with a 1-millimeter-thick cross-section. The standard number of cross-sections was 19 ± 3 per sequence. InVesalius then converted the DICOM images to the STL (stereolithography) file format, with MR scanning subtracting the imaged part. The images were then evaluated by a neurologist, radiologist or neurosurgeon.

        - Standardized volume was measured on each of the MRI scanners prior to the start of treatment. The exact reference volume was then imaged on an MRI scanner, and a 3D reconstruction was created. This provided evidence of its precision and accuracy.

        - Based on our observations, the standard deviation of magnetic resonance machine precision in Slovakia was calculated at about ±10%.

        - For the study, a ± 0.68% bias was accepted.

3. Neurological examination of tendon-periosteal reflexes. Reflexes are assessed on a scale of 1–7 (0 = reflexes not manifested, 3 = average reflexes, 6 = strong reflexes) [4].

4. Assessment of capillary blood lactate levels – complementary measurement. An indicator of fatigue is the level of lactate in the blood, where long-term increased concentration causes metabolic acidification in the body's internal environment. Because fatigue also decreases body performance, blood lactate levels were measured both at rest and during artificial exercise. The mean blood lactate levels displayed in **Table 2** are after 10–30 minutes of exercise (before and after

Spine	Gender	Aero		Rest	
		Before	After	Before	After
Lumbar	Male (N = 58)	7.4 (1.3)	5.3 (0.8)	3.3 (0.5)	1.5 (0.3)
	Female (N = 36)	7.9 (1.7)	5.5 (0.7)	3.1 (0.4)	1.4 (0.3)
Cervical	Male (N = 37)	7.9 (1.4)	5.5 (0.8)	3.3 (0.5)	1.4 (0.3)
	Female (N = 30)	7.9 (1.4)	5.3 (0.7)	3.2 (0.5)	1.4 (0.3)

Table 2.
Statistical analysis of lactate values.

enrollment in the study). The reference blood lactate level at rest is 0.7–1.8 mmol/L. A blood lactate value of 4 mmol/l during exercise is generally considered to be the limit of the body's efficiency for a patient used to exercising. Patients that are recreational athletes can push their blood lactate limit up to 5.5 mmol/l. Measuring blood lactate levels provides information for monitoring improvement in the body's physical condition from impedance therapy [4].

Design and flow of participants through the trial it shows in **Figure 1**.

4.3.3 Data analysis

Descriptive statistics, which compares input and output data, was used to process the data obtained. Information about the normal distribution of the data and the equality of variances was found from the Kolmogorov-Smirnov and Shapiro-Wilk normality tests and Levene's test of variances. If the significance of both tests at the alpha level is greater than 0.05, then the data and variances are normally distributed. Concurrently, the Student's t-test was used for evaluation. If the significance of the test of normality or variance at the alpha level is less than 0.05, it is a selection with a disrupted normal distribution of the data or variances, and so a nonparametric statistical significance test would be used for the evaluation, in this case, the Wilcoxon signed-rank test. A standard measure of the magnitude of our observations came from effect size. To process the data, MS Office Excel 2007 and SPSS 16 statistical software were used.

4.4 Results

Retrospective data were processed for 161 patients with an established ICD diagnosis of G54.0,1,2,4 and/or M54.2,4,5,12,16,17. There were 66 (41%) women and 95 (59%) men with a mean age of 50 (11) and 55 (13) years, respectively (**Table 1**). Due to the homogenized population, data from both the cervical and lumbar regions were statistically processed. Among the female patients, data was collected from the cervical and lumbar regions of 30 and the lumbar regions of 36. In the case of the male patients, data was taken from the cervical regions of 37 and from the lumbar region of the remaining 58.

The retrospective study for 2019 of the data obtained showed intervertebral disc volume to have risen in the men, due to DGU, at 3.2 cm^3 (21%) (95% CI) in the lumbar region and at 0.4 cm^3 (19%) (95% CI) in the cervical region. In the women, these figures were 2.2 cm^3 (16%) (95% CI) and 0.4 cm^3 (25%) (95% CI), respectively.

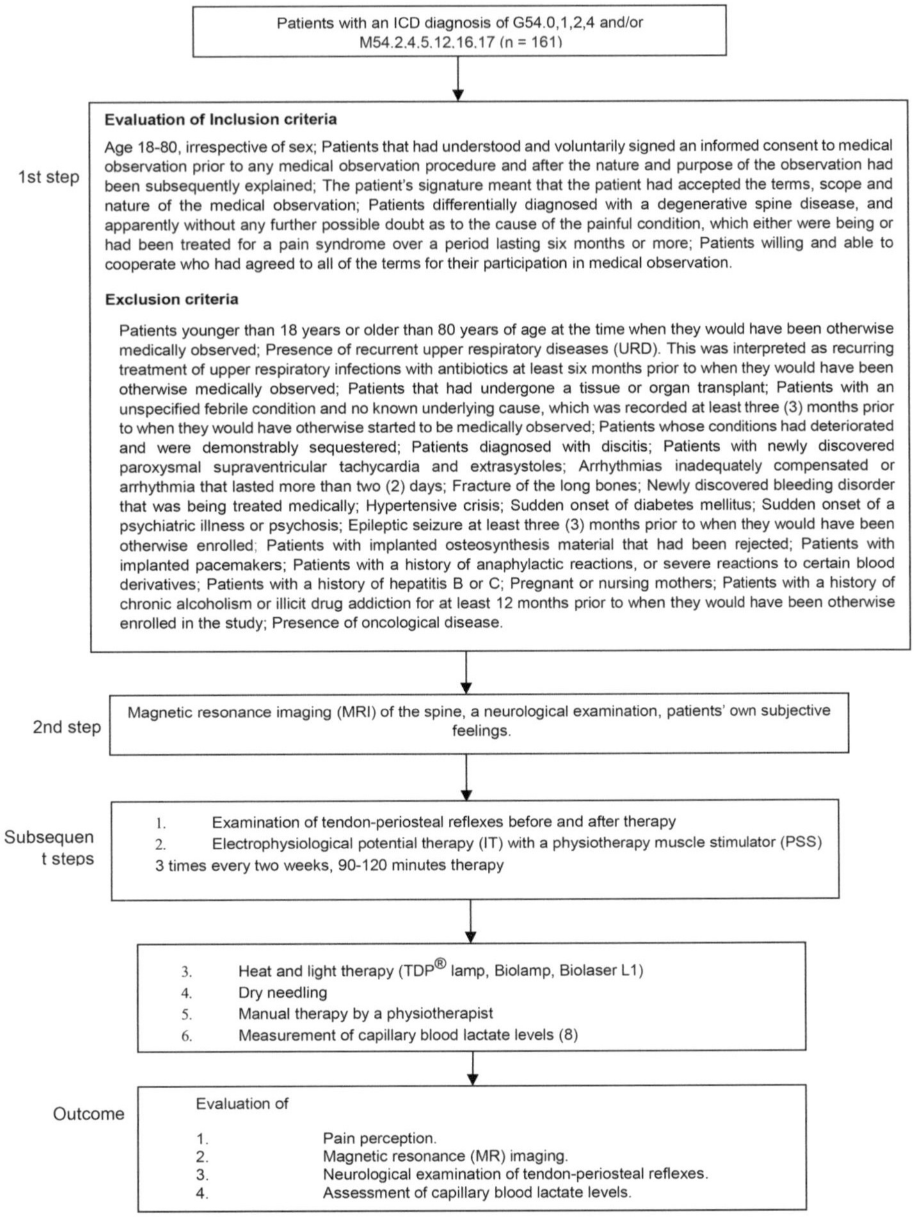

Figure 1.
Design and flow of participants through the trial.

Table 3 shows the increase in disc volume among both sexes and in both spinal regions studied to be highly statistically significant ($p < 0.001$). The pre- and post-IT magnetic resonance images in **Figures 2–7** objectify the treatment of patients with degenerative spine disease.

A reduction of pain was noted in the lumbar region by 4 points (78%) (95% CI) of the men and in the cervical region by 3 points (68%) (95% CI) of them. Among the women, 4 points (78%) (95% CI) of them experienced a reduction of pain in the cervical region and 4 points (73%) (95% CI) in the lumbar region. A highly

Spine	Gender	Disc volume (cm^3)	
		Before	After
Lumbar	Male (N = 58)	15.4 (4.9)	18.6 (5.1)
	Female (N = 36)	13.2 (4.3)	15.4 (4.5)
Cervical	Male (N = 37)	2.2 (0.5)	2.7 (0.5)
	Female (N = 30)	1.6 (0.3)	1.9 (0.30)

Table 3.
Mean (SD) of disc volume.

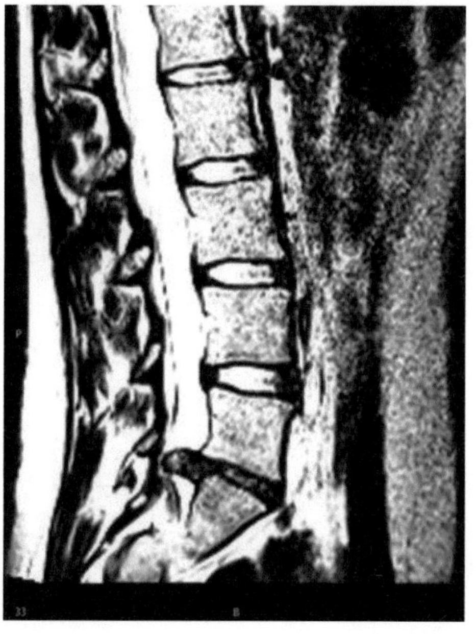

Figure 2.
MRI image of the lumbar spine before IT (female, 1997).

statistically significant reduction of pain ($p < 0,001$) was documented in both sexes and both study areas (**Table 4**).

Records obtained from entrance and exit neurological examinations, specifically in tendon-periosteal reflexes, showed highly statistically significant changes of $p < 0.01$ in both cohorts. The exception was among women who showed no normalized tendon-periosteal reflexes in the lumbar region, at a statistically significant $p = 0.064$ (**Table 5**). The processing of tendon-periosteal reflex data was based on optimizing their amenability, which equals a median value of 3.

The medical information obtained while examining the blood lactate level during the second block of planned long-term rehabilitation showed (**Table 2**) when DGU was confirmed in a patient, the blood lactate level could be adjusted to the second block's physiological parameters. This change in the lactate level is associated with the end of long-term rehabilitation and termination of treatment after the patient no longer requires medical care. **Table 6** summarizes the results from the monitoring of the entire population.

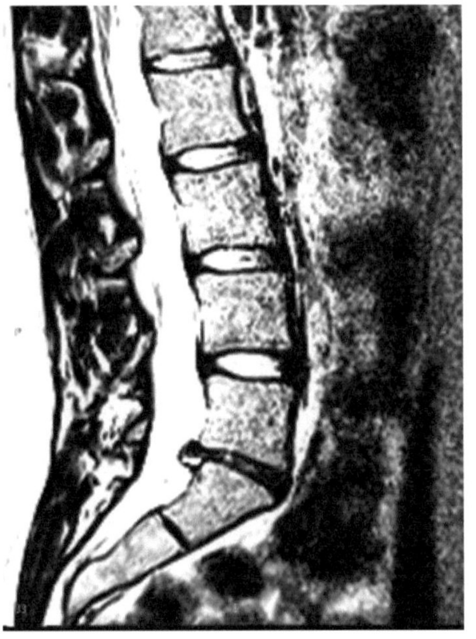

Figure 3.
MRI image of the lumbar spine after IT (female, 1997).

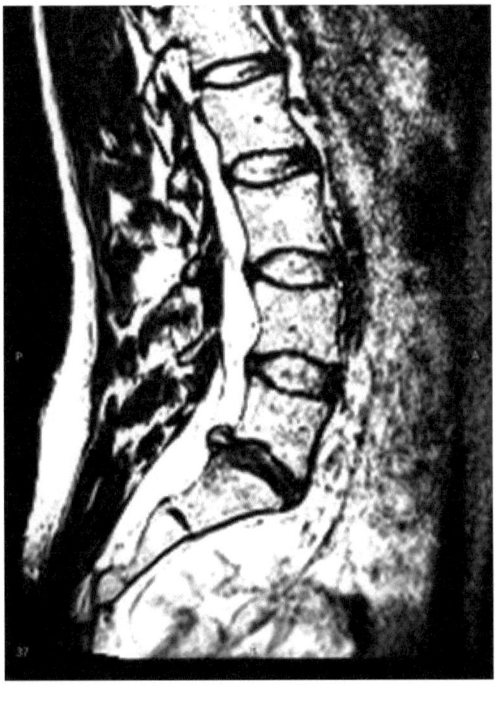

Figure 4.
MRI image of the lumbar spine before IT (female, 1982).

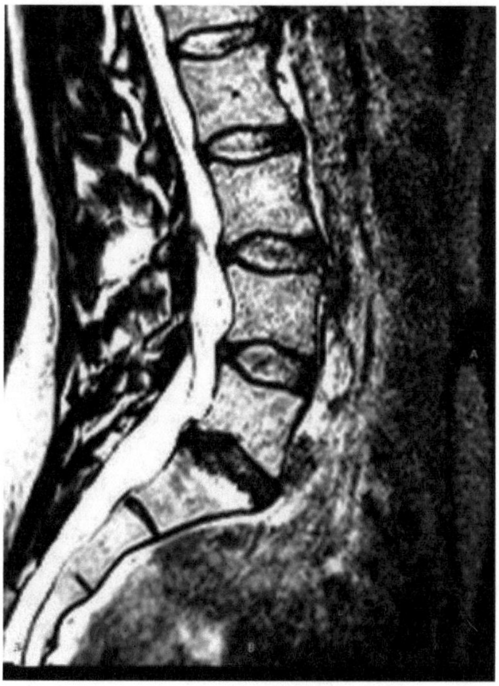

Figure 5.
MRI image of the lumbar spine after IT (female, 1982).

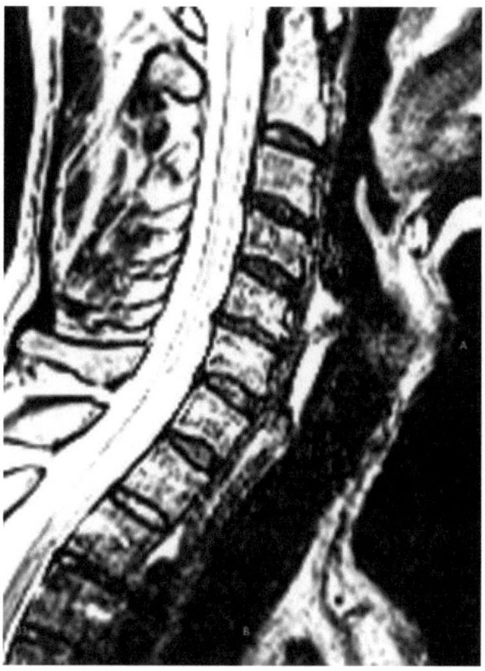

Figure 6.
MRI image of the cervical spine before IT (male, 1980).

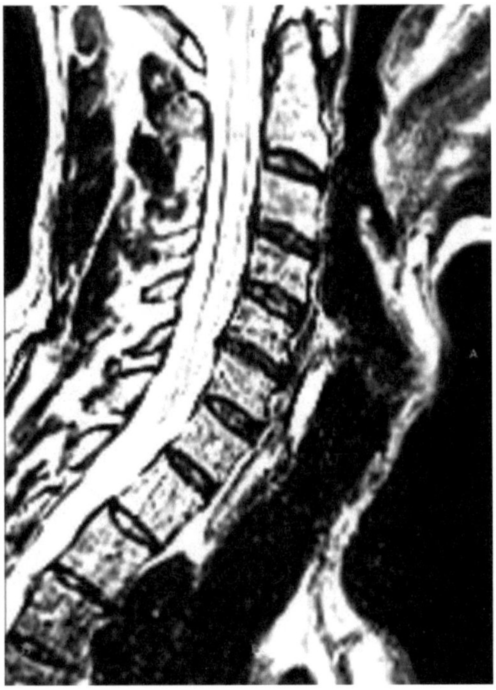

Figure 7.
MRI image of the cervical spine after IT (male, 1980).

Spine	Gender	Pain	
		Before	After
Lumbar	Male (N = 58)	5.3 (1.6)	1.2 (0.4)
	Female (N = 36)	6.1 (2.3)	1.7 (0.7)
Cervical	Male (N = 37)	4.5 (1.4)	1.4 (0.6)
	Female (N = 30)	5.5 (2.2)	1.2 (0.5)

1 = no pain, 10 = unbearable pain.

Table 4.
Mean (SD) of pain perception.

Spine	Gender	Tendon-periosteal reflexes	
		Before	After
Lumbar	Male (N = 58)	1.9 (1.1)	2.6 (0.5)
	Female (N = 36)	2.2 (1.3)	2.5 (0.6)
Cervical	Male (N = 37)	1.6 (0.8)	2.8 (0.4)
	Female (N = 30)	1.7 (1.0)	2.6 (0.5)

0 = reflexes not manifested, 3 = average reflexes, 6 = strong reflexes.

Table 5.
Mean (SD) of tendon-periosteal reflexes.

	N	Before	After
Disc volume (cm^3)	161	9.3 (7.2)	11.1 (8.4)
Pain (points)	161	5.3 (1.9)	1.4 (0.6)
PTR	161	1.8 (1.1)	2.6 (0.5)

Table 6.
Means (SD) of disc volume, tendon-periosteal reflexes and pain perception.

The outcome of treatment was considered to have been successful:

1. If conversion and comparison of DICOM magnetic resonance images before and after a patient underwent planned rehabilitation confirmed morphological changes in intervertebral discs caused by DGU.

2. If comparative neurological examinations showed improvement.

3. If the patient subjectively considered his or her condition to have improved because of the loss or significant reduction of pain complications, allowing him or her to return to original and not only self-supporting activities.

4.5 Discussion

The objective of the retrospective study was to monitor the effect of an innovative electrophysiological potential therapy, impedance therapy, on improving the condition of DDD patients and to confirm growth in intervertebral discs due to the DGU phenomenon. The outcome confirms the positive effect from impedance therapy in the enlargement and increased size of intervertebral discs. Evidence was provided by magnetic resonance imaging (MRI) scans of patients, which exactly demonstrated the disc grow-up (DGU) phenomenon.

Conservative treatment, rest and adequate medical therapy and rehabilitation are effective in 85–90% of patients at the level of their subjective symptoms. Surgery is indicated in 10% of the patients where radicular irritation persists and/or neurological deficit progresses with conservative treatment. Rare syndromes and progressive motor radicular deficits require urgent surgical treatment [15]. The remaining 5–10% of patients remain chronically disabled, especially with back pain, despite the treatment available. Surgery for patients with chronic back pain has not been very successful. Surgery is indicated when there is significant functional incapacity or pain is unresponsive to multidisciplinary conservative treatment. The prognosis for patients is influenced by the severity of the clinical manifestation, the possibility of providing rapid adequate treatment and psychosocial-economic factors. Degenerative changes of the spine as a disease of civilization could have been treated by standard medical or nonmedical treatment but never eliminated [4, 7, 16]. This reported retrospective study traces the emergence of the DGU phenomenon under the influence of IT. Evidence of intervertebral disc growth after SEIs because of DGU was first confirmed in "Impedance therapy in rehabilitation of degenerative disc disease a clinical randomized trial in a cohort composed of 55 patients with an ICD diagnosis of G54.0,1,2,4 and/or M54.2,4,5,12,16,17 and averaging 51 years of age. They were divided into monitored and control cohorts [4]. A total of 61 patients were enrolled in the study, from which six of the patients were excluded, four because of the exclusion criteria and two opted to discontinue their participation in the study. The first monitored cohort comprised 29 patients with a mean age of 57 (11) years. It had 22 (76%) men and 7 (24%) women whose average ages were 57 (12) and 55 (13) years, respectively. They received impedance therapy. This electrophysiological potential therapy produced changes in the health of the monitored cohort of patients when they followed the changes mapped out in the rehabilitation plan. Patients included in the cohort underwent a period of reverse transcription (RT) symptoms, which involved the reappearance of past difficulties, although they were less intensive. The presence of RT symptoms was a manifestation of DGU-caused intervertebral disc regeneration. The other control cohort consisted of 26 patients with a mean age of 46 (11) years. It had 10 women with the same average age as the control cohort and 16 men whose mean age of 46 (13) years. They received standard electrotherapy. There was a transient improvement in their condition noted during the first 3–4 weeks. Subsequently, it varied harmoniously between the painful conditions experienced before they were enrolled in the therapeutic block and periods of subjective feelings of good health.

In the monitored cohort, intervertebral disc growth was demonstrated in 76% of the patients, where the DGU phenomenon was confirmed in 22 patients (intervertebral disc volume increased by more than 10%). There was no evidence of the DGU phenomenon in 24% of the patients from the application of impedance therapy and no reduction in intervertebral disc volume either. DDD did not progress (intervertebral disc volume rose 0–5%) [4]. Existing available references list a number of studies that examined the use of physiotherapy in patients with degenerative spinal conditions, looking only at the impact on pain, range of motion in the spine and quality of life. In a review study, Kroeling [17] included 20 studies involving a total of 1239 patients, where the cohorts consisted of adult patients aged more than 18 years with both acute and chronic cervical spine pain or nonspecific pain, including degenerative changes, myofascial pain and headaches that originated from the cervical region. The outcomes from these studies could not be pooled because different populations had been examined, and there were different types and dosages of electrotherapy and comparative treatments with moderately different results measured. The CENTRAL, MEDLINE, EMBASE, MANTIS, CINAHL and ICL databases were searched with no language restrictions until August 2012. The results from these searches indicated that transcutaneous electrical nerve stimulation (TENS) had a more significant effect on pain reduction in patients with acute pain than electrical stimulation, exercise, infrared light, manual therapy and ultrasound. Efficacy was not statistically significant for combinations of infrared light therapy, thermotherapy and kinesiotherapy, nor the combination of cervical collar, exercise and pharmacotherapy. In patients with chronic cervical spine pain, TENS probably relieved pain as well or better than a placebo or electrical muscle stimulation, although not as well as exercise and infrared light. However, a similar effect was obtained with a combination of manual therapy, mobilization techniques and ultrasound [17]. Lau [18] published a randomized trial describing two physiotherapy phases, where the first phase consisted of movement therapy and interferential currents were indicated in the second phase. In the acute stage of the disease, either pharmacotherapy or soft relaxation techniques are recommended for back pain [18]. Hayden [19] in review found evidence that Pilates, McKenzie therapy and functional restoration were more effective than other types of exercise treatment for reducing pain intensity and functional limitations. Nevertheless, people with chronic low back pain should be encouraged to perform the exercise that they enjoy to promote adherence. In addition to IT, rehabilitation in our study includes exercise and continued physical activity.

A retrospective study of electrophysiological potential therapy - impedance therapy in 2019 showed the following:

1. Statistically significant growth in intervertebral disc volume at 2.8 cm^3 (19%) ($p < 0.001$).

2. A 4 (75%) points reduction in pain perception after IT ($p < 0.001$), with an exit neurological examination specifically demonstrating statistically significant changes in tendon-periosteal reflexes ($p < 0.01$).

4.6 Medical observations from the study

1. Based on empirical findings, the success and effectiveness of impedance therapy were dependent on the degree of DDD and the dynamics of degenerative structural changes.

2. A necessary condition for inducing regenerative processes was the regular frequency of impedance therapy (optimally three times every 2 weeks with an assessment of DGU after the first block).

3. The records of patients that had received impedance therapy documented changes in their condition that followed the course of changes described in the long-term rehabilitation plan.

4. Patients enrolled in impedance therapy underwent a period of RT symptoms and this is evidence of correctly applied impedance therapy. A reverse transcription symptom marks the reappearance of past difficulties albeit with less intense pain and no objective change in the patient's level of mobility. The presence of RT symptoms is a manifestation of DGU-caused intervertebral disc regeneration. Their significance comes not only at the level of having analyzed a correctly applied therapy. The presence of these symptoms is confirmed by the following:

    - Changes in capillary blood lactate level

    - Change in tendon-periosteal reflexes

    - Changes in muscle tension

    Reverse transcription symptoms appeared at two separate time intervals:

    - The first set of RT symptoms are predominantly linked to SEI-induced changes in blood lactate levels and take place between four and 8 weeks into planned long-term rehabilitation.

    - The second set (between 14 and 18 weeks into planned long-term rehabilitation) is linked to rapid intervertebral disc decompression. It more markedly irritates other unmyelinated C-fibers, whose stimulation appears because of peripheral sensitization. After the second set of RT symptoms, an MRI of the patient was indicated, followed by evaluation and 3D visualization by InVesalius of the intervertebral disc. Confirmation of the DGU phenomenon translates into the completion of the first block of the long-term rehabilitation plan and the patient's continuation in the second block, which focuses on increasing his or her exercise capacity and adjusting weight.

5. The inability of the body to respond to IT with a harmonious change in resistance highlighted the body's own slowed capability to regenerative induction, slowing the increase in intervertebral disc volume (the DGU phenomenon).

6. The effect of IT on a patient's pain in confirmed DDD cases has been demonstrated in the controlled reduction in the number of new, unwanted protrusions of sensitive nerve fibers that have sprouted. These show increased irritability due to the increased concentration of sodium and calcium channels.

7. The effect on unmyelinated C-fibers was demonstrated when the following was observed:

    - Changes in skin conductance or the psychogalvanic reflex (PGR) [9, 13];
    - Increase in intervertebral disc volume, reduction and gradual disappearance of DDD-typical structural changes and reduction of discogenic pain where the source was black disc, a degenerative disc disease [8].

8. Unless there is an active feedback loop in the internal information system and pooling, the full therapeutic impact of IT on a patient's body cannot be ensured.

Other diagnostic criteria for enrollment into impedance therapy:

- Degenerative disc disease (DDD)
- Recurrent back pain and no proven degenerative spinal disease
- Hernia of the intervertebral disc up to 9 mm and extending into the spinal canal without sequestration
- Impaired aerobic and anaerobic thresholds and simultaneously confirmed degenerative disc disease without subjective symptoms
- Listhesis of the lumbar or cervical spine
- Spinal block with or without back pain
- Diabetic polyneuropathy in the lower extremities
- Tennis and golfer's elbow
- Gonarthrosis with no traumatic etiology
- Chronic fatigue syndrome

DOI: http://dx.doi.org/10.5772/intechopen.1001951

- Exhaustion
- Histamine imbalance

5. Conclusion

Impedance therapy, an electrophysiological potential therapy, offers a new perspective on the course, prognosis and therapy for a disease of civilization, namely degenerative disc disease. The probability of reversing these structural degenerative changes is documented in the outcome of this study. It confirmed the possible active intervention in the degenerative cascade of the three-joint complex in individual movement segments of the spine, described by Kirkaldy-Willis in the 1970s. We believe that the effect and exact results of impedance therapy have disproved the theory of irreversible degenerative changes in the spine.

1. The outcome confirms the positive effect from impedance therapy in the enlargement and increased size of intervertebral discs. Evidence was provided by magnetic resonance imaging (MRI) scans of patients that exactly demonstrated the DGU phenomenon.

2. Impedance therapy has been applied as an innovative treatment for degenerative disc disease with an objectively measurable result of recovery for a patient's body in active medical practice.

3. The feedback loop for the next SEI, once a response to the previous SEI has been evaluated after a defined time interval, is critical to the application of impedance therapy. The prerequisites for IT to be applied were meeting inclusion criteria and the diagnostic conditions for impedance therapy in the rehabilitation plan.

4. Applying SEIs in electrophysiological potential therapy actively contributed to the elimination of DDD-caused pain. The first step in the application of impedance therapy focuses on removing structural changes no one can influence at their own volition. Later, the burden of regeneration shifts more to the patient. Once the body's internal balance has been set in a lactate analysis picture, gradual withdrawal from the long-term rehabilitation plan could then be laid out. Recent medical analyses have confirmed stable pain-free and movement-limited conditions for patients for at least 10 years after they had been rehabilitated and their long-term planned rehabilitation ended.

Degenerative changes of the spine as a disease of civilization could have been treated by standard medical or nonmedical treatment but never eliminated [5, 20]. A new type of treatment in the practice of physical therapy is the Impedance Therapy method.

Conflict of interest

The authors declare no conflict of interest.

Author details

Pavol Kostka[1]*, Elena Ziakova[2], Marek Janitor[3], Nina Sladekova[4], Martin Janitor[5], Daniel Vrabel[3] and Paulina Chripkova[3]

1 Institute of Impedance Therapy, Prague, Czech Republic

2 Faculty of Nursing and Professional Health Studies, Department of Physiotherapy, Slovak Medical University in Bratislava, Slovak Republic

3 Institute of Impedance Therapy, Bratislava, Slovak Republic

4 Faculty of Health Sciences, Department of Physiotherapy, University of Ss. Cyril and Methodius in Trnava, Slovak Republic

5 Amplia s.r.o., Bratislava, Slovak Republic

*Address all correspondence to: pavol.kostka.dr@gmail.com

References

[1] Bednarik J, Kadanka Z. Vertebrogenni neurologicke syndromy. Praha: Triton; 2000. p. 38

[2] Bednarik J et al. Klinicka neurologie–cast specialni II. Praha: Triton; 2010. pp. 1077-1112

[3] Kirkaldy-Willis WH, Paine KW, Cauchoix J, McIvor G. Lumbar spinal stenosis. Clinical Orthopaedics and Related Research. 1974;**99**:30-50. DOI: 10.1097/00003086-197403000-00004

[4] Kostka P, Ziakova E. Impedance therapy in rehabilitation of degenerative disc disease. Bratislavske lekarske listy. 2020;**121**(2):137-142. DOI: 10.4149/BLL_2020_019

[5] Lurie JD et al. Reliability of readings of magnetic resonance imaging features of lumbar spinal stenosis. Spine (Phila Pa 1976). 2008; **33**(14):1605-1610. DOI: 10.1097/BRS.0b013e3181791af3

[6] WMA. 52nd WMA general assembly. In: WMA Declaration of Helsinki – Ethical Principles for Medical Research Involving Human Subjects. Edinburgh, Scotland: WMA; 2000. p. 2000

[7] Rubin DI. Epidemiology and risk factors for spine pain. Neurologic Clinics. 2007;**25**(2):353-371. DOI: 10.1016/j.ncl.2007.01.004

[8] Luoma K et al. Low backpain in relation to lumbar disc degeneration. Spine. 2000;**25**(4):487-492. DOI: 10.1097/00007632-200002150-00016

[9] Patel RV. In: Kishner S, editor. Lumbar Degenerative Disk Disease, eMedicine. Medscape; 2016. Available from: https://emedicine.medscape.com/article/309767-overview

[10] Kishner S. In: Gest TR, editor. Lumbar spine anatomy. Medscape; 2015. Available from: https://emedicine.medscape.com/article/1899031-overview

[11] Kostka P. Impedancna terapia, 180 str. 2017. Available from: https://www.liecbaplatniciek.sk/doc/impedancna-terapia_vnutro.pdf

[12] Sharan, Alok D, Tang Simon Y, Alexander V. R: Basic Science of Spinal Disease. Jaypee Brothers Medical Publishers (P) Ltd; 2013. p. 300. Available from: https://books.google.sk/books/about/Basic_Science_of_Spinal_Diseases.html?id=0SU5VVqT_I8C&redir_esc=y

[13] Kucera P, Goldenberg Z, Kurca E. Symphatetic skin responce: Review of the method and its clinical use. Bratislavske lekarske listy. 2004;**105**(3): 108-116

[14] Paulo HJ et al. In Vesalius: Software Livre de Imagens Médicas. Philadelphia: Lippincott-Raven; 2014

[15] Mcculloch JA, Young PH. Essentials of Spinal Microsurgery. 7Rev ed. Philadelphia: Lippincott Williams & Wilkins; 1998. p. 668

[16] Martin BI et al. Expenditures and health status among adults with back and neck problems. JAMA. 2008;**299**: 656-664. DOI: 10.1001/jama.299.6.656

[17] Kroeling P et al. Electro therapy for neck pain (review). Cochrane Database of Systematic Reviews. 2013;**2013**: CD004251

[18] Lau P et al. Early physiotherapy intervention in an accident and

emergency department reduces pain and improves satisfaction for patients with acute low backpain: A randomised trial. The Australian Journal of Physiotherapy. 2008;**54**:243-249

[19] Hayden J et al. Exercise in chronic low back pain. Journal of Physiotherapy. 2021;**67**(4):252-262. DOI: 10.1016/j.jphys.2021.09.004

[20] Kostka P et al. Impedancna terapia II - aplikacia v medicinskej praxi. Poptlač, Poprad. 2019. p. 204 str

Chapter 12

Rehabilitation in the ICU

Monica Chiş and Ruxandra Copotoiu

Abstract

Prolonged stay in the ICU comes with a variety of sequelae evolving toward chronic conditions rendering rehabilitation a challenge for the medical staff and patients' families. Functional impairment is physical (touching mainly mobility: weakness, atrophy), cognitive or beyond (dysphagia, chronic pain, risk of falls). Properly identifying the risk factors means addressing them in a preventive manner. The curative approach, due to fragmented trajectories and the controversies related to early mobilization and the dose of physical rehabilitation, is still subject to debate. Possible barriers to implementing rehabilitation protocols were identified as well as future research themes regarding new targets for interventions to be tested in large-scale randomized controlled trials.

Keywords: ICU, post intensive care syndrome, muscular weakness, physical rehabilitation, prevention

1. Introduction

Progress made in critical care throughout recent years lead to an increase in survival rates and a greater number of post- ICU patients to care for. Surviving ICU does not mean a full return to the patients' capacities before 'the injury' leading to admission. Critical care survivors, their caregivers and families are burdened with functional impairments (physical, psychological, cognitive and beyond), prompting the implementations of a rapid and challenging rehabilitation program.

Patients' trajectories are various and fragmented, due to the type of injury precluding the ICU admission and the structures in place for the post-ICU care.

Recent research did not merely focus on survival, but also on the critical care survivors' recovery in the subsequent months, potentially years to follow.

2. Outcomes after ICU stay

It comes naturally for the outcome of a critically ill patient to depend on the severity of his condition upon admission and before becoming critically ill, on the number of days he was cared for, but also heavily, on the type of ICU attendance he was submitted to, that is on the competency of the ICU in cause (be it an academic facility or not), on the professionalism (knowledge, training, skills, dedication, ethics) and the management of the facility.

Outcomes after being cared for in an ICU refer to: sequels, evolving toward a chronic critical condition, acquiring muscular asthenia or weakness, developing delirium or other forms of acute psychosis (which is reputed for being associated with a bad outcome), developing multiple organ system failure, sepsis or becoming a reservoir (a source) for hospital-acquired germs. And as if these were not enough, survivors complain also of joint stiffness, pain, loss of condition and hair loss, and more disturbing, of dysphagia, which is a real invalidating burden, very difficult to treat, often undiagnosed and leading to nutrition issues, to say nothing of loss of hearing, smell and taste. Moreover, the recovery phase could last for years [1].

Since 2012, "ICU-acquired weakness" was defined as "diffuse, symmetric, generalized muscle weakness detected by physical examination and meeting specific strength-related criteria, that develops after the onset of critical illness without other identifiable cause [2].

The pathophysiology of ICU-AW blames it on an inflammatory response, bioenergetic dysfunction, altered protein balance, neuronal axon degeneration, changes in muscle histology and muscle wasting. AW seems to be triggered by the critical condition and its severity is independent of the underlying primary condition. The rhythm of muscular mass loss due to bedrest of the critically ill is approximately 2% per day, a rate different between muscles and dependent upon the measurements taken [3].

A general term to comprise the syndrome that describes the clinical signs of suffering survivors of a lengthy admission in the ICU was coined as PICS (post-intensive care syndrome). PICS refers to a new or worsening disorder, be it physical (muscular weakness, diminished autonomy to cope with daily living), PTSD (posttraumatic stress disorder), depression or other neurocognitive disorder impeding the quality of life and being a significant financial burden for both individuals and the society as a whole [4]. It was established that about 22% of former critically ill patients develop PTSD while 28% will be taunted by depression (Davydow cited by 5). Long-term patient outcomes may include pulmonary, neuromuscular, psychiatric and cognitive impairments as well as alteration of the physical function. PA (physical activity) was suspected to have a positive impact on delirium outcomes in intensive care unit patients. Since delirium impacts 80% of MV patients, there were expectations for PA to positively impact delirium outcomes. Immobility and functional decline are considered as risk factors for delirium. In non-critical patients, PA seems to provide neuroprotective effects by increasing neurotransmitter and anti-inflammatory mediator release and to facilitate synaptic transmission. It also increases cerebral blood flow in older adults and oxygen extraction efficiency, improving cognition. Therefore, Jarman et al. performed a systematic review and meta-analysis to investigate the impact of PA interventions on delirium outcomes in ICU patients. Unfortunately, they found only low-quality evidence in favor of greater-intensity PA. They concluded that there was insufficient evidence to recommend PA as a stand-alone intervention to reduce delirium in the ICUs [5].

While pulmonary outcomes appear as impairment in spirometry, lung volume and diffusion capacity, the incriminated risk factors are the duration of mechanical ventilation and the diffusion capacity. Even if the pulmonary impairment is generally mild, it can persist for over five years.

The ICU-acquired weakness includes polyneuropathy and myopathy and blames the hyperglycemia, the SIRS, sepsis and MODS (multiple system organ dysfunction syndrome). Polyneuropathy can extend to five years, far more than myopathy. Disuse atrophy is attributable to immobility/bed rest. The impairment of physical function is described as disuse atrophy, an impairment in activity of daily living (ADL/IADL) and in 6-minutes walking distance. Systemic corticosteroids use, ICU-acquired illness, age, slow-resolution of lung injury and preexisting IADL impartment are selected risk factors. It is expected for ADL to improve within months, but the signs may persist for one year, while IADL is to disappear in two years. Long-term impairment for 6-min walk distance is to be expected.

Depression attributable to traumatic/delusional memories of ICU, sedation, psychiatric symptoms at discharge, and impairment of physical function might decrease over the first year. PTSD is to improve a little over the first year and is due to sedation, agitation, physical restraints and traumatic/delusional memories. Anxiety may persist for the first year and identifies as risk factors the following: unemployment, duration of mechanical ventilation, as well as overall risk factors, such as female gender, younger age, less education, pre-ICU psychiatric symptoms and personality. The cognitive function is affected by impairment in memory, alteration of the executive function, mental processing speed and visio-spatial ability. It blames for the occurrence of lower pre-ICU intelligence, ICU delirium, sedation, hypoxia and glucose dysregulation. Although it might significantly improve during the first year, residual deficits may last up to 6 years.

There is a toll on families as well, and they are but psychiatric, such as depression, PTSD, anxiety and complicated grief. When it comes to depression, among identical risk factors with the critically ill, distance to the hospital and restricted visiting emerge.

For PTSD, unsatisfactory communication along with dissatisfaction with a caring, passive preference for decision-making and a mismatch between involvement in decision-making and preferences contribute to the persistence of PTSD for four years or more after death or discharge.

Complicated grief is deepened by the knowledge gap of the patient's wishes, while when it comes for children, paternal stress after discharge is associated with child stress and may persist even past childhood.

To the complexity of the postcritically ill syndrome, we can add the sequelae of critical illness: multidimensional functional disability (prolonged MV, compromised ambulation, pharyngeal muscle weakness, dysphagia, increased risk of aspiration, reduced health-related quality of life, a nutritional compromise leading to compromise physical and neurocognitive recovery [6]. Entrapment neuropathy manifests as foot or wrist drop that compromises rehabilitation and recovery, or frailty. Mood disorders, pressure injuries that contribute to increased post-ICU mortality, oral complications (gingivitis, dental caries, tooth injury or loss, need for longer dental follow-up), endocrinopathies (thyroid gland, adrenal function derangements, disruptive endocrine homeostasis and sexual function), changes in appearance (frozen joints, alopecia, scarring, disfigurement, complicated social reintegration), taste changes, hearing or vision changes, procedure-related trauma (rectal, urethral injury, vocal cord dysfunction, tracheal stenosis) and chronic renal dysfunction sometimes needing RRT (renal replacement therapy increased health care use and 1-year mortality [6].

The SCCM (Society of Critical Care Medicine) recommends discharge to subacute rehabilitation facilities once the acute medical issues are resolved, or to long-term acute care hospitals when greater medical specialization is required [7].

As long as life expectancy improves in Europe and ICU lengths of stay also in order to achieve survival, since predominantly medical admissions consume over 50% of yearly ICU treatment days, and as countries over Europe further in debt, as human resource to care for the critically ill and to take over after discharge is scarcer, post ICU syndrome becomes more and more prominent [7, 8].

Thus, the solution for the survivors of an ICU long stay appears to be rehabilitation in a specialized unit. The USA took the initiative since the early eighties by opening the LTACHs (long-term acute care hospitals) dedicated to ICU survivors suffering from a large spectrum of problems, such as weaning from prolonged mechanical ventilation, and nonsurgical complicated wound care (decubitus). The requirements of LTACHs imply not only compliance with the legal requirements of hospitals delivering acute care, but also multidisciplinary physician-led teams to supervise and coordinate individual complex patient programs that take over 25 days [9].

Articles from Europe, Australia and New Zealand, Africa and Asia are increasingly dedicated to rehabilitation of the ICU survivors. Thus, Herridge et al. were able to identify acronyms relevant for studies on the outcome of the critically ill: ICAP, ALTOS, FROG-ICU, RECOVER, THRIVE, My ICU care and ICU steps to name a few. They concomitantly questioned the ethics of indefinite trials of MV or ECMO support [6].

In addition, Reid et al. identified important reporting deficiencies in ICU delivered PR interventions that limit clinical implementation and future trial development [10].

3. Best practices identified, validated or confirmed

We will try to highlight the best practices identified as being associated with patient satisfaction and also with caregiver fulfillment as a patient. Seo and al tried to assess the functional recovery and promoted the AM-PAC score (Activity Measure Post-Acute Care) [11]. They recognized the post-intensive care syndrome as an obstacle for full recovery, which if ever happening, will do so in no less than three years and came up with a check list to qualify for rehabilitation starting the 3rd day after admission to the SICU (Surgical Intensive Care Unit). The check list comprises: no more than 2 vasopressors, no recent shock event (<4 hours), a mean BP $\geq$60 mmHg, heart rate $\leq$ 120 bpm, respiratory rate $\leq$ 24/min, axillary temperature $\leq$ 38°C, no dysrhythmia, RASS -2 to +2, FiO2 $\leq$ 0.5 and a PEEP $\leq$10 mmHg [11].

They recommended a rehabilitation plan comprising five steps to be performed 20 to 30 minutes on week days. The first step would be PROM (Passive Range of Motion) and Postural change. Then follows the start of active rehabilitation, The AROM (Active Range of Motion), with the head elevation at $\geq$60°. Upper and lower extremity exercises follow, then a sit to stand attempt followed by marching on the spot. As we can see, the intensity of the effort gradually increases, as the complexity of the movements. Seo's article was preceded by Conradie et al. who in 2017 published their adapted early mobility readiness protocol, very similar to Seo's check-list [12]. They included the PaO_2/FiO_2 ratio of $\geq$250, $SpO_2 \geq 90\%$ and all the aforementioned hemodynamic parameters with overlapping values. They concluded that active rehabilitation in critically ill surgical patients was feasible and safe regardless of age provided the patients' safety was checked before. Standing activity in the ICU was not routine postoperative care [11].

Vollenweider R et al. studied the sedated and ventilated ICU patients and concluded that passive early motion reduced the nitrosative stress, although there was

DOI: http://dx.doi.org/10.5772/intechopen.1002614

no clear effect on cytokines. They advanced an early adapted mobility readiness protocol hoping to provide the healthcare professionals with an interim tool to identify the patients who would tolerate a therapeutic upright position. They aimed at incorporating the upright standing position into standard nursing care, which would be a huge step toward improving recovery [13]. Lang JK et al. performed a systematic review of the published clinical practice guidelines for early mobilization (EM) in the ICU and they found that there was agreement on the principle of implementing EM [14].

Verceles et al. ran a study on prolonged MV critically ill patients suffering of AW, comparing and measuring the outcome of the patients submitted to either UC (usual care) with those who underwent an additional progressive multimodal rehabilitation program (MRP). They found that the addition of an MRP improved strength, physical function and mobility and was associated with greater weaning success and discharge home [15].

Beach et al. used motion sensors to measure PA of the critically ill ventilated for more than 48 hours and expected to stay in the ICU for at least 5 days. They also measured energy expenditure. They found that PA levels during the first 5 days of admission in the ICU when measured using METs were low. Sedation was the main barrier reported by physiotherapists. Motion sensors are safe, but used early in the ICU have limited clinical utility since sepsis impacts on metabolic rate. Since the correlation of PA against ICU mobility scale was strong, motion sensors promise to be best exploited to monitor activity levels in interventional studies [16].

Lai et al. had previously demonstrated that twice daily EM sessions reduced days of MV of medical critically ill patients when introduced within the first 3 days of MV, by almost 3 days (from 7.5 to 4.7 days) and also diminishes the risk of prolonged MV (≥7 days). However, the differences did not reach statistical significance [17].

A recent study concluded that early exercise training using a bedside cycle ergometer in critically ill ICU survivors who received MV enhanced the recovery of gastrointestinal function and improved the patients' nutrition status at hospital discharge [18].

When it comes to thoroughly assessing the methodology used in the studies dealing with EM of MV patients, a systematic review included in the Cochrane database concluded that the evidence for the effectiveness of EM on measure of physical function and performance is inconsistent and uncertain due to its low quality [19]. The same applies to adverse effects. There is hope that better-designed ongoing studies will clarify the issue of EM. This harsh conclusion emerged from the sample sizes (judged too small), clearly reported interventions and control conditions, but also the blinded outcome assessment that usually lacked. There is an additional need for standardization of outcome measures and to disentangle early intervention from the intensity of intervention [19].

According to this trend of refining research, Collet et al. initiated a study including relevant articles comprised in the electronic databases for a decade (2012–2022). They will assess the functional and cognitive rehabilitation interventions during admission [20]. In depth knowledge is unlikely to benefit, but current understanding is expected to be uplifted.

Results of PR (physical rehabilitation) studies are tricky to compare since CG (comparator groups) are different, Still, as O'Grady and all showed, the most common type of CG is usual care [21]. There is a remarkable heterogeneity in planned activities and CERT (Consensus on Exercise Reporting Template; proportion of reported items/total applicable) reporting deficiencies [21].

In line with this trend of thoroughness, Connolly et al. described the PRACTICE (physical rehabilitation core outcomes in critical illness), a protocol for the development of a core outcome set) [22].

At the end of the day, even if protocols to care for the MV patients are proposed and used, there are no validated techniques to prevent post-mechanical ventilation injuries and sequels.

As for those who require or look forward to apply an already established protocol, Raurell-Torreda et al. publish an early mobilization algorithm for the critical patient. There is an algorithm of decision-making, but also IMS (ICU Mobility Scale) objective according to safety criteria [23]. Garcia-Perez-de-Sevilla also investigated the effectiveness of physical exercise and neuromuscular electrical stimulation interventions for preventing and treating ICU-acquired weakness and concluded that both methods should be used to prevent significant muscle loss. If patients can cooperate, they recommend to prioritize physical exercise against neuromuscular electrical stimulation, as it is superior for improving functionality [24].

4. Controversies

Controversies were almost completely pinned by Laghi [25].

There is no doubt that rest is paramount for recovery. Potential benefits of increased bedrest in ill humans are already well known: conservation of metabolic resources to be used for healing and recovery; reduce oxygen consumption by muscles and divert oxygen delivery toward injured tissues and organs in need; reduce requirements for ventilation and the risk of VILI (ventilation induced lung injury); reduce requirements for high FiO2 and the risk of oxygen toxicity; improve blood flow to the central nervous system; reduce harmful falls and the stress to the heart; prevent ischemia and dysrhythmias; avoid pain from additional injury and to injured body parts [26]. Despite these benefits, when prolonged over the usual 6–9 hours of sleep, bedrest is associated with no trivial complications: skeleton muscle atrophy and weakness, joint contractures, thromboembolic disease, insulin resistance, microvascular dysfunction, insulin resistance, systemic inflammation, atelectasis and pressure ulcers [26]. Nondamaging exercise is a major stimulus for IL-6 release while IL-1 and TNF-α concentrations do not substantially increase with exercise. IL-6 is also a strong inhibitor of TNF-α and IL-1. Moreover, exercise induced IL-6 release from muscles is associated with elevated concentrations in plasma of the IL-IRA and IL-10, both anti-inflammatory mediators. Regulated exercise decreases C-reactive protein levels also. Thus, atherogenesis might be prevented by decreasing vascular inflammation and insulin-sensitivity is increased. Prolonged bedrest opposed, annulled the benefits of muscle exercise. Overall, the prevalence of ICU-AW is 48% [3].

Knowing that critically ill patients can lose over 15% of their muscle mass within one week, one can expect long-term detrimental effects [3]. The dominant method to assess muscle waste is ultrasound, followed by CT scans.

The rationale for rehabilitation in the ICU is not always crystal clear. Questioning the clinicians as to the shortcomings of implementing rehabilitation exercises in the ICU, Nickels et al. found out that it was unlikely attributable to a lack of perceived importance by nursing, medical or physiotherapy clinicians, the most likely to influence rehabilitation practices in the ICU [27].

As of today, several controversies emerge and seem to be there to stay at least for a while.

Rehabilitation in the ICU is different in medical compared to surgical ICUs. Mobility is sometimes easier to achieve in surgical patients who became critically ill due to their surgery need. Once solved, their recovery is accelerated by early mobilization. The validation of selection criteria to identify the long-stay ICU patients susceptible to best benefit from an ICU rehabilitation facility should be addressed in further studies [9].

4.1 Different approaches to the same issue

Different conclusions or outcomes, different types of research articles, various experiences, different patients, different spatial coordinates and socio-economic issues account for the variability of the outcome in terms of duration of complete recovery or length of stay. As for those for whom the ICU is one bridge too far, gentle and humane care is advanced and should be provided [9].

Lime in 2014, Patel et al. completed a secondary analysis on all patients (N = 104) enrolled in an RCT of early occupational and physical therapy vs. conventional therapy, which evaluated the endpoint of functional independence. Every single patient benefited from ITT (intensive insulin therapy) and blinded muscular strength testing on hospital discharge to assess the incidence of ICU – AW (clinically apparent weakness). Logistic regression analysis showed that early mobilization and increasing insulin dose prevented the incidence of ICU-AW, independent on the risk factors. Still, insulin may be associated with reduced ICU-AW, but its safety profile cautions against using it for preventive reasons. Further on, the dual effect of early mobilization in reducing relevant ICU-AW and promoting euglycemia suggested its potential usefulness as an alternative to ITT [28].

In an attempt to understand the discordant results of ICU-based PR (physical rehabilitation), O'Grady et al. found that there was heterogeneity and underreporting of CG (comparator group), which perhaps contributed to discordant results. Not uncommon in rehabilitation research, these findings suggest a common barrier. For instance, fidelity, means the PR received relative to the planned one. The author favors the use of RTSS (Rehabilitation Treatment Specification System), which describes rehabilitation treatments according to their targets, ingredients and mechanisms of action [21].

Anchored in modernity, Fuest et al. used AI (artificial intelligence) in an attempt to characterize the optimal individual dosage (frequency and level of duration) of EM (early mobilization). AI was able to divide a heterogenous critical care cohort into 4 clusters very different in terms of clinical characteristics and mobilization parameters. The different mobilization strategies according to the cluster supported the likelihood of being discharged home, thus giving room to an "individualized and resource-optimized mobilization approach" [29].

There are also issues as to the dose of PR administered. It appears that indeed, mechanically ventilated patients subject to usual care develop less adverse effects during PR compared to those critically ill MV patients submitted to an increase in early active mobilization. The study comes from the TEAM study investigators and the ANZICS Clinical Trials Group [30]. One year earlier though, Paton et al. stated that mobilization during critical care provided at higher levels, but not increasing the number of active mobilization sessions improved health status at 6 months [31]. The dosage of mobilization was measured by ICMS (Intensive Care Mobility Scale).

5. The road ahead

a. ICU rehabilitation future – preventing ICU-related complications, the contribution of telemedicine and AI (algorhythms and clusters, AI to enhance our thinking or to merely increase the feeling of doing something the righteous way); low-cost physiotherapy strategies (balloon blowing exercise during pandemics. Tailored ICU rehabilitation programs are needed in order to humanize the approach of the post-ICU survivors [9].

b. Potential for development

c. Rehab for both patients, families and caregivers

Among the recommendations to improve patient and family-centered outcomes after critical illness, we enlist: provide broad education on ICU outcomes and the continuum of critical care construct; ensure accountability and reporting of multidimensional outcomes at one year; include ICU outcomes as part of informed consent, perform trials of limited treatment, engage families in week-end goals of care discussions; prioritize basic and translational science inquiry into multisystem tissue injury and repair, risk stratification, role of nutrition and rehabilitation, and determination of outcome trajectories; integrate longitudinal, granular data on ICU outcomes into administrative data sets as the ongoing standard for patient-and family-centered data collection, foster local, national and international programs focused on ICU care continuum and advocate for permanent funding as a timely and urgent public health priority; ensure optimal, consistent and timely communication by the multidisciplinary team with family members; provide respectful and compassionate care for the patient and family and encourage their involvement at bedside and on a mandatory basis in end-of life decisions [6].

A metanalysis and systematic review on physical rehabilitation in the ICU concluded that it improved physical function and reduced ICU and hospital LOS (length of stay), although it failed to impact other outcomes [32]. However, PR (physical rehabilitation) had no impact on muscle strength, duration of MV, mortality and health-related quality of life, while rehabilitation delivered for less than five days per week was less effective than higher dosages [25]. Driven by the results of Wang's research, Laghi advanced the hypothesis that peripheral muscle weakness in the ICU was a marker of disease severity rather than the proximate mechanism contributing to poor clinical outcomes. Moreover, it was already shown that there was a limited association between the diaphragm dysfunction and the limb muscle weakness in mechanically ventilated patients [25]. Finally, it appears that PR and including functional exercises delivered 5 days per week to the critically ill is worth the effort.

Swallowing function in the ICU is often severely impaired, mainly to the intubated patients, but not confined to them. A new entry in the ICU is the speech-language pathologist (SLP) who additionally provides expertise in cognitive communication and swallowing functions during and after MV, endotracheal tube in place or not, to say nothing of tracheostomy. SLPs role was increasingly growing since the COVID-2 pandemic, so the expertise they provided was highly appreciated [33].

It appears that occupational therapists as well became sensitive to critically ill patients. Thus, a study by Costigan et al. established that "there could be opportunities for occupational therapists to expand their role and spearhead original research investigating an enriched breath of ICU interventions" [34].

There are barriers blocking the recovery of the patients surviving an ICU stay, such as the regulatory requirements for acute inpatient rehabilitation, or funding-related issues due mainly to limited or no-insurance coverage. Research gaps and sources do not really help, but they have to be overcome by a joint effort of clinicians and researchers. Nurses also identified barriers to implementing protocols of rehabilitation, and they included staffing levels, lack of resources, poor care coordination, concerns about personal and team safety, lack of knowledge or training, invasive lines and medical instability, fear of dislodgement, neurological limitations and sedation, low priority, presence of endotracheal tubes, poor communication such as contradictory information which is a definite source of disbelief and loss of confidence, inadequate equipment, increased workload, fatigue, self-injury and time [6, 35].

According to Herridge, the ICU community can and should define our next priorities as mitigation of suffering and the sense of futility in the ICU and disability after discharge [6].

The ideal setting for survivors would be the comprehensive multidisciplinary outpatient ICU-follow-up clinics [8].

6. Conclusion

Balancing the potential beneficial effects of bed rest against muscle exercise is a challenging task. The large variety in the design of interventions renders any evidence-based conclusion impossible. The positive impact on functionality is undeniable and physical therapists must be involved. Although technical difficulties and questions remain, the pertinence of tailored rehabilitation regimens is not an issue. A multidisciplinary approach organized in outpatient post-ICU clinics with a broad referral network of specialists could be an answer for all ICU survivors, not only for those issued from the last pandemic.

Author details

Monica Chiş[1*] and Ruxandra Copotoiu[2]

1 Emergency County Hospital of Tg.Mures, University of Medicine and Pharmacy, Science and Technology GE Palade Tg.Mures, Romania

2 Department of Anesthesia, Intensive Care and Peri-operative Medicine, Nouvel Hôpital Civil, Strasbourg, France

*Address all correspondence to: monicacopotoiu@gmail.com

References

[1] Brown SM, Bose S, Banner-Goodspeed V, et al. Approaches to post intensive care syndrome: A narrative review. Annals of the American Thoracic Society. 2019;**16**(8):947-956. DOI: 10.1513/AnnalsATS.201812-913FR

[2] Needham DM, Davidson J, Cohen H, et al. Improving long-term outcomes after discharge from intensive care unit: Report from stakeholders' conference. Critical Care Medicine. 2012;**40**(2):502-509. DOI: 10.1097/CCM. Ob013e318232da75

[3] Fazzini B, Markl T, Costas C, et al. The rate and assessment of muscle wasting during critical illness: A systematic review and meta-analysis. Critical Care. 2023;**27**:2. DOI: 10.1186/s13054-022-04253-0

[4] Rousseau AF, Prescott HC, Brett SJ, et al. Longterm outcomes after critical illness: Recent insights. Critical Care. 2021;**25**:108. DOI: 10.1186/s13054-021-03535-3

[5] Jarman A, Chapman K, Vollam S, et al. Invetigating the impact of physical activity interventions on delirium outcomes in intensive care unit patients: A systematic review and meta-analysis. Journal of International Care Society. 2023;**24**(1):85-95. DOI: 10.1177/17511437221103689

[6] Herridge MS, Azoulay E. Outcomes after critical illness. The New England Journal of Medicine. 2023;**388**:913-924. DOI: 10.1056/NEJMra2104669

[7] Needham DM, Dowdy DW, Mendez-Tellez PA, Herridge MS, Pronovost PJ. Studying outcomes of intensive care unit survivors: Measuring exposures and outcomes. Intensive Care Medicine. 2005;**31**:1153-1160

[8] Schoffelen AF, Hofhuis JGM, Posthouwer D, Rommes JH, Spronk PE. Consumption of ICU resources by long-stay patients does not change over time: 9-year observation in a teaching hospital in the Netherlands. Journal of Critical Care. 2010;**14**(5):313-317

[9] Spronk PE. Don't stand there, but deliver tailored ICU rehabilitation services. Acta Anesthesiology Scandinavian. 2022;**66**:305-306. DOI: 10.1111/aas.14016

[10] Reid JC, Unger J, McCaskel D, et al. Physical rehabilitation interventions in the intensive care unit: A scoping review of 117 studies. Journal of Intensive Care. 2018;**6**:80. DOI: 10.1186/s40560-018-0349-x

[11] Seo YJ, Park SR, Lee JH, Jung C, Choi KH, Hong S-K, et al. Feasability, safety, and functional recovery after active rehabilitation in crirically ill surgical patients. Australian Critical Care. 2020;**33**:281-286

[12] Conradie E, Fourie CE, Hanekom SD. Investigating the clinical feasability of an adapted early mobility readiness protocol for critically ill patients: A anon-randomized experimental pilot trial. Intensive and Critical Care Nursing. 2017;**42**:44-50. DOI: 10.1016/j.iccn.2017.04.004

[13] Vollenweider R, Manettas AI, Häni N, de Bruin ED, Knols RH. Passive motion of the lower extremities in sedated and ventilated patients in the ICU - a systematic review of early effects and replicability of interventions. PLoS One. 2022;**17**(5):e0267255. DOI: 10.1371/journal.pone.0267255

[14] Lang JK, Paykel MS, Haines KJ, et al. Clinical practice guidelines for early mobilization in the ICU: A systematic review. Critical Care Medicine. 2020;**2020**:e1121-e1128. DOI: 10.1097/CCM.0000000000004574

[15] Verceles AC, Wells CL, Sorkin JD, et al. A multimodal rehabilitation program for patients with ICU acquired weakness improves ventilator weaning and discharge home. Journal of Critical Care. 2028;**47**:204-210. DOI: 10.1016/j.jcrc.2018.07.006s

[16] Beach LJ, Fetterplace K, Edbrooke L, et al. Measurement of physical activity levels in the intensive care unit and functional outcomes: An observational study. Journal of Critical Care. 2017;**40**:189-196. DOI: 10.1016/j.jcrc.2017.04.006

[17] Lai C-C, Chou W, Chan K-S, et al. Early mobilization reduces duration of mechanical ventilation and intensive care unit stay in patients with acute respiratory failure. Archives. 2017;**98**:931-939. DOI: 10.1016/j.apmr.2016.11.007

[18] Yu T, Cai F, Jiang R. Effects of early bedside cycle exrcise on gastrointestinal function in intensive care unit patients receiving mechanical ventilation. Frontiers in Medicine. 2022;**9**:B23067. DOI: 10.3389/fmed.2022.823067

[19] Doiron KA, Hoffman TC, Beller EM. Early intervention (mobilization or active exercise) for critically ill adults in the intensive care unit (Review). Cochrane Database of Systematic Reviews. 2018;**3**:CD010754. DOI: 10.1002/14651858.CD010754.pub2

[20] Collet MO, Laerkner E, Jensen J, et al. Functional and cognitive rehabilitation interventions during intensive care admission: A protocol for a systematic integrative review. Acta Anesthesiology Scandinavian. 2013;**67**:670-674

[21] O'Grady HK, Farley C, Hanna QEB, et al. Comparator groups in ICU-based studies of physical rehabilitation: A scoping review of 125 studies. Critical Care Explotrations. 2023;**5**(5):1-12. DOI: 10.1097?CCE.0000000000000917

[22] Connolly B, Denehy L, Hart N, et al. Physical rehabilitation core outcomes in critical illness (PRACTICE): Protpcol for development of a core outcome set. Trials. 2018;**19**:294. DOI: s13063-018-2678-4

[23] Raurell-Torreda M, Regaira-Martinez E, Planas-Pascual B, et al. Early mobilisation algorithm for the critical patient. Expert recommendations. Effermeria Intensiva. 2021;**32**:153-163. DOI: 10.1016/j.enfi.2020.11.001

[24] Garcia-Perez-de Sevilla G, Sanchez-Pinto PB. Effectiveness of physical exercise and neuromuscular electrical stimulation interventions for preventing and treating intensive care-unit acquired weakness: A systematic review of randomized controlled trials. Intensive Critical Care Nursing. 2023;**74**:103333. DOI: 10.1016/j.iccn.2022.103333

[25] Laghi F, Shaik H. Physical rehabilitation in the ICU: Is it worth the effort? Critical Care Medicine. 2022;**50**(3):504-507. DOI: 10.1097/CCM.0000000000005289

[26] Brower RG. Consequences of bed rest. Critical Care Medicine. 2009;**37**(10):S422-S428. DOI: 10.1097/CCM.0b013e3181b6e30a

[27] Nickels M, Aitken LM, Walsham J, et al. Clinicians' perception of rtionales for rehabilitative exercise in a critical care setting: A cross sectional study.

Australian Critical Care. 2017;**30**:79-84. DOI: 10.1016/j.aucc.2016.03.003

[28] Patel BK, Pohlman AS, Hall J, et al. Impact of early mobilization on glycemic control and ICU-acquired weakness in critically ill patients who are mechanically ventilated. Chest. 2015;**146**(3):583-589. DOI: 10.1378/chest.13-2046

[29] Fuest KE, Ulm B, Daum N, et al. Clustering of critically ill patients using an individualized learning approach enables dose optimization of mobilization in the ICU. Critical Care. 2023;**27**(1):1. DOI: 10/1186/s13054-022-04291-8

[30] TEAM Study Investigators and the ANZICS Clinical Trials Group. Early active mobilization during mechanical ventilation in the ICU. The New England Journal of Medicine. 2022;**389**(19): 1747-1758. DOI: 10.1056?NEJMoa2209083

[31] Paton M, Lane R, Paul E, et al. Mobilization during critical illness: A higher level of mobilization improves health status at 6 months, a secondary analysis of a prospective cohort study. Critical Care Journal. 2012;**49**(9):e860-e869. DOI: 10.1097/CCM.0000000000005058

[32] Wang YT, Lang JK, Haines KJ, et al. Physical rehabilitation in the ICU: A systematic review and meta-analysis. Critical Care Medical Journal. 2021:375-388. DOI: 10.1097/CCM.0000000000005285

[33] Freeman-Sanderson A, Ward EC, Miles A, et al. A consensus statement for the management and rehabilitation of communication and swallowing function in the ICU: A global response to COVID-19. Archives Physical Medical Rehabilitation. 2012;**102**:835-842. DOI: 10.1016/j.apmr.2020.10.113

[34] Costigan FA, Duffett M, Harris JE, et al. Occupational therapy in the ICU: A scoping review of 221 documents. Critical Care Medicine. 2019;**47**(12):e1014-e1021. DOI: 10.1097?CCM.0000000000003999

[35] Popoola M, Dingle M, MacLaren J, et al. Ware what are the barriers to nurses mobilizing adult patients in intensive care units? An integrative review. Australian Critical Care. 2022;**35**:595-603. DOI: 10.1016/j.aucc.2021.09.002

Chapter 13

An Evidence-Based Approach to Non-Invasive Ventilation in Cardiac Rehabilitation after Coronary Artery Bypass Grafting (CABG)

Om Prakash Palanivel, Sanjay Theodore,
Senthil Purushothaman, Ali Albshabshe,
Nasser Mohammed Alwadai and Mohammed Abdu Rajhi

Abstract

Pulmonary impairment and decreased functional capacity are significant concerns following cardiovascular surgery, leading to extended hospital stays and mortality. Non-invasive ventilation (NIV) can provide significant prophylactic and therapeutic benefits in pre-operative and postoperative respiratory failure following coronary artery bypass grafting (CABG) surgery. Despite scant data, non-invasive ventilation outcomes are promising in phase I cardiac rehabilitation. There exists evidence that validates the utilization of non-invasive ventilation in the acute phase of cardiac rehabilitation and its application in patients following CABG; this context continues to be a subject of controversy within the existing body of literature. The purpose of this chapter is to demonstrate the efficacy of non-invasive ventilation as a prophylactic and therapeutic intervention for patients undergoing coronary artery bypass grafting (CABG) surgery, with the obvious aim of mitigating the occurrence of postoperative pulmonary dysfunction and decreased functional capacity.

Keywords: coronary artery bypass graft (CABG), non-invasive ventilation (NIV), post operative pulmonary complications (PPC), acute respiratory failure (ARF), continuous positive pressure support (CPAP), pressure support (PS), bilevel positive pressure (BiPAP)

1. Introduction

According to the World Health Organization (WHO), cardiovascular illnesses are responsible for a total of 17.9 million deaths annually. This figure is equivalent to around 32% of the overall world mortality rate. It is anticipated that coronary artery disease (CAD) will be the dominant contributor to morbidity and death in the realm of cardiovascular illness by the year 2030, resulting in about 23 million people losing their lives as a direct consequence of the condition [1]. Coronary artery

IntechOpen

bypass grafting (CABG) is a surgical procedure that has been found to enhance lifelong longevity and improve the overall individual's standards of life afflicted with moderate to severe coronary artery disease. In contrast to the transient respiratory and functional capacity impairment experienced in the immediate aftermath of CABG surgery, the enduring advantages of CABG confer a lifelong benefit that enhances functional mobility and facilitates independent engagement in daily living activities. Almost all individuals who had CABG surgery experienced transient acute postoperative pulmonary complications (PPC). Nevertheless, when suitable preventive measures are implemented in the acute phase of cardiac rehabilitation, these short-time acute respiratory and functional abnormalities often exhibit favorable responses. The severity of PPC encompasses a spectrum of manifestations, including pain, weakness of the respiratory muscles, atelectasis, collapse of the lungs, reduced lung volume, profound hypoxia, and skeletal muscle weakness. In more severe cases, PPC may cause respiratory compromise and acute respiratory distress syndrome (ARDS), both of which are linked to escalated healthcare costs and excessive utilization of resources [2]. CABG's mechanism often causes transient, acute postoperative pulmonary impairment. Many aspects must be considered during intraoperative procedures. These parameters include median sternotomy, anesthesia, surgery time, cardiopulmonary bypass (CPB), administration of blood-related substances, local hypothermia for heart protection, and harvesting of the internal mammary artery. Postoperative mechanisms encompass various factors that contribute to heightened pain resulting from the median sternotomy, intercostal drainage tubes, phrenic nerve impairment, augmented respiratory effort, compromised cough reflex, hypoxemia, and skeletal muscle weakness associated with diminished functional mobility. Additionally, specific preoperative variables exert an influence on postoperative pulmonary dysfunction, encompassing pre-existing lung diseases, smoking habits, advanced age, obesity, obstructive sleep apnea (OSA), heart failure, and inadequate nutritional status. During the process of rehabilitation, a notable proportion of patients who undergo heart surgery, specifically 10%, experience considerable pulmonary dysfunction. The occurrence of this condition is subject to variation, contingent upon the severity of the pulmonary complications that arise after the surgical procedure. During the initial days following cardiac surgery, three prevalent postoperative pulmonary complications that may endure are atelectasis, pleural effusion, and pneumonia [3, 4]. Furthermore, it is worth noting that hypoxia is observed in approximately 79% of cases, while hypercapnia is observed in approximately 38% of cases, typically within the first 24 h following the transition from the critical care unit. Despite the utilization of modern surgical techniques and improved postoperative care, postoperative pulmonary complications following CABG continue to exist and remain a significant cause of both mortality and morbidity. For the past two decades, NIV has been the commonly employed initial treatment for acute respiratory failure characterized by hypoxia or hypercapnia, which is often observed during chronic obstructive pulmonary disease exacerbations, cardiogenic pulmonary edema, and pneumonia. Due to the positive outcome observed with non-invasive ventilation, there has been a decrease in the necessity for endotracheal intubation. Nevertheless, there is a limited body of scientific research that has investigated therapeutic approaches aimed at preventing or mitigating pulmonary complications after cardiac surgery. Historically, chest physical therapy and the utilization of an incentive spirometer have been employed as methods to mitigate and manage postoperative pulmonary complications. While reintubation and mechanical ventilation

DOI: http://dx.doi.org/10.5772/intechopen.1002854

are frequently utilized in the therapeutic care of patients experiencing respiratory failure and they are accompanied by various adverse outcomes including pneumonia, infections, increased expenses, morbidity, and mortality. Numerous modern clinical research has examined NIV efficacy in the prevention or reduction of postoperative complications in the acute phase of cardiac rehabilitation among individuals undergoing cardiac surgery. However, it is worth noting that there is limited research available on the potential benefits of non-invasive ventilation in reducing pulmonary complications and increasing functional capacity after extubation following CABG surgery.

The objective of this chapter is to demonstrate the efficacy of NIV as a prophylactic and therapeutic intervention for patients undergoing CABG surgery, with the specific aim of mitigating the occurrence of postoperative pulmonary dysfunction and decreased functional capacity. Additionally, this chapter aims to provide insights into the potential benefits of utilizing NIV in the acute phase of cardiac rehabilitation as an alternative therapeutic approach in the post-CABG population. Specifically, it will explore the potential effects of NIV on various aspects such as atelectasis, functional capacity, tissue perfusion, pulmonary function, reintubation rates, length of hospitalization, and overall functional capacity. The objective of this chapter is to furnish physiotherapists and healthcare providers with a comprehensive outline of NIV in the subsequent headings. These aspects must be taken into account in the management of inpatient clinical settings to guarantee the safety and efficacy of NIV therapy.

1. Physiology of non-invasive ventilation

2. The physiological mechanisms underlying respiratory failures after cardiac surgery

3. The application of non-invasive ventilation in prophylactic and therapeutic settings in cardiac surgery

4. Modalities of non-invasive ventilation (NIV)

5. Failure of non-invasive ventilation (NIV)

6. NIV interfaces and start-up

7. Untapped opportunities in the non-invasive ventilation (NIV)

8. Non-invasive ventilation (NIV) as an aid to cardiac rehabilitation (phase-I)

9. Future research

2. Physiology of non-invasive ventilation

NIV refers to a respiratory life support device that utilizes positive pressure and mask interfaces, eliminating the need for invasive ventilation methods such as the use of an endotracheal breathing tube. The primary importance of non-invasive ventilation (NIV) lies in its ability to alleviate the workload on the respiratory muscles and uphold adequate levels of arterial blood oxygen (PO_2) and carbon dioxide (PCO_2).

The physiological effects of non-invasive ventilation (NIV) bear a resemblance to those of invasive ventilation, which involves the use of an artificial airway. However, several physiological effects distinguish non-invasive ventilation (NIV). Firstly, it is crucial to acknowledge that while there are advanced leak compensation NIV machines available, only a limited number of NIV machines are capable of delivering complete pre-determined pressure and volumes that are comparable to invasive ventilation. These leaks can have an impact on the sensitivity of triggering during flow delivery and the breath cycle, consequently affecting the synchrony between the patient and the ventilator. Non-invasive ventilation (NIV) is administered to the oronasal pharynx, which serves as connection between the esophagus and the trachea. Although gastroesophageal sphincters are present, the occurrence of elevated positive pressures in the esophagus can result in the expansion of the stomach. Hence, there is a notable risk of aspiration for the trachea when it is not adequately protected. The effectiveness of pulmonary hygiene techniques, such as pulmonary toilets and airway suctioning, is impeded. To mitigate exhalation leaks, the utilization of a single-limb circuit can potentially result in heightened carbon dioxide (CO_2) retention, commonly referred to as re-breathing, particularly when flow delivery settings are set at lower levels. Non-invasive ventilation (NIV) also offers notable benefits in comparison to invasive ventilation. The maintenance of glottic function in NIV results in a minimal risk of aspiration. The potential for non-invasive ventilation (NIV) breaks to enable patients to engage in speech and swallowing is a noteworthy aspect to consider. Furthermore, the level of irritation experienced by the airway due to trans-laryngeal intervention is relatively low, which could enhance patient comfort and potentially reduce the requirement for sedation when compared to invasive ventilation. NIV has been shown to effectively maintain upper respiratory tract patency in individuals diagnosed with obstructive sleep apnea. Additionally, in patients suffering from congestive heart failure, NIV has demonstrated the potential to mitigate the occurrence of pulmonary edema and reduce venous return. Improper administration of NIV can result in lung damage, similar to the adverse effects observed with invasive ventilation. The application of non-invasive ventilation (NIV) exerts a positive pressure, thereby alleviating the strain on the inspiratory muscles. It enhances pulmonary compliance by facilitating the dilation of obstructed alveoli, thereby enabling enhanced efficiency in the exchange of gases within the lungs, specifically oxygenation, and ventilation. Consequently, there is an enhancement in respiratory mechanics, potentially leading to the prevention of reintubation. The application of NIV during the acute phase of cardiac rehabilitation in post-cardiac surgery patients has been found to yield several direct advantages, such as the prevention of atelectasis and pneumonia, enhancement of functional capacity and pulmonary function, improvement in tissue perfusion, reduction in hospitalization duration, as well as decreased morbidity and mortality rates. One notable advantage of NIV in the context of post-cardiac surgery is its ability to prevent the need for reintubation. Reintubation carries various risks, involving prolonged invasive ventilation, pneumonia, infection, shock, ICU and hospital stays, and death. Non-invasive ventilation (NIV) has been found to optimize heart function after extubation by reducing inspiratory effort and left ventricular (LV) afterload. Moreover, NIV can be administered both as a prophylactic and as a therapeutic intervention. Additionally, it has the effect of normalizing or reducing the stress response and discomfort experienced after surgery, while also minimizing the occurrence of complications and enhancing the overall outcomes associated with cardiac surgical procedures [5–7].

3. The physiological mechanisms underlying respiratory failure after cardiac surgery

Acute respiratory failure, characterized by hypoxic and/or hypercapnic respiratory failure, can manifest in a significant proportion of individuals who have undergone cardiac surgery. This occurrence can be attributed to various factors, including pre-existing comorbidities such as advanced age, restrictive or obstructive lung disease, and heart failure, as well as perioperative and postoperative influences such as general anesthesia, duration of surgery, atelectasis, pleural effusion, and incisional pain. Hypoxemic respiratory failure can manifest following cardiac surgery due to postoperative pulmonary dysfunction, which encompasses various conditions such as aspiration, atelectasis, pneumonia, pulmonary edema, and acute respiratory distress syndrome. These aforementioned conditions collectively hinder the efficient transfer of oxygen across the alveolar-capillary membrane in the pulmonary system, resulting in a partial pressure of oxygen (PaO_2) below the threshold of 60 mmHg. In the context of clinical environments, the established approach to managing hypoxemic respiratory failure involves the administration of oxygen therapy in conjunction with chest physical therapy. Similar to what was mentioned earlier, hypercarbia respiratory failure (hypoventilation) can occur after cardiac surgery when there is insufficient removal of carbon dioxide from the distal alveoli. This leads to respiratory acidosis, characterized by an elevation in the partial pressure of carbon dioxide ($PaCO_2$) above 45 mmHg, along with concurrent hypoxemia. Nevertheless, the primary factors contributing to hypercarbia encompass prolonged neuromuscular blockade after cardiac surgery, excessive sedation, and respiratory exhaustion [8–10].

4. The application of non-invasive ventilation in prophylactic and therapeutic settings in cardiac surgery

As mentioned earlier, individuals who undergo cardiac surgery face an increased susceptibility to experiencing pulmonary complications and decreased functional capacity following the procedure. Despite the limited availability of data, the use of NIV in the acute phase of cardiac rehabilitation as a preventive and therapeutic intervention has the potential to reduce or prevent postoperative pulmonary complications, including atelectasis, reintubation rates, impaired tissue perfusion, and skeletal muscle weakness associated with decreased functional capacity.

4.1 Atelectasis

Atelectasis is a medical condition distinguished by the partial or complete collapse of a lung or a specific segment of a lung. Atelectasis frequently occurs following cardiac surgery and is a prevalent contributor to hypoxia and impaired gas exchange. Atelectasis is a common finding in postoperative chest radiographs following cardiac surgery, with a prevalence ranging from 30% to 72%. It is considered a significant factor in the development of respiratory dysfunction after surgery [11, 12]. Specifically, basal atelectasis is observed in 94% of patients within the initial 48-hour period after CABG surgery. Irrespective of the administration method, be it intravenous or inhalational, it is observed that the majority of patients undergoing general anesthesia encounter atelectasis during both spontaneous respiration and following the administration of muscle paralytics [13]. CABG surgery induces changes in respiratory mechanics, leading to diminished expiratory flow, reduced ciliary rate, and impaired cough reflex, ultimately resulting in atelectasis and pneumonia. These complications can subsequently contribute to heightened respiratory effort and diminished lung capacity. Failure to appropriately treat and manage atelectasis may result in compromised pulmonary function, the development of pneumonia hospital-acquired, and an extended duration of hospitalization. Typically, conventional postoperative physiotherapy after CABG involves the integration of an incentive spirometer and respiratory exercises. In a randomized controlled study comprising 26 patients who underwent CABG, the control group (CG) exhibited an atelectasis rate of 61.5%, while the NIV group demonstrated a rate of 54% (P = 0.691). Following the surgical procedure, it was observed that the group receiving NIV exhibited a significantly greater vital capacity (P 0.015). This study demonstrates that NIV is highly favored by patients who experience heightened discomfort as a result of pain perception [14]. In a study conducted by Matte et al. [15], it was observed that 30% of patients who underwent treatment with incentive spirometry and 15% of patients who received treatment with CPAP or BIPAP exhibited mild or moderate atelectasis on the second day following their surgery. The study sample consisted of 96 patients. Nevertheless, there was a notable enhancement in oxygenation and a decreased decline in lung volumes. According to Pasquina et al. [16]. A study found that 60% of patients who underwent non-invasive ventilation (NIV) with BIPAP experienced an improvement in their radiological atelectasis score, while only 40% of patients who underwent NIV with CPAP showed a similar improvement. Similarly, the application of continuous positive airway pressure (CPAP) to individuals who encountered post-operative atelectasis after cardiac procedures (as indicated by radiographic evidence) resulted in a notable enhancement of the condition, as assessed through radiological scoring. According to a study conducted by researchers [16], it has been observed that atelectatic lung zones have the potential to reduce functional residual capacity and elevate pulmonary shunt, even in cases where heart surgery has been performed successfully without any complications. The presence of unventilated atelectatic lung zones can contribute to nearly 20% of the overall lung capacity, resulting in hypoxemia following CABG [17]. According to this perspective, the initiation of NIV serves to prevent the collapse of alveoli and facilitate improved recruitment of alveoli, thereby mitigating the occurrence of atelectasis and augmenting functional residual capacity.

4.2 Pulmonary function assessment

The presence of a limited capacity to produce autonomous deep inhalations leads to the manifestation of restrictive breathing patterns, and the etiology of this restrictive breathing pattern is characterized by multiple contributing factors. While CABG surgery has proven to be a successful method for coronary revascularization, it is frequently linked to a restrictive breathing pattern and declined pulmonary function, which in turn may result in adverse health outcomes and even death. The etiology of impaired pulmonary function after CABG surgery is multifactorial, encompassing various factors such as a reduced expansion of the rib cage and disorganized movement of the chest wall, dysfunction of the diaphragmatic dysfunction due to phrenic nerve injury, accumulation of pleural fluid, and the occurrence of basal atelectasis. Nevertheless, it is worth noting that a decrease in pulmonary function can also be attributed to respiratory muscle dysfunction, characterized by a reduction in both functional residual capacity (FRC) and vital capacity (VC). In the initial week following coronary artery bypass graft (CABG) surgery, there is a notable decline of 30–60% in slow vital capacity. This reduction persists at a diminished level of 12% even after a duration of up to 1 year. A significant decrease in preoperative functional residual capacity (FRC) values, amounting to 70%, is observed for a duration of at least 7–10 days. Additionally, there is a reduction of 40–50% in vital capacity (VC) compared to preoperative levels, which persists for a period of 10–14 days. Nevertheless, in the context of postoperative cardiac surgery, the occurrence of a restrictive breathing pattern and hypoxemia is predominantly inevitable, although subject to potential modification [14]. According to Stell et al. [18], the utilization of NIV in the postoperative acute phase of cardiac rehabilitation has been found to enhance vital capacity, a critical metric for assessing the likelihood of reintubation. Additionally, NIV can decrease the load on the respiratory system and enhance pulmonary functions through the activation of closed alveoli, thereby opening up the atelectasis lung. Consequently, NIV demonstrates superiority over alternative techniques in facilitating deep breaths, leading to enhanced lung volume and capacities among patients who exhibit uncooperative behavior, excessive sedation, or an inability to engage in deep breathing due to pain, particularly in the immediate postoperative phase following cardiac surgery [18, 19]. Franco et al. [14] discovered notable disparities in vital capacities among two cohorts of patients who underwent heart surgery. The measured values in the NIV group were 2.64, 0.99, 1.53, and 1.94 before the operation, immediately after extubation, and 24 and 48 hours after extubation, respectively. In contrast, the control group had values of 2.11, 0.90, 0.90, and 0.97 [20]. The NIV group exhibited superior performance as a result of the patient's active engagement in generating deep breaths, thereby mitigating discomfort experienced during physical exertion. Furthermore, this intervention is advantageous for patients who exhibit reluctance in performing deep inhalations after cardiac surgery.

4.3 Reintubation rate

Reintubation may occur in critically ill postoperative cardiac surgery patients, despite adherence to the recommended weaning protocols. The rates of reintubation in a critical care unit following general surgical procedures vary between 1% and 13%, while the rate after cardiac surgery is approximately 6.6%. The act of reintubation has been found to increase the duration of mechanical ventilation, which in turn leads to an extension of both the length of stay in the intensive care unit (ICU) and the overall hospital stay. Reintubation has been widely recognized as an independent factor contributing to elevated mortality rates. Therefore, it can be inferred that patients who necessitate reintubation exhibit an unfavorable prognosis, as evidenced by a mortality rate ranging from 30% to 40%. A cohort of 1640 patients admitted to the intensive care unit (ICU) underwent a retrospective analysis and revealed a reintubation rate of 7.3% (n = 119), with 36 patients (30.3%) undergoing CABG surgery. The majority of patients undergoing cardiovascular surgery exhibit a range of medical conditions, including hypertension, diabetes, hyperlipidemia, as well as comorbidities such as pneumonia and renal failure. Additionally, there is an increased likelihood for these individuals to necessitate re-intubation, as well as exhibit inferior scores in terms of SOFA, APACHE II, and Euro SCORE. Remarkably, the cohort that did not undergo non-invasive ventilation before reintubation exhibited a greater mortality rate. Consequently, a multitude of studies advocates for the prompt implementation of non-invasive ventilation (NIV) following extubation as a proactive approach to mitigate the risk of extubation failure, mitigate complications, and reduce the duration of hospitalization. Based on a recent extensive analysis, the utilization of NIV after cardiothoracic surgery has been shown to enhance individuals' oxygenation levels, decrease the likelihood of postoperative complications, and diminish the need for endotracheal intubation [21, 22].

4.4 Tissue perfusion

Tissue perfusion refers to the process by which blood is delivered to and circulated within the various tissues of the body. Blood lactate and central-venous oxygen saturation ($ScvO_2$) have been identified as important and separate factors that can predict the occurrence of complications and death after cardiac surgery, especially in patients with left ventricular failure. Nevertheless, there exists a correlation between tissue hypoxia and negative postoperative outcomes, including skeletal muscle weakness, systemic acute inflammation, septic shock, and acute renal failure. Postoperative complications are often exacerbated by low $ScvO_2$ levels and elevated blood lactate values, leading to prolonged hospitalization and heightened rates of morbidity and mortality. A deviation from normal $ScvO_2$ levels, such as a lower value of 68% or a higher value exceeding 80%, may suggest an augmented rate of oxygen extraction to fulfill the metabolic requirements of organs. Additionally, this condition may be accompanied by an elevation in anaerobic energy production and the accumulation of blood lactate. The potential benefits observed after the implementation of NIV in individuals with left ventricular (LV) dysfunction can be attributed to its ability to improve cardiac function by reducing inspiratory effort and LV afterload. There is empirical evidence suggesting that NIV can potentially improve cardiac function through the modification of cardiac morphology. Elevated pleural pressure, subsequently leading to a decrease in transmural pressure, results in a reduction in both left-ventricle preload and afterload. This phenomenon induces an instantaneous impact on cardiac function in response to positive pressure. As a result of this observation, a proposition has been put forth suggesting that the application of positive pressure could potentially augment cardiac function and myocardial contractility. The utilization of bi-level positive airway pressure is advised due to the findings of a randomized controlled trial, which indicated that it yielded a greater improvement in left ventricular ejection fraction compared to continuous positive airway pressure in individuals diagnosed with systolic dysfunction [23]. According to Ranucci et al., blood lactate levels exhibited an increase of over threefold when the central venous oxygen saturation (CvO_2) reached a value of 68%. The combined assessment of blood lactate levels and $ScvO_2$ has the possibility to serve as a valuable clinical tool in distinguishing the etiology of elevated lactate levels, specifically whether they are attributed to hypoperfusion or other causative factors. In comparison to the cessation of mechanical ventilation (extubation), the initiation of NIV resulted in an increase in $ScvO_2$. Conversely, the termination of mechanical ventilation (extubation) led to a decrease in $ScvO_2$ [24]. Nevertheless, there was no alteration observed in arterial blood oxygenation (SaO_2). The findings indicate that enhanced distribution of blood flow, resulting in improved tissue perfusion, has a positive impact on heart function. Furthermore, the utilization of NIV contributes to a reduction in the effort required for respiration, primarily due to its assistance in supporting the function of the inspiratory muscles [25]. The occurrence of dyspnea in the early stages of heart failure can be ascribed to a redistribution of blood circulation toward the peripheral muscles during periods of physical exertion. Even during periods of inactivity, the reduced capacity of the respiratory and peripheral muscles to undergo oxidation processes may result in an elevation in oxygen consumption and an inadequate provision of oxygen to meet the body's demands. NIV utilization has been demonstrated to decrease the effort required for respiration, leading to enhanced blood flow distribution and subsequent improvement in the perfusion of tissues and improved skeletal muscle weakness [26]. The application of non-invasive ventilation (NIV) in different clinical scenarios resulted in a significant decrease in blood lactate levels and an increase in central venous oxygen saturation ($ScvO_2$). The utilization of NIV in the acute phase of cardiac rehabilitation following CABG surgery can effectively promote tissue perfusion.

4.5 Functional capacity

Functional capacity refers to an individual's capability for executing tasks and engaging in activities in an approach that aligns with functional objectives. The occurrence of a significant decrease in functional capacity after undergoing heart surgery is well-documented in the literature. Several factors have been identified as contributors to this decline in functional capacity, including respiratory compromise, tissue perfusion, peripheral muscle dysfunction, and reduced cardiac function. Consequently, the utilization of non-invasive ventilation (NIV) in the acute phase of cardiac rehabilitation shortly after the removal of an endotracheal tube can effectively enhance pulmonary function and oxygenation. This, in turn, facilitates the peripheral muscle's blood flow, ultimately resulting in enhanced physical functional performance [27]. Additionally, the use of non-invasive ventilation (NIV) reduces the elevated workload on the respiratory system and enhances the delivery of blood to tissues by augmenting the left ventricular afterload function, ultimately leading to optimal cardiac output. In their study, Cordeiro et al. [28] demonstrated that the immediate implementation of NIV in the acute phase of cardiac rehabilitation following extubation yields a significant enhancement in pulmonary function. However, it is worth noting that an enhancement in circulatory function and peripheral muscle perfusion has been shown to have a positive impact on walking and physical exercise performance [28]. Based on data obtained from the Brazilian Registry of Clinical Trials, the 6-minute walk test showed that the control group averaged 264.34 m and the experimental group 334.07 m. Three NIV sessions with a positive pressure of 10 cmH_2O for 1 h within 26 h after extubation yielded these outcomes. A 0.002 p-value showed a significant difference between the groups [29].

4.6 Acute respiratory failure (ARF)

Acute respiratory failure (ARF) is a medical condition categorized by the insufficient ability of the respiratory system to effectively oxygenate the blood and eliminate carbon dioxide. ARF is a commonly observed condition that occurs after cardiac surgery, particularly among individuals with pre-existing lung disease and undergoing major heart surgery. The study revealed that individuals who underwent cardiac surgical procedures that involved a combination of factors such as low ejection fraction and severe SAPS II scores were identified as being at the greatest susceptibility for the development of ARF following the surgery. In a study conducted by Filsoufi et al. [30], a cohort of 5798 individuals who underwent heart surgery within a six-year timeframe was examined. The researchers found that the incidence of acute renal failure (ARF) reached its peak at 9.1%, with a total of 529 cases [30]. ARF is predominantly observed in patients undergoing both valve and CABG procedures, with a prevalence rate of 14.8%. In a study conducted over a span of 4 years, Kilger et al. [31] examined a cohort of 2261 individuals who underwent cardiac surgery. The findings of the study revealed that 35% of the patient population experienced post-extubation ARF. Furthermore, it was observed that intermittent NIV treatment proved beneficial for 33% of these patients. ARF following extubation is a significant complication that has the possibility to elevate both morbidity and mortality rates [31]. The administration of early NIV therapy in the acute phase of cardiac rehabilitation after extubation demonstrated efficacy in mitigating the occurrence of respiratory compromise following extubation in a population at high risk. Patients diagnosed with hypoxemic ARF have the potential to successfully circumvent the need for endotracheal intubation. In a clinical study involving 94 patients with ARF, it was observed that 89 individuals (94%) were able to successfully avoid the need for endotracheal intubation through the implementation of NIV. Notably, initiating NIV within a timeframe of 3 h following a minor decline in the proportion of arterial oxygen partial pressure to fractional inspired oxygen (PaO_2/FIO_2) was found to be advantageous for patients with moderate hypoxemic respiratory failure after cardiovascular surgery. This finding holds a significant interest. Nevertheless, it is imperative to prioritize early intubation and exercise caution when selecting patients for NIV. Additionally, it is important to note that a 24-h interval between extubation and NIV initiation poses a substantial risk for NIV failure [32, 33]. In a randomized controlled trial, it was determined that a score exceeding 20 on the Acute Physiologic Assessment and Chronic Health Evaluation (APACHE) II is an independent risk factor for NIV failure in patients who undergo extubation for acute respiratory failure (ARF) [34]. Nevertheless, the occurrence of reintubation ranges from 6% to 52% among patients who undergo NIV following cardiac surgery [17]. After undergoing cardiothoracic surgery, the implementation of NIV therapies demonstrated enhanced oxygenation and a decreased necessity for reintubation. The use of NIV proved to be a secure and effective strategy for managing postoperative ARF in a cohort of 83 patients. These individuals were discharged to their homes after receiving NIV to treat respiratory failure after heart surgery, which took place outside of the critical care department [35]. According to the available evidence, individuals diagnosed with hypoxemic ARF have the possibility to successfully circumvent the need for endotracheal intubation. In a clinical study involving a cohort of 94 patients diagnosed with ARF, it was observed that 89 individuals (94%) were able to successfully avoid the need for endotracheal intubation through the implementation of NIV. NIV in the acute phase of cardiac rehabilitation has been identified as a secure and feasible alternative for managing cases of postoperative ARF in settings outside of the critical care department, provided that careful monitoring is maintained.

5. Modalities of non-invasive ventilation

Non-invasive positive pressure ventilation (NIPPV) refers to oxygen delivery through a face mask, utilizing either constant or variable pressures. Examples of NIPPV include bi-level positive airway pressure (BiPAP) and constant positive airway pressure (CPAP). A significant proportion of medical practitioners opt for uncomplicated and easily transportable NIV devices. BiPAP (IPAP and EPAP) devices have been specifically engineered to provide two adjustable pressure levels. There are two types of positive airway pressure: inspiratory positive airway pressure (IPAP) and expiratory positive airway pressure (EPAP). CPAP is administered exclusively through the use of expiratory positive airway pressure (EPAP). A limited number of machines possess time modes that allow for the delivery of pressure support (PS) at pre-established intervals [36]. In addition to their primary function, invasive ventilators can deliver NIV. However, it should be noted that older models of ventilators may generate frequent alarms related to "air leaks" when used for NIV ventilation. This is primarily because these older models cannot adequately adjust for changes in airflow. The more recent iterations of ventilators have addressed the issue of leakage in the ventilator circuit through the implementation of microprocessors. These microprocessors are responsible for monitoring the variations in inspiratory and expiratory tidal volumes during the initial breath cycle. Consequently, the peak inspiratory flow experiences an increase without a concomitant increase in the inspiratory time. CPAP modes are frequently employed in conventional ventilators to deliver NIV. Currently, the chosen CPAP and PS levels align with the IPAP and EPAP configurations of the conventional portable NIV. It is advisable to consider that the PS setting on the conventional ventilator provides an additional level of PS beyond the specified CPAP level. In contrast, the pressure support of the IPAP in a typical portable NIV machine incorporates the configured EPAP. Therefore, the PS provided by a portable device, measured at 14 and 8 cm H_2O, is equivalent to the delivery of 6 and 8 cm H_2O by a standard ventilator. If the patient requires supplementary breaths, the utilization of the synchronized intermittent mandatory ventilation (SIMV)-pressure control mode may be considered. The inclusion of non-invasive ventilation pressure support (NIV PS) has become prevalent in contemporary ventilators. In the present scenario, the inspiratory pressure and positive end-expiratory pressure (PEEP) are adjusted to meet the required breaths, while the PS and CPAP are adjusted to regulate the patient's ventilation during spontaneous breaths.

6. Failure of non-invasive ventilation

Endotracheal intubation (ETI) becomes necessary in situations where NIV proves ineffective, as the alternative outcome would be the patient's demise. The study results specify that there is a distinct association between NIV failure and mortality specifically in patients with ARF. This observation suggests that the utilization of NIV applications should be approached cautiously. The primary factors contributing to the failure of NIV in the acute phase of cardiac rehabilitation of postoperative CABG patients are characterized by inadequate monitoring and a lack of attentiveness toward the patients' response to NIV therapy. NIV failure can be categorized into three distinct time periods: immediate failure, which occurs within minutes to less than 1 hour; early failure, which transpires between one and 48 h; and late failure, which manifests after 48 h. Simultaneously, it is important to take into account additional factors such as the size of the mask, circuit leaks, and inadequate trigger levels. These aspects can be adjusted according to the patient's comfort to achieve the most favorable outcome. Nevertheless, despite these interventions, if respiratory distress persists, it is advisable to contemplate discontinuing NIV and instead opt for elective intubation and mechanical ventilation. The ratio of arterial oxygen (PaO_2) to inspired oxygen (FiO_2), commonly referred to as the PaO_2/FiO_2 ratio, along with baseline indicators such as heart rate and respiratory rates, serve as prognostic factors for determining the success or failure of NIV in cases of acute respiratory failure [37–39]. In a separate investigation on acute postoperative respiratory insufficiency, it was observed that the PaO_2/FiO_2 ratio exhibited a decline after 1 hour of NIV therapy. Several randomized controlled trials (RCTs) conducted on patients in intensive critical care units have made predictions about the failure of NIV in cases of postoperative ARF. These predictions include factors such as the worsening of pre-existing diseases, high scores on the Simplified Acute Physiology Score (SAPS) II, scores on the Acute Physiology and Chronic Health Evaluation (APACHE) II, presence of multiple organ dysfunctions, acute respiratory distress syndrome (ARDS), community-acquired pneumonia, and shock [40, 41]. Evidence-based research insists on the cautious selection of patients or the avoidance of NIV therapies in CABG patients experiencing severe acute respiratory failure. Recent studies have indicated a correlation between delays in the intubation process and adverse outcomes, as well as heightened mortality rates in the affected population.

7. NIV Interfaces and start-up

The crucial factor contributing to the success of NIV in the acute phase of cardiac rehabilitation is purely based on the careful selection of an appropriate mask, encompassing considerations of patient comfort, optimal fit, and tolerance. Currently, there are various interfaces for NIV, including oronasal masks, nasal masks, nasal pillows, full-face masks, and helmets. However, there is not much actual data to show that one technique is better than the other. The utilization of a full-face mask has been observed to result in oronasal dryness and claustrophobic sensations. However, it effectively mitigates the occurrence of air leaks in the vicinity of the eyes and mouth, while also alleviating discomfort experienced above the nasal bridge. Oronasal masks, conversely, are frequently employed in clinical settings [42]. Proper monitoring of non-invasive ventilation (NIV) following extubation is essential. It is crucial to engage in preoperative discussions with the patient regarding the significance and procedural techniques associated with NIVs. This proactive approach is vital as it contributes to the patient's postoperative comfort. It is recommended that patients receive an adequate dosage of analgesics and be positioned at an inclination of no less than 35 degrees before initiating non-invasive ventilation (NIV). The initiation of the NIV (CPAP Mode) involves the implementation of low-pressure support (PS) to facilitate the patient's prompt adaptation to the administered pressure, thereby synchronizing with their respiratory pattern. Once the patient has achieved a satisfactory level of respiration comfort, progressively increase the pressure support (PS) and secure the head straps as necessary. The increment of the PSs should be tailored to the individual patient to achieve a reduction in breathing effort and ensure appropriate synchronization. To ascertain the veracity of clinical alterations, it is recommended to procure arterial blood gas measurements within a time frame of 1–2 h. The subsequent step involves the utilization of an inspiratory volume trigger, which can vary between 1 and 2 L/min, or an inspiratory pressure trigger, ranging from 1 to 2 cm of water. This trigger is implemented with a moderate to maximal slope. Typically, in the initial stages of utilizing the NIV mode known as BiPAP, it is common practice to apply minimal levels of expiratory positive airway pressure (EPAP) at 4 cm of water and inspiratory positive airway pressure (IPAP) at 8 cm of water, which is 4 cm higher than the EPAP level. The EPAP and IPAP levels can be incrementally increased by 1–2 cm of H_2O until reaching a maximum of 10 cm of H_2O for EPAP and 25 cm of H_2O for IPAP. If there is a need for increased pressure, it may be required to make adjustments to the interface, optimize the fit of the mask, or consider the option of intubation [43].

8. Untapped opportunities in the non-invasive ventilation (NIV)

Irrespective of the benefits ascribed to the utilization of NIV in the acute phase of cardiac rehablitation, there exists considerable heterogeneity in the approaches employed for its implementation across different healthcare institutions worldwide. A significant proportion, specifically 30%, of medical practitioners/respiratory physiotherapists do not perform an initial blood gas analysis before initiating non-invasive ventilation (NIV). In a study involving a sample of 3000 physicians, it was found that 648 individuals, constituting 21.6% of the participants, reported utilizing NIV in the critical care unit setting. Among these respondents, 469 physicians, accounting for 72.4% of the NIV users, reported incorporating NIV into their clinical practice, representing approximately 68.4% of their overall patient care. Furthermore, it was observed that a significant proportion of physicians, specifically 71.4%, reported employing NIV frequently for managing chronic obstructive pulmonary disease (COPD) exacerbations [44]. The routine utilization of NIV for the prevention or treatment of respiratory failure after CABG surgery was not observed. According to a retrospective analysis spanning 6 years, it was observed that among patients with acute respiratory failure who satisfied the eligibility criteria for the NIV trial, only 34% received NIV, while a significant majority of 66% required endotracheal intubation [45]. One evident factor contributing to the underutilization of the NIV is the presence of inadequate comprehension and insufficient training among medical practitioners, including doctors and respiratory therapists. To optimize the results of NIV in the acute phase of cardiac rehabilitation, it is recommended to seek virtual tutoring and training as a means to mitigate failures and enhance the utilization of NIV during the postoperative period [46].

9. Non-invasive ventilation (NIV) as an aid to cardiac rehabilitation (phase-I)

In healthy elderly people, 10 days of bed rest reduces quadriceps strength by 20% [47]. After CABG surgery, pulmonary function and skeletal muscle weakness are the main factors reducing ADLs. Despite early mobilization and chest physiotherapy, cardiac surgery patients often develop pulmonary dysfunction and muscular weakness. This might worsen post-operative outcomes if preoperative variables such as loss of body tissue, physical inactivity, altered metabolism, multiple comorbidities, decreased LV functions and age were present. Generally, pulmonary dysfunction and muscular inactivity are caused by surgical stress and pain which is the most reversible component after cardiac surgery [48]. In this context, cardiac rehabilitation is an effective therapy for patients with cardiovascular disease that improves pulmonary, functional capacity, and quality of life, as well as reducing hospital admissions and health care costs. Cardiac rehabilitation consists of three phases: phase-1 (clinical phase), phase-2 (outpatient cardiac rehabilitation), and phase-3 (post-cardiac rehabilitation maintenance). Phase 1 cardiac rehabilitation starts in the critical care units (if the patient is stable). Rehabilitation intensity depends on the patient's medical state and acute illness complications. Following CABG and after extubation NIV could be considered as a prophylactic and therapeutic tool to improve pulmonary gas exchange in postoperative patients. This, in turn, facilitates the peripheral muscle's blood flow, ultimately resulting in enhanced physical mobility. The frequency and duration of non-invasive ventilation (NIV) treatment, regardless of its prophylactic or therapeutic nature, are exclusively determined by the patient's medical condition and their level of participation.

Despite evidence of extensive research supporting the advantages of NIV associated with cardiac rehabilitation, the level of patient participation in such programs remains notably deficient. According to data obtained from Medicare and the Centers for Disease Control and Prevention (CDC), it has been shown that around 31% of patients who had coronary bypass grafting surgery participated in or were enrolled in cardiac rehabilitation or secondary prevention programs. Qualitative research done in 2017 on how patients felt about cardiac rehabilitation showed that the severity of the cardiovascular illness or incident, the presence of pre- and post-psychological obstacles, such as time constraints and exercise-related apprehension in phase I cardiac rehabilitation, and the patient's future goals were some of the things that affected the patients' feelings about cardiac rehabilitation and their participation in the program [49]. Hence, the cardiac rehabilitation team needs to consider NIV as prophylactic or therapeutic, based on the patient's medical conditions and other factors, when formulating phase I cardiac rehabilitation programs for patients.

10. Future research

Previous research investigations have highlighted the potential advantages of NIV for individuals undergoing cardiovascular surgery, both before and after the procedure. However, there is a dearth of empirical evidence to substantiate this assertion. Further investigation is warranted to ascertain the appropriate recipients, timing, and methodologies for treatment. It is observed that individuals who undergo cardiac surgery have a higher propensity for developing pulmonary complications. Consequently, the timely administration of NIV in selected patients has the potential to substantially reduce the duration of hospitalization and demonstrate cost-effectiveness. Unfortunately, there is currently a lack of available data about the economic aspects of the subject matter. It would be beneficial to undertake additional comprehensive research to examine the complexities associated with non-invasive ventilation (NIV). Moreover, it is imperative to undergo training to ensure the efficacy and safety of NIV. To facilitate the implementation of non-invasive ventilation (NIV) interventions, the cardiac thoracic intensive care unit (CTICU) must establish a consistently available NIV service and employ a skilled team comprising of a physician and a respiratory physiotherapist who possess extensive knowledge and expertise in NIV techniques [50].

11. Conclusions

The use of established guidelines, evidence-based training, and practical application have together enhanced the efficacy of non-invasive ventilation (NIV) in phase-I of cardiac rehabilitation. The involvement of a healthcare practitioner, such as a physician or respiratory physiotherapist, who has the requisite knowledge and is ready to dedicate extra time to the initiation and execution of non-invasive ventilation (NIV) therapy is essential for the initiation of NIV therapy. Nevertheless, more research using randomization is required to demonstrate empirical support for the use of non-invasive ventilation (NIV) in patients who have had coronary artery bypass graft (CABG) surgery, particularly during the phase-I cardiac rehabilitation.

Author details

Om Prakash Palanivel[1], Sanjay Theodore[2], Senthil Purushothaman[1*], Ali Albshabshe[3,4], Nasser Mohammed Alwadai[5] and Mohammed Abdu Rajhi[6]

1 Chettinad School of Physiotherapy, Chettinad Hospital and Research Institute, Chettinad Academy of Research and Education (CARE), Kelambakkam, Tamil Nadu, India

2 Department of Cardiovascular and Cardio-thoracic surgery, Institute of Cardiovascular Disease, Chettinad Super Speciality Hospital, Chettinad Academy of Research and Education (CARE), Kelambakkam, Tamil Nadu, India

3 Medicine/Adult Critical Care, King Khalid University, Abha, KSA

4 Adult Critical Care Medicine, Aseer Central Hospital, Abha, KSA

5 Aseer Central Hospital, Abha, KSA

6 Ahad Al-Masaraha General Hospital, Ahad Al-Masaraha, Saudi Arabia

*Address all correspondence to: senthilp101010@gmail.com

References

[1] Alwan A, Armstrong T, Bettcher D, Branca F, Chisholm D, Ezzati M, et al. Burden: Mortality, morbidity and risk factors. In: Global Status Report on Noncommunicable Diseases 2010. Geneva, Switzerland: World Health Organization; 2011. pp. 9-31. ISBN 978. Available from: www.who.int/nmh/publications/ncd_report2010/en/

[2] Guarracino F, Ambrosino N. Noninvasive ventilation in cardio-surgical patients. Minerva Anestesiologica. 2011;**77**(7):734-741

[3] Al Jaaly E, Fiorentino F, Reeves BC, Ind PW, Angelini GD, Kemp S, et al. Effect of adding postoperative noninvasive ventilation to usual care to prevent pulmonary complications in patients undergoing coronary artery bypass grafting: A randomized controlled trial. The Journal of Thoracic and Cardiovascular Surgery. 2013;**146**(4):912-918. DOI: 10.1016/j.jtcvs.2013.03.014. Epub 2013 Apr 11

[4] Jensen L, Yang L. Risk factors for postoperative pulmonary complications in coronary artery bypass graft surgery patients. European Journal of Cardiovascular Nursing. 2007;**6**(3):241-246. DOI: 10.1016/J.EJCNURSE.2006.11.001. Epub 2007 Mar 7

[5] MacIntyre NR. Physiologic effects of noninvasive ventilation. Respiratory Care. 2019;**64**(6):617-628. DOI: 10.4187/respcare.06635

[6] Hess DR. Noninvasive ventilation for acute respiratory failure. Respiratory Care. 2013;**58**(6):950-972. DOI: 10.4187/respcare.02319

[7] Squadrone V, Coha M, Cerutti E, Schellino MM, Biolino P, Occella P, et al. Piedmont intensive care units network (PICUN). Continuous positive airway pressure for treatment of postoperative hypoxemia: A randomized controlled trial. Journal of the American Medical Association. 2005;**293**(5):589-595. DOI: 10.1001/jama.293.5.589

[8] García-Delgado M, Navarrete-Sánchez I, Colmenero M. Preventing and managing perioperative pulmonary complications following cardiac surgery. Current Opinion in Anaesthesiology. Apr 2014;**27**(2):146-152. DOI: 10.1097/ACO.0000000000000059

[9] Hedenstierna G. Alveolar collapse and closure of airways: Regular effects of anaesthesia. Clinical Physiology and Functional Imaging. 2003;**23**(3):123-129. DOI: 10.1046/j.1475-097x.2003.00483.x

[10] Canet J, Gallart L. Predicting postoperative pulmonary complications in the general population. Current Opinion in Anaesthesiology. 2013;**26**(2):107-115. DOI: 10.1097/ACO.0b013e32835e8acd

[11] Jindani A, Aps C, Neville E, Sonmez B, Tun K, Williams BT, Tung K, Tung K. Postoperative cardiac surgical care: An alternative approach. British Heart Journal. 1993;**69**(1):59-63; discussion 63-4. DOI: 10.1136/hrt.69.1.59. Erratum in: Br Heart J 1994;**71**(2):207.

[12] Jain U, Rao TL, Kumar P, Kleinman BS, Belusko RJ, Kanuri DP, et al. Radiographic pulmonary abnormalities after different types of cardiac surgery. Journal of Cardiothoracic and Vascular Anesthesia. 1991;**5**(6):592-595. DOI: 10.1016/1053-0770(91)90013-j

[13] Gunnarsson L, Tokics L, Gustavsson H, Hedenstierna G. Influence

of age on atelectasis formation and gas exchange impairment during general anaesthesia. British Journal of Anaesthesia. 1991;**66**(4):423-432. DOI: 10.1093/bja/66.4.423

[14] Franco AM, Torres FC, Simon IS, Morales D, Rodrigues AJ. Assessment of noninvasive ventilation with two levels of positive airway pressure in patients after cardiac surgery. Revista Brasileira de Cirurgia Cardiovascular. 2011;**26**(4):582-590. English, Portuguese. DOI: 10.5935/1678-9741.20110048

[15] Matte P, Jacquet L, Van Dyck M, Goenen M. Effects of conventional physiotherapy, continuous positive airway pressure and non-invasive ventilatory support with bilevel positive airway pressure after coronary artery bypass grafting. Acta Anaesthesiologica Scandinavica. 2000;**44**(1):75-81. DOI: 10.1034/j.1399-6576.2000.440114.x

[16] Pasquina P, Merlani P, Granier JM, Ricou B. Continuous positive airway pressure versus noninvasive pressure support ventilation to treat atelectasis after cardiac surgery. Anesthesia and Analgesia. 2004;**99**(4):1001-1008. DOI: 10.1213/01.ANE.0000130621.11024.97

[17] Pieczkoski SM, Margarites AGF, Sbruzzi G. Noninvasive ventilation during immediate postoperative period in cardiac surgery patients: Systematic review and meta-analysis. Brazilian Journal of Cardiovascular Surgery. 2017;**32**(4):301-311. DOI: 10.21470/1678-9741-2017-0032

[18] Stell IM, Paul G, Lee KC, Ponte J, Moxham J. Non-invasive ventilator triggering in chronic obstructive pulmonary disease. A test lung comparison. American Journal of Respiratory and Critical Care Medicine. 2001;**164**(11):2092-2097

[19] Rezaiguia S, Jayr C. Prévention des complications respiratoires après chirurgie abdominale [Prevention of respiratory complications after abdominal surgery]. Annales Françaises d'Anesthèsie et de Rèanimation. 1996;**15**(5):623-646. French. DOI: 10.1016/0750-7658(96)82128-9

[20] Siddiqui KM, Samad K, Jonejo F, Khan MF, Ahsan K. Factors affecting reintubations after cardiac and thoracic surgeries in cardiac intensive care unit of a tertiary care hospital. Saudi Journal of Anaesthesia. 2018;**12**(2):256-260. DOI: 10.4103/sja.SJA_631_17

[21] Zhu G, Huang Y, Wei D, Shi Y. Efficacy and safety of non-invasive ventilation in patients after cardiothoracic surgery: A PRISMA-compliant systematic review and meta-analysis. Medicine (Baltimore). 2016;**95**(38):e473

[22] Shoji CY, Figuereido LC, Calixtre EM, Rodrigues CDA, Falcão ALE, Martins PP, et al. Reintubation of patients submitted to cardiac surgery: A retrospective analysis. Revista Brasileira de Terapia Intensiva. 2017;**29**(2):180-187. DOI: 10.5935/0103-507X.20170028

[23] Khayat RN, Abraham WT, Patt B, Roy M, Hua K, Jarjoura D. Cardiac effects of continuous and bilevel positive airway pressure for patients with heart failure and obstructive sleep apnea: A pilot study. Chest. 2008;**134**(6):1162-1168. DOI: 10.1378/chest.08-0346. Epub 2008 Jul 18

[24] Ranucci M, Isgrò G, Carlucci C, De La Torre T, Enginoli S, Frigiola A, et al. Central venous oxygen saturation and blood lactate levels during cardiopulmonary bypass are associated with outcome after pediatric cardiac surgery. Critical Care. 2010;**14**(4):R149. DOI: 10.1186/cc9217. Epub 2010 Aug 4

[25] Marcondi NO, Rocco IS, Bolzan DW, Pauletti HO, Begot I, Anjos NR, et al. Noninvasive ventilation after coronary artery bypass grafting in subjects with left-ventricular dysfunction. Respiratory Care. 2018;**63**(7):879-885. DOI: 10.4187/respcare.05851. Epub 2018 Jun 12

[26] Kallet RH, Diaz JV. The physiologic effects of noninvasive ventilation. Respiratory Care. 2009;**54**(1):102-115

[27] Reis HV, Borghi-Silva A, Catai AM, Reis MS. Impact of CPAP on physical exercise tolerance and sympathetic-vagal balance in patients with chronic heart failure. Brazilian Journal of Physical Therapy. 2014;**18**(3):218-227. DOI: 10.1590/bjpt-rbf.2014.0037

[28] Cordeiro A, LL, Silva C, Santana M, et al. Impact of non-invasive ventilation immediately after extubation on clinical and functional outcomes in patients submitted to coronary artery bypass grafting: Clinical trial. Authorea. 2020:1-9. DOI: 10.22541/au.160813098.85693657/v1

[29] de Araújo-Filho AA, de Cerqueira-Neto ML, de Assis Pereira Cacau L, Oliveira GU, Cerqueira TCF, de Santana-Filho VJ. Effect of prophylactic non-invasive mechanical ventilation on functional capacity after heart valve replacement: A clinical trial. Clinics (São Paulo, Brazil). 2017;**72**(10):618-623. DOI: 10.6061/clinics/2017(10)05

[30] Filsoufi F, Rahmanian PB, Castillo JG, Chikwe J, Adams DH. Predictors and early and late outcomes of respiratory failure in contemporary cardiac surgery. Chest. 2008;**133**(3):713-721. DOI: 10.1378/chest.07-1028. Epub 2008 Feb 8

[31] Kilger E, Möhnle P, Nassau K, Beiras-Fernandez A, Lamm P, Frey L, et al. Noninvasive mechanical ventilation in patients with acute respiratory failure after cardiac surgery. The Heart Surgery Forum. 2010;**13**(2):E91-E95. DOI: 10.1532/HSF98.20091116

[32] Nakazato K, Takeda S, Tanaka K, Sakamoto A. Aggressive treatment with noninvasive ventilation for mild acute hypoxemic respiratory failure after cardiovascular surgery: Retrospective observational study. Journal of Cardiothoracic Surgery. 2012;**7**:41. DOI: 10.1186/1749-8090-7-41

[33] García-Delgado M, Navarrete I, García-Palma MJ, Colmenero M. Postoperative respiratory failure after cardiac surgery: Use of noninvasive ventilation. Journal of Cardiothoracic and Vascular Anesthesia. 2012;**26**(3):443-447. DOI: 10.1053/j.jvca.2011.11.007. Epub 2012 Jan 17

[34] Lindberg P, Gunnarsson L, Tokics L, Secher E, Lundquist H, Brismar B, et al. Atelectasis and lung function in the postoperative period. Acta Anaesthesiologica Scandinavica. 1992;**36**(6):546-553. DOI: 10.1111/j.1399-6576.1992.tb03516.x

[35] Cabrini L, Zangrillo A, Landoni G. Preventive and therapeutic noninvasive ventilation in cardiovascular surgery. Current Opinion in Anaesthesiology. 2015;**28**(1):67-72. DOI: 10.1097/ACO.0000000000000148

[36] Olper L, Cabrini L, Landoni G, Rossodivita A, Nobile L, Monti G, et al. Non-invasive ventilation outside the intensive care unit after cardiac surgery. Minerva Anestesiologica. 2010;**76**:1-6

[37] British Thoracic Society Standards of Care Committee. Non-invasive ventilation in acute respiratory failure. Thorax. 2002;**57**(3):192-211. DOI: 10.1136/thorax.57.3.192

[38] Agarwal R, Handa A, Aggarwal AN, Gupta D, Behera D. Outcomes of noninvasive ventilation in acute hypoxemic respiratory failure in a respiratory intensive care unit in North India. Respiratory Care. 2009;**54**(12):1679-1687

[39] Singh VK, Khanna P, Rao BK, Sharma SC, Gupta R. Outcome predictors for non-invasive positive pressure ventilation in acute respiratory failure. The Journal of the Association of Physicians of India. 2006;**54**:361-365

[40] Wallet F, Schoeffler M, Reynaud M, Duperret S, Workineh S, Viale JP. Factors associated with noninvasive ventilation failure in postoperative acute respiratory insufficiency: An observational study. European Journal of Anaesthesiology. 2010;**27**(3):270-274. DOI: 10.1097/EJA.0b013e32832dbd49

[41] Antonelli M, Conti G, Moro ML, Esquinas A, Gonzalez-Diaz G, Confalonieri M, et al. Predictors of failure of noninvasive positive pressure ventilation in patients with acute hypoxemic respiratory failure: A multi-center study. Intensive Care Medicine. 2001;**27**:1718-1728

[42] Holanda MA, Reis RC, Winkeler GF, Fortaleza SC, Lima JW, Pereira ED. Influence of total face, facial and nasal masks on short-term adverse effects during noninvasive ventilation. Jornal Brasileiro de Pneumologia. 2009;**35**(2):164-173. DOI: 10.1590/s1806-37132009000200010

[43] Mathai AS. Non-invasive ventilation in the postoperative period: Is there a role? Indian Journal of Anaesthesia. 2011;**55**(4):325-333. DOI: 10.4103/0019-5049.84829

[44] Chawla R, Sidhu US, Kumar V, Nagarkar S, Brochard L. Noninvasive ventilation: A survey of practice patterns of its use in India. Indian Journal of Critical Care Medicine. 2008;**12**(4):163-169. DOI: 10.4103/0972-5229.45076

[45] Sweet DD, Naismith A, Keenan SP, Sinuff T, Dodek PM. Missed opportunities for noninvasive positive pressure ventilation: A utilization review. Journal of Critical Care. 2008;**23**:1117

[46] Elena B, Tommaso P, Gianluca F, et al. The importance of education and training for noninvasive ventilation: Suggestions from the literature. Egyptian Journal of Internal Medicine. 2019;**31**:435-441. DOI: 10.4103/ejim.ejim_45_19

[47] Kortebein P, Ferrando A, Lombeida J, Wolfe R, Evans WJ. Effect of 10 days of bed rest on skeletal muscle in healthy older adults. Journal of the American Medical Association. 2007;**297**(16):1772-1774. DOI: 10.1001/jama.297.16.1772-b

[48] Iida Y, Yamazaki T, Arima H, Kawabe T, Yamada S. Predictors of surgery-induced muscle proteolysis in patients undergoing cardiac surgery. Journal of Cardiology. 2016;**68**(6):536-541. DOI: 10.1016/j.jjcc.2015.11.011. Epub 2016 Jan 14

[49] Cabrini L, Zangrillo A. Non-invasive ventilation after cardiac surgery. HSR Proceedings in Intensive Care & Cardiovascular Anesthesia. 2011;**3**(1):5-7

[50] Cabrini L, Plumari VP, Nobile L, Olper L, Pasin L, Bocchino S, et al. Non-invasive ventilation in cardiac surgery: A concise review. Heart, Lung and Vessels. 2013;**5**(3):137-141

Chapter 14

Physiotherapy in Chronic Venous Disease

Margit Eidenberger

Abstract

Chronic venous disease is a highly prevalent disorder. Risk factors are obesity, smoking, orthostasis, and family history. Pathophysiology encompasses changes such as venous hypertension, reflux, valve incompetencies, and calf-muscle weakness. Patients complain about skin changes, leg edema, pain, and ulcers. Possible recurrence of varicoses and surgery complications shift the focus on conservative approaches. The mainstay is compression therapy, applied by using multi-layer compression bandages or adequate compression stockings. Active exercises tackle muscle pump weakness, ankle joint restrictions, and physical activity. Aerobic exercises focus on lower limb activities (walking, cycling, aqua exercises) and are complemented by resistance exercises and muscle stretching. The gait pattern needs analysis and adaptation. Breathing exercises and manual lymphatic drainage act as a supplement. A critical factor for success is the patient's adherence to lifestyle changes and health behavior. Therapists must motivate, guide, and educate their patients. They advise them on clothes/shoes and activities of daily life.

Keywords: chronic venous disease, post-thrombotic syndrome, venous ulcer, compression therapy, exercise training, breathing exercises, manual lymphatic drainage

1. Introduction

Chronic venous disease (CVD) is a highly prevalent morbidity, affecting up to 17% in male and 40% in female gender, respectively [1]. Well-known risk factors are obesity, older age, smoking, orthostasis, and specific family history [2, 3]. CVD pathophysiology encompasses morphological and functional changes such as venous hypertension, venous reflux, valve incompetencies [1], and calf muscle weakness or failure [4]. Patients complain about skin changes, leg edema, pain, and recurrent ulcers all of which impact quality of life (QoL) negatively [5].

CVD can be staged by using the Clinical condition, Etiology, Anatomic location, Pathophysiology (CEAP) classification (C0–C6), involving clinical condition, etiology, anatomic location, and pathophysiology as denominators, ranging from no clinical signs to active ulcer [6].

Conservative (compression therapy [CT], physiotherapy) and invasive/operative treatment methods (endovenous sclerosis, valvuloplasty) [7] are available and are applied based on the disease's severity. Possible recurrences of varicose veins after surgery and surgery complications (infection, scarring, and nerve injury) [1] shift the focus to the beforementioned conservative approaches. Various current scientific evidence hints at the successful implementation of physiotherapeutic treatment methods for CVD [8].

The mainstay of treatment is CT [9]. Multi-layer compression bandages including padding, if necessary, or compression stockings in the long-term can be used. Active exercise training strives at counteracting muscle pump weakness, ankle joint restrictions, and patients' overall often diminished physical activity [3]. As an adjunctive component, breathing exercises and manual lymphatic drainage are applied to enhance venous backflow [8]. In this chapter, it was decided to not mention other possible therapies, such as drugs or surgery, as this would deviate from the primary intention of physiotherapeutic approaches.

A critical factor for therapy success is the patient's therapy adherence hindered by a need to change lifestyle and health behavior as well as a perceived discomfort with the CT [10]. Patients with more advanced health literacy adhere better to their prescribed therapies. So, therapists must motivate for exercise and CT, guide, and educate their patients to change their daily life, and wear proper clothes and shoes in order to achieve long-term results. Lifestyle changes need first time, second, support and advice, and finally tailoring to the patient's needs to succeed [3].

This chapter will give an overview of different physiotherapeutic approaches, guiding the patient through different stages of CVD disease, i.e., varicoses, chronic venous insufficiency, deep venous thrombosis, and venous ulcer by showing the latest evidence for physiotherapeutic protocols and regimes.

2. Physiology and pathophysiology

2.1 Vein and tissue physiology and pathophysiology

A total of 90% of the venous blood flow is executed in the deep venous system, lying subfascial in the musculature. The remaining 10% of blood is transported by the superficial veins. Under physiological conditions (normal vein diameter, sufficient valves, no obstacles) during a muscle contraction, the venous blood from the deep veins is promoted forward to the heart against gravity. Both systems are interconnected by the so-called communicating, i.e. perforating veins. During muscle relaxation, more blood is sucked from the superficial system on the surface into the deep system [8] and from the distal parts of the leg to the more proximal ones. This kind of microcirculation is the reason for instructing dynamic exercises, which combine both, contraction and relaxation alternatingly.

CVD pathophysiology encompasses morphological and functional changes such as venous hypertension, venous reflux, and valve incompetencies [1]. CVD is differentiated in primary venous insufficiency, characterized by a reduced elastin component in venous walls. Primary venous insufficiency is more common in women than in men. Secondary venous insufficiencies are the consequence of previous deep venous thrombosis (DVT) leading to inflammatory responses and valve destruction at the thrombus site. Inflammation further leads to increased permeability of venous walls [11]. It has been shown that ongoing inflammation is a considerable part of CVD. Inflammatory-related cells such as neutrophils, inflammation-related proteins [12], and the neutrophil-lymphocyte ratio were elevated in patients with CVD [13]. If CVD is not treated accordingly, the disease will progress to increasing morbidity and higher stages [1].

Post-thrombotic syndrome (PTS) develops with an incidence of about 25–50% in the first 2 years after DVT [14, 15]. This wide range can be explained by the thrombus length and location as well as patient characteristics (age) and other existing comorbidities. Patients develop chronic venous hypertension, which cannot be reduced with walking or exercise alone, as the primary morbidity leads to damaged venous valves and subsequently venous reflux. The vein is also constricted because of incomplete thrombus removal and inner wall scarring [15]. Besides this, a significant number of DVTs remain unrecognized and therefore undiagnosed and untreated [16]. A vicious cycle develops with venous hypertension leading to further endothelial permeability of plasma and proteins into the interstitial space [4, 17].

A considerable number of patients develop venous leg ulcer (VLU) with a total prevalence of 1.5% [18]. Superficial skin trauma (e.g., after scratching because of the itchy condition) is often the reason for VLU or its recurrence. Ulcers are highly prone to recurrence with a 60–70%-rate within 10 years [19]. Ulcers are most likely located cranially of the medial malleolus, where the Cockett perforator veins connect the superficial and the deep venous system, and a high pressure is exerted on the superficial venous system. Additional symptoms are pruritus, atrophic skin changes, atrophy blanche, hyperpigmentation from hemosiderin deposition, eczema, and lipodermatosclerosis [4, 20]. Persistent VLUs for more than 3 months, with a length of ≥10 cm or combined with obesity or advanced age have a poor prognosis in healing. For proper therapy VLUs must be differentiated from other ulcers, e.g. caused by peripheral arterial disease, diabetes mellitus, or malignancies [20]. Though not showing any vein obstruction or reflux at ultrasonography, obese patients (stage 1–3 = BMI 35—≥ 40) can develop VLUs, indicating a correlation between CVD and obesity because of increased intraabdominal pressure [21]. It was confirmed that obesity contributes to hindered venous backflow [22].

Patients complain about skin changes, leg edema, pain, itching night cramps [11], and recurrent VLUs, all of which reduce QoL gravely [5]. The more skin manifestations are present as symptoms, the higher the reported pain was in a sample of 250 patients from CEAP stages C2 to C6 [6]. Loss of work productivity, sick leaves, dependences, and limited self-esteem can follow. The economic and social burden of CVD should not be underestimated. It was calculated that the cost of treating VLU per year reaches 3 billion dollars in the USA [18]. These costs are mainly attributed to the intensive wound care requirements [15], but also to hospital admissions.

2.2 Clinical assessment

After taking a detailed patient's history (including family history) a physical examination including inspection and palpation of both legs follows. During this examination, patients are undressed in the lower body and remain in a standing position. Visible varicose veins are documented on the body chart. Palpation or more precise infrared thermometers can determine elevated leg/foot temperature [23]. Ulcers are photographed with a measurement ruler lying nearby for later comparison. Their location is also documented on the body chart.

Poor knee alignment is another indicator for reduced venous backflow as knee recurvation pushes the veins at knee level against the upper dorsal part of the tibia. Orthopedic comorbidities, such as osteoarthritis or several foot alignment disorders (pes valgus, hallux valgus, flat foot, etc.) can afflict efficient stance phase and muscle force meanwhile and should be targeted later by e.g. insoles, foot muscle exercises, and joint reharmonization techniques. To exclude other circulatory diseases, distal pulses

(*A. poplitea*, *A. tibialis* posterior, *A. dorsalis* pedis), and an ankle-brachial index should be taken. The patient's common sitting position should be evaluated. Knee flexion of more than 90° should be avoided because of vein constriction in the popliteal area and further to avoid stocking material wrinkles giving pressure. Patients should also avoid a cross-legged position while sitting for the very same reasons.

A test of possible indentation (pressing the thumb into the patient's forefoot/lower limb tissue gives a first hint of pitting edema. This is followed by a Stemmer's sign, where the assessor takes a skinfold between his thumb and index finger at the second toe, the forefoot, the ankle, and the lower limb. Stemmer's sign is an easily applicable, quick, but sensitive means for edema detection [24]. Physiotherapists should measure leg and foot circumference at certain predefined points: forefoot (4 cm/8 cm above little toenail, ankle (lateral malleolus), 10/20/30 cm above ankle level (**Figure 1**). The figure-of-eight measurement can be used to specify ankle proportions.

For gait analysis patients are asked to walk through the room while the assessor is watching for step/stride length, foot, and joint mobility. Video apps can assist in re-watching the gait sequence, also at low speed. It should be noticed if patients are using some kind of cane, crutches, or rollator. The easiest way to assess patients' QoL is by employing the Visual Analog Scale (0 = very low, 100 = very high). Physical activity can be assessed with e.g. the International Physical Activity Questionnaire [25, 3].

2.3 Muscle status

Lower limb muscle strength is very often reduced in CVD patients. Physiotherapists are measuring muscle strength from 0 (no muscle activity at all) to 5 (full exhibition against maximal resistance). This symptom worsens with CVD severity. Possible explanations are the inactivity/reduced physical activity level [25] in combination with obesity and pain. Physical activity is also correlated to QoL, both declining with progressing disease [26], resulting in compromised active social participation. Muscle strength measurements with an isokinetic dynamometer showed significant reductions in lower limb muscle strength of the plantar flexion muscle groups in comparison to healthy controls [27]. Muscle strength, measured with a heel-rise test capability, was reduced in more severe cases of CVD [28].

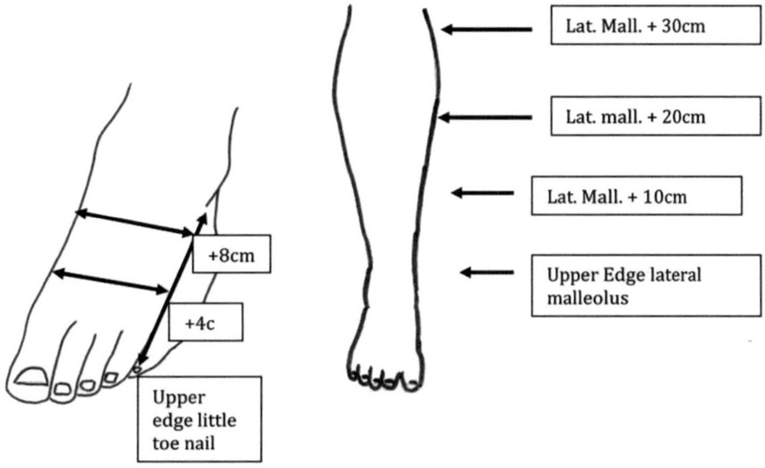

Figure 1.
Foot/lower leg measurement.

Lower limb muscle strength is connected to limited ankle range of motion (ROM) which does not allow full joint movements and therefore inhibits muscle strength enforcement at different angles and an altered gait pattern while walking. The latter leads to a reduction of bodily counter-acting of ground reaction forces in the transition from terminal stance to pre-swing. During this gait phase, the foot should actively push off the ground. The gastrocnemius muscle (M. triceps surae) is responsible for the important calf muscle pump. Additional muscles (M. flexor hallucis longus, M. flexor digitorum longus) are responsible for the so-called "sole-pump". Impossibility or restriction (bedrest, plaster cast) of muscle pump activity, therefore, results in reduced muscle strength and venous flow.

2.4 Ankle range of motion

Ankle ROM measurement in physiotherapy practice is taken with a (digital) goniometer. More sophisticated devices such as inclinometers are available, but not commonly used in everyday practice. A normal ROM is ranged at 20/0/50.

Although adjusted for age, gender, obesity, and previous trauma, Tavares et al. documented a significant loss in ankle ROM in individuals with CVD (n = 810) of about 14° which represents a loss of 20% of the total ROM. This reduction was applied to legs with active VLUs compared to healthy legs. The authors could not detect significant differences in ROM between legs with confirmed CVD, but no ulcer and healthy legs [29]. A very recent meta-analysis was able to show that both, dorsiflexion, and plantarflexion is impaired in patients with VLU when comparing healthy subjects and patients with CVD without ulcer [30]. As more women are affected by CVD, also high-heeled shoes can be a predisposing factor for loosing full ankle ROM because of the pronounced plantarflexion during standing and walking.

ROM and muscle strength are in close connection: without full ROM the muscle is unable to develop its force at different joint angles. The calf muscle efficacy depends on the ankle joint, i.e. talocrural mobility as well as on muscular force [8]. Furthermore, without sufficient dorsiflexion during the swing phase, while walking, the calf muscles are not pre-stretched in the same way as they would have been with normal ROM. This results in a diminished muscle force capacity in the upper-next contraction while walking, that is the following transition from mid-stance to pre-swing, where the calf and plantar foot muscles should push off the ground effectively.

2.5 Assessments and staging tools

Duplex ultrasonography is an efficient means to evaluate the venous system and the gold standard for imaging CVD and confirms the diagnosis. It can provide an assessment of vein anatomy and its function. It is widely used because of its low costs, non-invasiveness, and good reliability. It serves for treatment planning as well as for evaluation [31].

The CEAP classification stages CVD into 7 different categories. It uses denominators such as clinical condition, etiology, anatomic location, and pathophysiology. Stage C0 is characterized by not visible or palpable signs of CVD, C1 by teleangiectasia or varicoses <3 mm, C2 by varicoses >3 mm, C3 by edema, C4a/b by stasis dermatitis and lipodermatosclerosis, C5 by a healed venous ulcer, and finally C6 by active ulcer [6]. Clinical signs given as cutaneous symptoms and disease severity measured with CEAP and pain are significantly correlated [6].

The Venous Clinical Severity Score (VCSS) uses pain, varicoses, edema, skin pigmentation, inflammation, induration, number of active ulcers, their duration, size, and whether CT is applied as denominators. The scale is given as a 4-point Likert description (absent = 0, mild =1, moderate = 2, severe =3). The results range from 0 to 30, the more points, the severe the CVD is [6].

The CICIQ (Chronic Lower Limb Venous Insufficiency Questionnaire) is a validated questionnaire to check health-related quality of life in CVD with several cross-cultural adaptations. Two versions are available: 14 or 20 items (4 dimensions: physical, psychological, social aspects, pain). Both versions display adequate psychometric properties and can differentiate between various levels of CVD [32].

The Villalta classification is recommended to stage and diagnose PTS. It shows better sensitivity than comparable tools. Symptoms such as pain, cramps, heaviness, paresthesia, and pruritus are self-rated by the patient. The clinical signs (pretibial edema, skin induraion, hyperpigmentation, redness, venous ectasia, pain on calf compression, and ulcer) are rated by the physician with a scale of 0–3, except ulcer (present vs. absent) [33].

2.6 Six-minute-walk test

The Six-Minute-Walk Test can depict functional capacity and treatment efficacy over time in CVD patients. This test is easy to execute for physiotherapists with only a corridor with a minimum walking length of 30 or 50 m, several plastic cones to subdivide the distance into smaller units and a watch. For safety reasons, the blood pressure, heart rate, oxygen saturation, and the patient's level of fatigue after completing the test are also measured. In CVD patients the 6MWT distance was significantly reduced when compared with healthy controls [25]. When assessed with their preferred walking speed, CVD patients choose to walk significantly slower than healthy controls (1.25 m/sec ± 0.31 vs. 1.44 m/sec ± 0.015 [34].

3. Compression therapy

The mainstay of treatment is CT [9]. Physiological reasons for compression encompass improvement of valve function, reduction of fluid filtration into the interstitial tissue, support of insufficient muscle pump, increase of blood flow velocity, and pain reduction [35]. After endovenous thermal ablation CT could reduce pain in the first 10 days after surgery and enforce a quicker return to normal activities of daily life (ADL) [36]. During walking CT can improve venous hemodynamics by reducing venous reflux [37]. Because of a reduction of several inflammation-associated proteins CT could improve endothelial function [12]. Contraindications to be considered are peripheral arterial disease with an ankle-brachial index of <0.6, heart failure class III and IV, severe sensitivity disorders, e.g. neuropathy accompanying diabetes mellitus as well as allergy to the material used.

CT can be applied by using multi-layer compression bandages or compression stockings in the long term. Four different compression stocking classes with pressures from 18 to >47 mm Hg are prescribed in different lengths according to the patient's symptoms and needs. They exert a graduated pressure, the highest at the ankle level, subsequently decreasing up to the knee or thigh, ensuring upward blood flow. Flat-knitted customized stockings are recommended for patients with greatly varying leg diameters or CVD in combination with lymphedema. Over-the-counter sold round-knitted stockings are prescribed in CVD.

Although CT is strongly recommended for CVD, patients' adherence is rather poor. Given reasons are discomfort, difficulties with donning/doffing (e.g. limited mobility, finger/hand arthritis), feelings of claustrophobia, etc. Several donning aids such as handy gloves or more sophisticated devices (slippery sleeves, stocking donning butlers, or the Doff N′ Donner, a soft silicone sleeve) can easily CT use. To overcome the donning problems for elderly patients, compression wrapping systems can be an alternative [38]. It was stated that achieving a good adherence to CT is "*more important than choosing the highest possible compression class*" [39]. Stockings are worn daily, donned after morning hygiene, and doffed shortly before going to bed. After 6 or 9 months at the most, they need to be exchanged for a new pair because of tension loss with wearing and washing [4, 20]. Two sets of stockings are prescribed for hygienic reasons.

Even for skilled and trained medical staff, applying a thorough multi-layer compression bandage remains a challenge. To overcome the difficulties with applying the pressure warranted and needed to support venous backflow, various pressure sensor devices such as the Kikuhime are recommended for bandage practice [40]. Bandages with optic marks that indicate optimal elongation can support healthcare staff and even lay persons in reaching an effective pressure [41].

After a mean wear time of 9.66(±1.7) hours of different CT (tights, knee-high) in CEAP class 3 for 6 months, a recent study showed significant improvements in CEAP class, pain, and QoL (measured with CIVIQ-20). The authors strongly support the physicians' task to educate patients on the importance of CT and to prescribe CT. Otherwise they "*are also partly to blame*" [42] for outcome failure.

Makedonov et al. recommend elastic compression stockings immediately after DVT, as they have the potential to prevent PTS development. It may not be necessary to apply these stockings for 2 years (which was a long-followed tradition). If a period of symptom stability is reached after just 1 year, this also may be enough. They also recommend early mobilization after DVT to diminish the risk of PTS [43]. Early mobilization also applies to patients after endovascular recanalization techniques [17] and superficial thrombophlebitis. Interestingly, patients with PTS who have a good adherence to their compression stockings showed similar scores in QoL as patients without PTS, underlining the importance of this intervention [44]. Below-knee stockings are better tolerated than above-knee stockings. The pressure should be selected at 20–40 mm Hg for patients with leg edema and discomfort after DVT [33]. After VLU healing, good adherence to CT is crucial for the prevention of a recurrence [39]. Additionally, intermittent pneumatic compression may be an option for CVD and VLU. It should not come as a stand-alone treatment in VLU but can be used to amend conventional CT [20]. Multiple chamber devices should be preferred with a pressure set at 20–70 mm Hg.

4. Exercise therapy

Active exercise training strives at counteracting muscle pump weakness, ankle joint restrictions, and patients' overall diminished physical activity. This influences microcirculation and venous hypertension by regulating bodily fluid balance [45] and is accompanied by losing body weight. Patients can combine exercise and CT effects by wearing their stockings during exercise. PTS patients should never exercise without CT. This ensures proper heart-directed venous backflow and led to higher transcutaneous oxygen partial pressure measurements than exercise alone [18].

Different therapy approaches (aerobic, resistance, stretching) are combined for rehabilitative goals. Aerobic exercises with a focus on lower limb activities such as walking, cycling, running, aqua exercises, and swimming are complemented by lower limb resistance exercises and muscle stretching.

A systematic review scrutinized the effectiveness of therapeutic exercises for CVD patients. 11 studies with different therapy regimes were included. Aside from hemodynamic benefits (venous reflux, ejection fraction, residual volume), higher production of nitric oxide was described. Nitric oxide is a neuromodulator of venous tone which can prevent hypoxia injury [46].

The gait pattern needs to be therapeutically analyzed and changed, if necessary, for an improvement of muscle pump activity during walking. Patients need to adhere to a physiologic foot axis, that is a slight divergent line from the center of the heel to the proximal joint of the great toe. While climbing stairs, patients should not use the handrail, if possible. Furthermore, maximal muscle strength while ascending stairs can be achieved if the person puts only her/his forefoot on the next stair. This reduces the contact surface to the ground and subsequently leads to increased muscle deployment.

In PTS, exercise therapy has the capacity to reduce swelling and via an improvement of the calf muscle pump alleviate the patients' pain and discomfort. A systematic review that scrutinized exercise therapy in PTS was only able to include one study meeting their inclusion criteria (exercise therapy, Villalta score as outcome measurement). Supervised and unsupervised exercise for 6 months (aerobic, strength, stretching) was compared with an educational session. Unfortunately, this study with only 39 participants bears a high risk of bias and failed to show significant differences. The paucity of evidence on this topic calls for further high-quality studies, as the authors could not give recommendations for exercise in PTS [15].

Mutlak et al. performed a 4-armed study (n = 80, exercise only, compression only, combination of both, control) to explore easy-to-perform dynamic exercises (10 dorsiflexions every wakening hour). After 3 months ulcers had increased in diameter in the control group and stayed equal in the compression group. Both, exercise and exercise plus CT reduced ulcer size. The reduction was more noticeable in the combined group [18].

4.1 Aerobic exercises

Each rehabilitation protocol must be tailored to patients' capabilities and needs. Therefore, a thorough assessment, a therapy protocol, and patient education are crucial. This approach facilitates patients' motivation and can advance healthcare literacy for improving self-care management [47]. To enhance venous backflow, dynamic muscle contractions are recommended. The actual full joint ROM should be exploited during exercise.

The easiest exercise is the venous pump which can be applied in active and bedridden weak patients. As longer bed rest deteriorates venous capacity [48], countermeasures are warranted to avoid DVT. Patients are lying supine, legs elevated, and are wearing their CT if prescribed any. The ankle is moved in full range plantar- and dorsiflexion for 20 to 30 repetitions in 3 series with a short break (30 secs) in between ideally every wakening hour. The toes should be involved in the movement as well because plantar veins contribute to the physiology of venous return [49]. The venous pump exercise could reduce edema significantly better in a group of CVD patients

(CEAP C3–C5) in comparison to leg-elevated bed rest [50]. To enhance effectiveness, patients can use rubber bands for resistance or tight pillows to push the feet against. Pedal ergometers are small practical transportable training devices to be placed at the lower end of the bed for lying patients or on the floor in front of sitting patients (**Figure 2**). Patients can exercise with the pedal ergometer at different predefined resistances. Short training sessions for weak patients can start at 5–10 minutes of continuous training and progress to 20–30 minutes.

Walking/treadmill walking or bicycle exercises are useful means to employ great parts of lower limb musculature. They are also recommendable because of their familiar movement pattern, the low need for additional exercise equipment, and their easy compatibility with everyday life. Patients should walk at a moderate velocity, that is 3–4 km/h for at least 30 minutes daily wearing trainers or other comfortable flat shoes.

4.2 Resistance training

Strength/resistance training (RT) is indicated because of the before-mentioned muscle pump weakness [4]. RT should involve different lower limb muscle groups with a focus lying on ankle plantarflexion, i.e. the gastrocnemius muscle to ensure an active calf-muscle pump. Additionally, also ankle dorsiflexion, knee flexion, and extension components need to be integrated into the training sequence. To decipher the correct number of repetitions, patients are subjected to a multiple repetition maximum test of the latter resistance exercise. Training is executed with a submaximal number of the repetitions possible, e.g. 70%. The core exercise is the so-called "calf-raises" or "heel-rises" in different positions, at different muscle lengths, and by employing various muscle enforcements: dynamic-isotonic, concentric, and eccentric muscle contraction (**Figure 3**). For progressive training, it is important to re-evaluate the muscle strength and consequently adapt the number of repetitions and level of difficulty. Exercises should be accomplished daily.

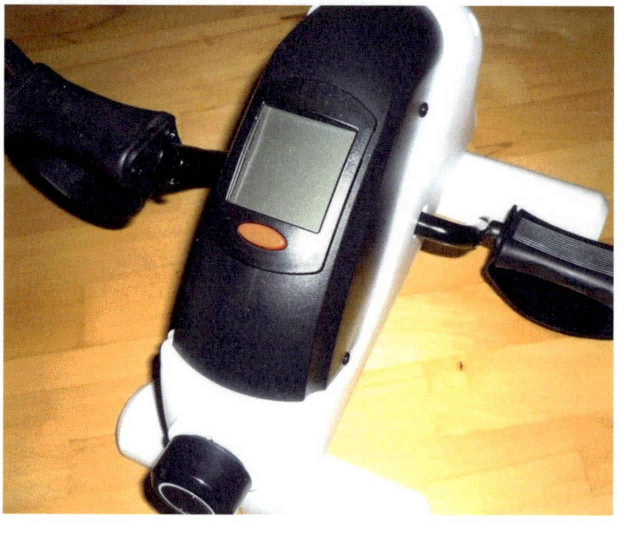

Figure 2.
Pedal ergometer.

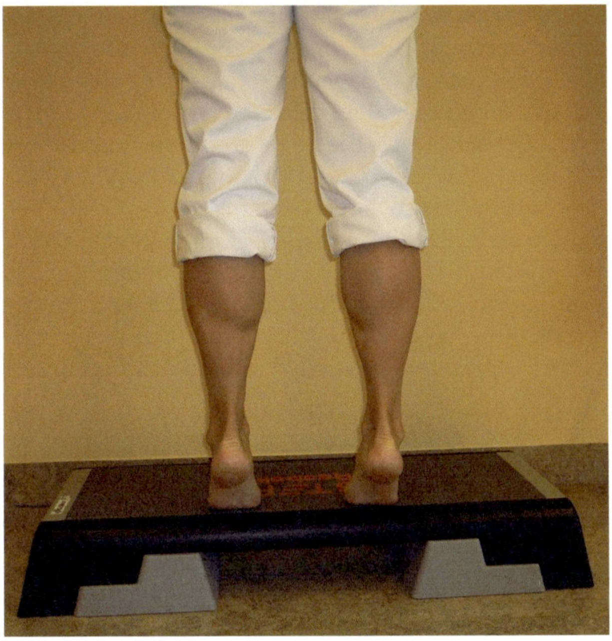

Figure 3.
Calf raises

As muscle strength can be heavily compromised, RT sometimes needs to start at low levels, that is heel-rises in a sitting position. With time, the position moves on to standing on both legs and finally to a single-leg stance. A randomized controlled trial (n = 63) therapy protocol (10 repetitions, increased every 3 days per 5 repetitions until 25 reps were reached; changing from sitting to double-stance and finally to single-stance) led to a trend of complete ulcer healing ($p = 0.09$; 77% vs. 53%) compared to usual care. Healing rates were better in the subgroup of patients who adhered at least to 75% of the therapy protocol [51]. O'Brien et al. confirmed similar findings. Their study protocol included a daily to perform progressive RT of calf muscle strength. The study had not enough power to significantly show a difference between this regime of 12 weeks and usual care. Nevertheless, there was a 24% difference in healing rates in favor of the exercise group, which was considered clinically significant. Patients who adhered to >75% of the program reached a significant improvement in ankle ROM [52].

To further aggravate the training circumstances, flexible surfaces, e.g. rolled-up gymnastic mats or balance pads can be used. Aside from strength, this also improves ankle ROM and balance capabilities.

4.3 Aqua exercises

Aquatic exercises bear several advantages in comparison to dry-land activities [53]. Firstly, the hydrostatic pressure of water executes pressure similar to CT. Hydrostatic pressure at 0.5 m below surface level is equivalent to 0.05 bar and 37.5 mm Hg, i.e. compression class level III. Secondly, during swimming or similar underwater movements, the nearly prone or supine position removes parts of the gravitational force hindering venous backflow. Thirdly, additional leg and foot movements activate the muscle pump. Lastly, it represents the possibility of exercise for obese patients without too much joint load. Unfortunately, patients with active ulcers cannot enter the pool for obvious reasons. Menegatti et al. subjected a group of 17 patients to an aqua exercise protocol (5 sessions per 30 minutes) aiming at mobilization and muscle activation of the lower limbs. Though lacking a control group, they showed a significant reduction of extracellular water content as well as a significant reduction of leg volume (−15.7%). The special water properties containing different chemical ingredients, e.g. Natrium or Kalium, may have played a role in these results [54]. A randomized controlled trial involved 201 patients for aqua exercises (walking in water, swimming) vs. control. All patients were instructed to wear knee-high compression stockings (30–40 mm Hg) the other time. 28% of aqua exercisers displayed a reduction of ≥4 points in the Venous Clinical Severity Score (significant in comparison to the control group). Leg circumference decreased significantly in favor of aqua exercise [55]. A systematic review of Kneipp therapy (walking in calf-high cold water, lower leg cold water gushes) looked for evidence for this traditional therapy. 64% of the implemented studies reported significant enhancements for the Kneipp therapy [56].

4.4 Breathing exercises

As an adjunctive component, breathing exercises (supine, legs elevated, and combined with CT) can assist the other remedies. Several physiological reasons imply their effectiveness. The diaphragm enhances the blood flow from the lower extremities to the heart by executing a suction effect on the inferior vena cava [8]. In a 3-armed trial, inspiratory muscle training (IMT; 2×15 min per day for 8 weeks; 5 days per week) plus CT was compared to CT alone or calf muscle exercise training. Although the sample size was small (n = 32), the authors observed a significant increase in venous refill time in both legs after IMT. Consequently, they recommended the implementation of this approach to the therapy regime in CVD [8]. It should be noted that patients were sitting during IMT, maybe results would have been more pronounced if patients would have been lying supine, as suggested before. Kwon et al. measured blood flow velocity in the femoral vein during quiet breathing, deep breathing, and both, combined with ankle exercises in 20 healthy males in a supine position. Deep breathing accelerated the velocity from 10.1 cm/sec (±4.2) to 15.5 (±3.9) cm/sec. The highest velocity was reached with deep breathing combined with ankle exercises (plantar-dorsiflexion; 26.6 (9.4). If these results also apply to individuals with CVD need further confirmation [57].

4.5 Additional measures

Additional measures include leg elevation to counteract gravity and body weight management. Short, repeated periods of lying supine during the day (5–10 minutes) relieve swelling and pain. If activities of daily life do not permit lying sequences, patients should at least put their leg(s) on a second chair for some time, e.g. during office hours. Patients should be educated on proper clothes (no socks with tight rubber bands, flat-soled shoes). Furthermore, they are encouraged to exercise regularly and keep an active lifestyle [1] to lose weight. Whenever possible, they should give preference to taking the stairs instead of the elevator, taking the bike instead of the car for short distances, etc. The physiotherapist is part of a multidisciplinary team, consisting of other healthcare professionals such as wound care nurses, surgeons, and dieticians, if needed. Patient-centered therapeutic education can alleviate CVD

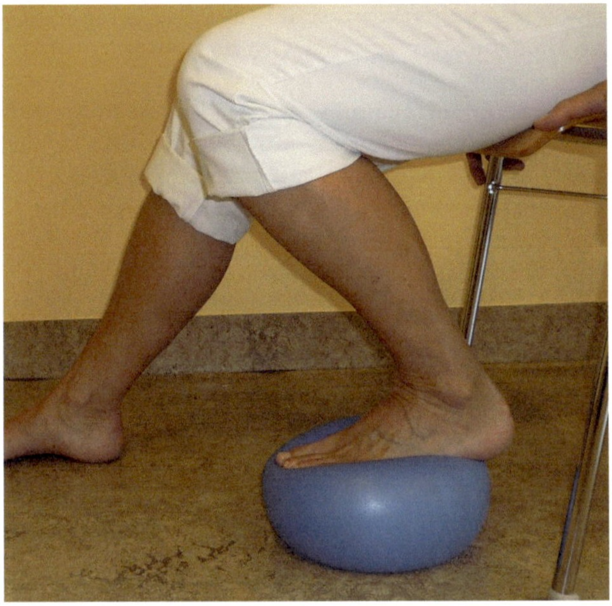

Figure 4.
Redondo ball exercise.

symptoms and enhance QoL [58]. It is crucial that therapy protocols are tailored to the different needs of individual patients and fit into their life.

Calf muscle stretching (20–30 seconds, standing position, heel remains on the surface) after endurance and/or strength training aims at relaxing and elongating muscles. Additionally, during the stretching maneuver, the ankle joint is mobilized into dorsiflexion [52]. Simultaneously, deep veins are stretched in a longitudinal direction, producing a reduction in venous diameter, better valve closure, and enhanced venous backflow [59]. Stretching after active exercise and predominantly after strength training also prevents training-related muscle soreness.

To improve ankle ROM patients can use a belt or strap to passively pull their own foot in dorsiflexion. This exercise is best being taken while sitting on a mat on the ground, knees extended, and hips 90° flexed. Patients having difficulties moving to the floor sit on a stool, leaning on the backrest, hip nearly extended, and knee extended. The stretching position should be held for at least 20–30 seconds, giving passive structures the possibility to relax. During the exercise patients can report a feeling of stretched tissue, but no pain. Another possibility employs a Redondo ball while sitting on a chair (**Figure 4**). The affected foot is placed on the ball and the patient is instructed to roll the ball backward by flexing the knee which leads to enlarged dorsiflexion. The final position is held for several seconds, followed by a rolling back until the foot is placed underneath the knee. 10–20 repetitions are recommended for this exercise.

5. Manual lymphatic drainage

Manual lymphatic drainage (MLD) in CVD involves the neck, possibly the abdomen, and one or both lower limbs in approximately 45 minutes to 1 hour time. The therapy is completed by CT, patient education, and active exercises [60].

A few studies have explored MLD within CVD. In 2014 a study group compared MLD in a cohort of CVD patients (CEAP C1-5) and healthy controls. They showed an increase of blood flow in both, the femoral and the great saphenous vein after MLD in both groups. However, this flow was less accentuated in patients with a higher stage of the disease. They recommended MLD as a viable strategy for CVD [61]. Another group tested 10 MLD sessions for the lower limb vs. disease education in 41 CVD patients. They concluded that MLD improves venous edema (measured with the VCSS) and heaviness at the follow-up after 4 weeks and 2 months, respectively [62]. A small patient group with VLU was subjected to complex decongestive therapy (MLD + compression + skincare + exercise) for 5 (n = 8) or 10 days (n = 9) and a control group (n = 9) who received CT alone. This resulted in significantly improved ulcer healing for the 10-day course in comparison to CT (p = 0.039) [63]. Mosti et al. treated 38 patients with 10×20min MLD in advance of their venous surgery and compared them to a control group (n = 42). This protocol led to a significant reduction of foot volume post-surgery in favor of the MLD group. No significant group differences were observed in QoL or venous refilling time [64].

6. Conclusion

CVD is a highly prevalent disorder. It can be treated with various kinds of exercise therapy on dryland and underwater. Aerobic exercises focus on lower limb activities (walking, cycling, aqua exercises) and are complemented by resistance exercises and muscle stretching. Breathing exercises, leg elevation, and manual lymphatic drainage act as a supplement. A critical factor for success is the patient's adherence to lifestyle changes and health behavior. Compression therapy is an indispensable part of CVD. Patient education aims at health literacy and patients' adherence to exercise and compression therapy. In CVD, the physiotherapist is part of a multidisciplinary team. The enhancement of various patients' complaints (pain, leg edema, ankle range of motion, venous reflux) allows for an improvement of quality of life and a better degree of participation in activities of daily life.

Author details

Margit Eidenberger
University of Applied Sciences for Health Professions Upper Austria, Steyr, Austria

*Address all correspondence to: margit.eidenberger@fhgooe.ac.at

References

[1] Patel SK. Venous insufficiency. In: Surowiec SM, editor. Drugs Used in Treatment of Venous Insufficiency. Treasure Island: Stat Pearls Publishing; 2022. https://www.statpearls.com/point-of-care/31060

[2] Nawaphan T. Risk factors for and treatment of chronic venous disease in Thai patients. Vascular Health and Risk Management. 2022;**18**:667-676. DOI: 10.2147/VHRM.S382726

[3] Kiloatar H et al. An evaluation of quality of life, physical activity level and symptoms in patients with early stages of chronic venous disease. Journal of Vascular Nursing. 2021;**39**(4):108-113. DOI: 10.1016/j.jvn.2021.07.007

[4] Eberhardt RT, Raffetto JD. Chronic venous insufficiency. Circulation. 2014;**130**(4):333-346. DOI: 10.1161/CIRCULATIONAHA.113.006898

[5] Mejia-Gonzales M et al. Prevalence of chronic venous disease in health staff and its impact on quality of life at 6 months. Cirugia y Cirujanos. 2022;**90**(3):332-337. DOI: 10.24875/CIRU.20001245

[6] Caballero Escuti G, Ruiz Lascano A, Tabares AH. Correlation between cutaneous manifestations and functional alterations in chronic venous disease of the lower extremities. Actas Dermo-Sifiliográficas. 2022;**113**(9):856-865. DOI: 10.1016/j.ad.2022.05.013

[7] Goel RR, Hardy SC, Brown T. Surgery for deep venous insufficiency. Cochrane Database of Systematic Reviews. 2021;**9**(9):CD001097. DOI: 10.1002/14651858.CD001097.pub4

[8] Aydin G et al. Effects of inspiratory muscle training versus calf muscle training on quality of life, pain, venous function and activity in patients with chronic venous insufficiency. Journal of Vascular Surgery. Venous and Lymphatic Disorders. 2022;**0**(5):1137-1146. DOI: 10.1016/j.jvsv.2022.04.012

[9] De Maeseneer MG et al. Editor's Choice—European Society for Vascular Surgery (ESVS) 2022 clinical practice guidelines on the Management of Chronic Venous Disease of the lower limbs. European Journal of Vascular and Endovascular Surgery. 2022;**63**(2):184-267. DOI: 10.1016/j.ejvs.2021.12.024

[10] Coral FE et al. Chronic venous insufficiency and graduated compression stockings: Analysis of public health system patients' adherence to treatment. Journal of Vascular Bras. 2021;**20**:e20200034. DOI: 10.1590/1677-5449.200034

[11] Yetkin E et al. Symptoms in dilating venous disease. Current Cardiology Reviews. 2020;**16**(3):164-172. DOI: 10.2174/1573403X16666200312101245

[12] Moñux G et al. Compression stockings attenuate the expression of proteins associated with vascular damage in human varicose veins. Journal of Vascular Surgery. Venous and Lymphatic Disorders. 2021;**9**(2):428-434. DOI: 0.1016/j.jvsv.2020.05.020

[13] Mosmiller LT et al. Evaluation of inflammatory cell biomarkers in chronic venous insufficiency. Phlebology. 2017;**32**(9):634-640. DOI: 10.1177/0268355517701806

[14] Chaitidis N et al. Management of Post-thrombotic Syndrome: A comprehensive review. Current Pharmaceutical Design.

2022;**28**(7):550-559. DOI: 10.2174/1381612828666220131094655

[15] Jasionowska S et al. Systematic review of exercise therapy in the management of post-thrombotic syndrome. Phlebology. 2022;**37**(10):695-700. DOI: 10.1177/02683555221129738

[16] Urbanek T, Labropoulos N. Can we predict and prevent the postthrombotic syndrome? VASA. 2021;**50**(1):11-21. DOI: 10.1024/0301-1526/a000932

[17] Schleimer K et al. The treatment of post-thrombotic syndrome. Dt Ärtzebl International. 2016;**113**:863-870. DOI: 10.3238/arztebl.2016.0863

[18] Mutlak O, Aslam M, Standfield N. The influence of exercise on ulcer healing in patients with chronic venous insufficiency. International Angiology. 2018;**37**(2):160-168. DOI: 10.23736/S0392-9590.18.03950-0

[19] Kolluri R et al. An estimate of the economic burden of venous leg ulcers associated with deep venous disease. Vascular Medicine. 2022;**27**(1):63-72. DOI: 10.1177/1358863X211028298

[20] Bonkemeyer Millan S, Gan R, Townsend PE. Venous ulcers: Diagnosis and treatment. American Family Physician. 2019;**100**(5):298-305

[21] Scholl L, Dörler M, Stücker M. Ulcers in obesity-associated chronic venous insufficiency. Der Hautarzt. 2017;**68**(7):560-565. DOI: 10.1007/s00105-017-3971-y

[22] Willenberg T et al. The influence of abdominal pressure on lower extremity venous pressure and hemodynamics: A human in-vivo model simulating the effect of abdominal obesity. European Journal of Vascular and Endovascular Surgery. 2011;**41**(6):849-855. DOI: 10.1016/j.ejvs.2011.02.015

[23] Krishnan S, Nicholls SC. Chronic venous insufficiency: Clinical assessment and patient selection. Seminars in Interventional Radiology. 2005;**22**(3):169-177. DOI: 10.1055/s-2005-921961

[24] Brenner E, Putz D. 30 Jahre Stemmersches Zeichen. Vasomed. 2006;**4**:153

[25] Erdal ES et al. Evaluation of physical activity level and exercise capacity in patients with varicose veins and chronic venous insufficiency. Phlebology. 2021;**36**(8):636-643. DOI: 10.1177/02683555211002339

[26] Espeit L et al. Fatigue, physical activity, and quality of life in people self-reporting symptoms of chronic venous disease. Journal of Vascular Surgery. Venous and Lymphatic Disorders. 2022;**10**(5):1147-1154.e1. DOI: 10.1016/j.jvsv.2022.04.016

[27] Ercan S et al. Evaluation of the isokinetic calf muscle strength and the range of motion of joint in C3 chronic venous insufficiency. Vascular Specialist International. 2019;**35**(2):95-100. DOI: 10.5758/vsi.2019.35.2.95

[28] Pereira DAG et al. Association between heel-rise test performance and clinical severity of chronic venous insufficiency. Phlebology. 2020;**35**(8):631-636. DOI: 10.1177/0268355520924878

[29] Tavares PA et al. Association of venous leg ulcers with ankle range of motion in people attending chiropractic mobile clinics in the Dominican Republic. Journal of Chiropractic Medicine. 2017;**16**(4):263-270. DOI: 10.1016/j.jcm.2017.08.004

[30] Nepomuceno de Souza I et al. Impairments in ankle range of motion, dorsi and plantar flexors muscle strength and gait speed in patients with chronic venous disorders: A systematic review and meta-analysis. Phlebology. 2022;**37**(7):496-506. DOI: 10.1177/02683555221094642

[31] Hong KP. Correlation of clinical class with duplex ultrasound findings in lower limb chronic venous disease. Journal ofJ Chest Surgery. 2022;**55**(3):233-238. DOI: 10.5090/jcs.22.010

[32] De Almeida ILGI et al. Reliability and validity of specific quality of life assessment questionnaires related to chronic venous insufficiency: A systematic review. Journal of Vascular Bras. 2022;**1**:e20210229. DOI: 10.1590/1677-5449.202102292

[33] Rabinovich A, Kahn SR. How I treat the postthrombotic syndrome. Blood. 2018;**131**(20):2215-2222. DOI: 10.1182/blood-2018-01-785956

[34] Van Uden CJ et al. Gait and calf muscle endurance in patients with chronic venous insufficiency. Clinical Rehabilitation. 2005;**19**(3):339-344. DOI: 10.1191/0269215505cr809oa

[35] Gianesini S et al. Volume control of the lower limb with graduated compression during different muscle pump activation conditions and the relation to limb circumference variation. Journal of Vascular Surgery. Venous and Lymphatic Disorders. 2020;**8**(5):814-820. DOI: 10.1016/j.jvsv.2019.12.073

[36] Ma F et al. Compression therapy following endovenous thermal ablation of vaicose veins: A systematic review and meta-analysis. Annals of Vascular Surgery. 2021;**80**:302-312. DOI: 10.1016/j.avsg.2021.09.035

[37] Ibegbuna V et al. Effect of elastic compression stockings on venous hemodynamics during walking. Journal of Vascular Surgery. 2003;**37**(2):420-425. DOI: 10.1067/mva.2003.104

[38] Balet F et al. Limitations to self-management of adjustable compression wraps in the elderly: Results of a prospective cohort study. International Angioplasty. 2021;**40**(3):261-266. DOI: 10.23736/S0392-9590.21.04580-6

[39] Kroeger K et al. Prophylaxis of recurrent venous leg ulcer. Zentralblatt für Chirurgie. 2017;**142**(3):306-311. DOI: 10.1055/s-0042-109977

[40] Karafa M, Karafova A. Kikuhime device in the management of venous leg ulcers. Clinical Interventions in Aging. 2020;**15**:1533-1539. DOI: 10.2147/CIA.S264567

[41] Weindorf M et al. Einfluss visueller Kontrollsysteme auf den Druck von Kompressionsverbänden. Phlébologie. 2012;**41**:18-24. DOI: 10.1055/s-0037-1621797

[42] Berszakiewicz A et al. The effect of compression therapy on quality of life in patients with chronic venous disease: A comparative 6-month study. Postepy Dermatology Alergology. 2021;**38**(3):389-395. DOI: 10.5114/ada.2020.92277

[43] Makedonov I, Kahn SR, Galanaud J-P. Prevention and management of the post-thrombotic syndrome. Journal of Clinical Medicine. 2020;**9**:923. DOI: 10.3390/jcm9040923

[44] Silva JC et al. Determinants of quality of life in patients with post-thrombotic syndrome. Annals of Vascular Surgery. 2022;**85**:253-261. DOI: 10.1016/j.avsg.2022.03.002

[45] Marini E et al. Combined aerobic and resistance training improves microcirculation in metabolic syndrome. The Journal of Sports Medicine and Physical Fitness. 2019;**59**(9):1571-1576. DOI: 10.23736/S0022-4707.18.09077-1

[46] Souza Silva KL et al. The impact of exercise training on calf pump function, muscle strength, ankle range of motion, and health-related quality of life in patients with chronic venous insufficiency at different stages of severity: A systematic review. Journal of Vascular Bras. 2021;**20**:e20200125. DOI: 10.1590//1677-5449.200125

[47] Downie S, Shnaigat M, Hosseinzadeh H. Effectiveness of health literacy- and patient activation-targeted interventions on chronic disease self-management outcomes in outpatient settings: A systematic review. Australian Journal of Primary Health. 2022;**28**(2):83-96. DOI: 10.1071/PY21176

[48] Van Duijnhoven NTL et al. The effect of bed rest and an exercise countermeasure on leg venous function. European Journal of Applied Physiology. 2008;**104**(6):991-998. DOI: 10.1007/s00421-008-0854-z

[49] Uhl JF, Gillot C. Anatomy of the foot venous pump: Physiology and influence on chronic venous disease. Phlebology. 2012;**27**(5):219-230. DOI: 10.1258/phleb.2012.012b01

[50] Quilici BC et al. Comparison of reduction of edema after rest and after muscle exercises in treatment of chronic venous insufficiency. International Archives of Medicine. 2009;**2**(1):18. DOI: 10.1186/1755-7682-2-18

[51] Bolton L. Exercise and chronic wound healing. Index Wounds. 2019;**31**(2):65-67

[52] O'Brien J et al. Evaluating the effectiveness of a self-management exercise intervention on wound healing, functional ability and health-related quality of life outcomes in adults with venous leg ulcers: A randomised controlled trial. International Wound Journal. 2017;**14**:130-137. DOI: 10.1111/iwj.12571

[53] Bissacco D et al. Rationale and current evidence of aquatic exercise therapy in venous disease: A narrative review. Vascular. 2022;**2022**:1708. DOI: 10.1177/17085381221102783

[54] Menegatti E et al. The effects of thermal water physical exercise in patients with lower limb chronic venous insufficiency monitored by bioimpedance analysis. Diagnostics (Basel). 2020;**10**(11):889. DOI: 10.3390/diagnostics10110889

[55] Sharifi M et al. The randomized, controlled ATLANTIS trial of aquatic therapy for chronic venous insufficiency. Journal of Vascular Surgery. Venous and Lymphatic Disorders. 2021;**9**(4):961-970. DOI: 10.1016/j.jvsv.2020.10.016

[56] Stier-Jarmer M et al. Effekte der Kneipp-Therapie: Ein systematischer Review der aktuellen wissenschaftlichen Erkenntnisse. Complementary Medical Research. 2021;**28**(2):146-159. DOI: 10.1159/000510452

[57] Kwon OY et al. Effects of ankle exercise combined with deep breathing on blood flow velocity in the femoral vein. The Australian Journal of Physiotherapy. 2003;**49**(4):253-258. DOI: 10.1016/s0004-9514(14)60141-0

[58] Thibert A et al. Systematic review of adapted physical activity and therapeutic education of patients with chronic venous disease. Journal of

Vascular Surgery. Venous and Lymphatic Disorders. 2022;**10**(6):1385-1400. DOI: 10.1016/j.jvsv.2022.05.004

[59] Reich-Schupke S. Warum kann eine Kompressionstherapie bei Immobilität sinnvoll sein? Vasomed. 2016;**28**(6):278-284

[60] Miller A. Lymphedema-clinical picture and therapy. Der Hautarzt. 2020;**71**(1):32-38. DOI: 10.1007/s00105-019-04523-z

[61] Dos Santos Crisostomo RS et al. Manual lymphatic drainage in chronic venous disease: A duplex ultrasound study. Phlebology. 2014;**29**(10):667-676. DOI: 10.1177/0268355513502787

[62] Dos Santos Crisostomo RS et al. Influence of manual lymphatic drainage on health-related quality of life and symptoms of chronic venous insufficiency: A randomized controlled trial. Archives of Physical Medicine and Rehabilitation. 2015;**96**(2):283-291. DOI: 10.1016/j.apmr.2014.09.020

[63] Szolnoky G et al. Adjunctive role of manual lymph drainage in the healing of venous ulcers: A comparative pilot study. Lymphology. 2018;**1**(4):148-159

[64] Molski P et al. Manual lymphatic drainage improves the quality of life in patients with chronic venous disease: A randomized controlled trial. Archives of Medical Science. 2013;**9**(3):452-458. DOI: 10.5114/aoms.2013.35343